ATLAS OF
OPERATIVE DENTISTRY

ATLAS OF
OPERATIVE DENTISTRY

WILLIAM W. HOWARD, B.S., D.M.D., F.A.C.D., F.A.G.D.

Professor and Chairman, Department of Fixed Prosthodontics,
School of Dentistry, University of Oregon Health Sciences Center;
Editor, Journal of the Academy of General Dentistry;
Past President and former Member, Oregon State Board of Dental Examiners;
Staff Member, Shriners Hospital for Crippled Children, Portland, Oregon

RICHARD C. MOLLER, D.D.S.

Vancouver, Washington; former Assistant Professor,
Department of Operative Dentistry, School of Dentistry,
University of Washington, Seattle, Washington

THIRD EDITION

With **1533** illustrations

The C. V. Mosby Company

ST. LOUIS • TORONTO • LONDON   1981

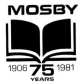

MOSBY

1906 **75** 1981
YEARS

A TRADITION OF PUBLISHING EXCELLENCE

THIRD EDITION

Previous editions copyrighted 1968, 1973

Printed in the United States of America

The C. V. Mosby Company
11830 Westline Industrial Drive, St. Louis, Missouri 63141

Library of Congress Cataloging in Publication Data

Howard, William W
    Atlas of operative dentistry.

    Includes bibliographical references and index.
    1. Dentistry, Operative—Atlases.   I. Moller,
Richard C., 1946-   joint author.   II. Title.
[DNLM: 1. Dentistry, Operative—Atlases.   WU 17
H853a]
RK501.H65   1981   617.6′059   80-25063
ISBN 0-8016-2282-4

C/VH/VH 9 8 7 6 5 4 3 2 1   03/B/368

To
Emma-Jane and **Lisa**

FOREWORD
to third edition

After twenty-three years of private practice, William W. Howard accepted the Chairmanship of the Crown and Bridge Department of the University of Oregon, with private practice privileges.

Need for more detailed instruction for undergraduates thus became apparent to him. He called on Richard Moller with nine years of undergraduate teaching experience at the University of Washington to add the detailed material that undergraduates need.

This in no way detracts from the value of this book for graduates. It adds one more dedicated authorship and dimension to the text. Moller's experience and his interpretation of the literature is thus superimposed on the original editions.

Undergraduates must be taught *a way* to do things, meanwhile being alerted to the realities of other methodology. Once acquiring a degree and a right to practice, he or she must resolve to explore *other* disciplines and technology with a growing awareness of the magnitude of service possible in dentistry. G. V. Black said, "No professional person has a right to be other than a continual student."

Before undertaking this foreword for the third edition, I was invited to make detailed comments on the drafts in preparation. Some of my ideas were accepted and incorporated. But the result should in no way be construed as being my textbook. This newest version has been influenced also by the many other references in the text that will become a valuable addition to any dental library.

Miles R. Markley, D.D.S.

FOREWORD
to first and second editions

The *Atlas of Operative Dentistry* by Dr. Howard will thrill both the undergraduate and the continual student, regardless of his age and ability.

Dr. Howard's text is unique because it is written by a practicing dentist, one with a tremendous background of personal experience. Therefore everything in the text is *practical* and is aimed at providing the superb restorative service for which he is noted.

His illustrations are dramatic and are in themselves well worth the cost of this masterpiece publication. Countless hours of his own time went into carving casts of working situations and into supervising the artist who translated them to paper.

Dr. Howard has been teaching practicing dentists in operative study clubs for years and brings this fund of knowledge and experience to us in book form.

Miles R. Markley, D.D.S.

PREFACE

One of the most frequent criticisms of the first two editions pertained to their limited scope of information. Through both lack of time and procrastination, I had not moved far toward correcting the deficiencies identified until last year when I met Dr. Richard Moller.

As a former faculty member in the Restorative Dentistry Department at the University of Washington for nearly ten years, he has developed and written many innovative teaching manuals and self-instructional guides on operative dentistry. Dr. Moller has an impressive understanding of operative dentistry and great talent to execute his knowledge. Through his contribution we have greatly expanded many subject areas toward our objective of making this book more comprehensive. It is our purpose to make the book useful to all levels of teaching of operative dentistry.

W.W.H.

We do not claim to be the originators of the techniques and procedures herein included but are deeply grateful to those whose fine minds and professional attitudes toward sharing scientific information have contributed the knowledge and techniques that are available to the dental profession. We would like to give credit by acknowledging each contribution, but to do so would be time consuming and of doubtful value for our purposes.

The last three chapters include restorations not as frequently performed as those presented in earlier chapters. However, an operator truly skilled and knowledgeable in all aspects of the field will be equally adept in the subject matter presented in the last part of the book.

The exclusion of any procedure or technique is in no respect to imply its inferiority. The field of operative dentistry is in fact so complex that time and space limits do not permit a complete collection of procedures.

Preventive dentistry, a topic riding a wave of justified popularity, sometimes tends to imply overly simple conceptions of its techniques. Essential components of a truly prevention-oriented philosophy are many, some of them intricately complex. Fine operative dentistry continues to be one of the major essential components of preventive dentistry.

Patients receptive to the ideals of a good prevention program deserve highly refined conservative restorative procedures. The contents of this atlas are designed to inspire those who accept such a philosophy to strive continually to improve their skills. Our dental schools must place renewed emphasis on the teaching of operative techniques.

Continued emphasis must remain on conservation of tooth structure, a concept greatly enhanced by modern cutting instruments and high-speed handpieces. All procedures presented are predicated on the use of the rubber dam and vacuum for protection of the patient, dentist, and assistant.

Dr. Moller has produced the majority of the added illustrations and much of the text is adapted from his copyrighted manual *Restorative Dentistry Technique*, which he published in 1977. From this manual many illustrations are also included. Portions of this text are from William W. Howard's *Review of Operative Dentistry*, published by The C. V. Mosby Company in 1973.

Lori Unis Ryland has assisted with modifications of many of the original illustrations drawn by Clarice Francone (that is, new rotary instruments) and has drawn several new ones.

William W. Howard
Richard C. Moller

CONTENTS

ATLAS OF
OPERATIVE DENTISTRY

CHAPTER 1

OPERATIVE DENTISTRY

Definition of operative dentistry

Current Clinical Dental Terminology defines *operative dentistry* as "The branch of oral health service concerned with operations to restore or reform the hard dental tissues; e.g., operations that are necessitated by caries, trauma, impaired function, and the improvement of appearance."*

For the purposes of this atlas the field of operative dentistry will be limited to the *restoration or treatment of faulty, missing, or diseased parts of the clinical crowns of natural teeth.* Restorations as extensive as three-quarter crowns are included.

---

*From Boucher, C. O., editor: Current clinical dental terminology, ed. 2, St. Louis, 1974, The C. V. Mosby Co.

Overview

To be successful, the practice of operative dentistry must be closely related to preventive dentistry. This relationship can be attributed to the fact that, even under highly favorable conditions, restorations begin to deteriorate to some degree immediately on exposure to the oral environment. In the absence of effective preventive or personal care on the part of a patient, this deterioration is accelerated to such an extent that a decision to initiate clinical measures to control disease should be postponed until the patient can demonstrate personal ability to maintain an acceptable level of oral health. A further factor in this relationship can be seen as the influence of the level of excellence of restorative treatment on the patient's ability to care for his or her mouth. Improper restoration or poor quality restoration of teeth can preclude any chance that an acceptable level of dental health will be attained. Indeed, only a continuing high degree of excellence in dental treatment will provide for a continuing high standard of oral health.

General terms (Fig. 1-1)

The following terms and definitions are used to describe teeth and are essential to the field of operative dentistry.

Median line, sometimes referred to as the midline, is defined as the intersection of the midsagittal plane and the maxillary and mandibular dental arches. The median line divides the central body surface into right and left.

Anterior teeth are the incisors and canines.

Posterior teeth are the premolars and molars.

Mesial designates the surface or component of a tooth toward the median line as oriented in the dental arch.

Distal designates the surface or component of a tooth away from the median line as oriented in the dental arch.

Occlusal refers to the surface or component of a posterior tooth toward the masticating surface.

Lingual designates the surface or component of a tooth toward the tongue.

Labial refers to the surface or component of an anterior tooth toward the lips.

Buccal refers to the surface or component of a posterior tooth toward the cheeks.

Facial is sometimes used in place of *labial* or *buccal.*

Incisal refers to the cutting edge of anterior teeth or a component toward that edge.

Proximal refers to the surface or component nearest an adjacent tooth.

Gingival denotes the portion of a tooth surface or component near or toward the gingival attachment.

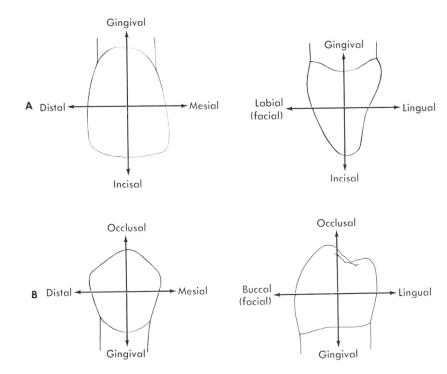

Fig. 1-1. A, Surfaces of anterior teeth (tooth No. 8 illustrated). **B,** Surfaces of posterior teeth (tooth No. 29 illustrated).

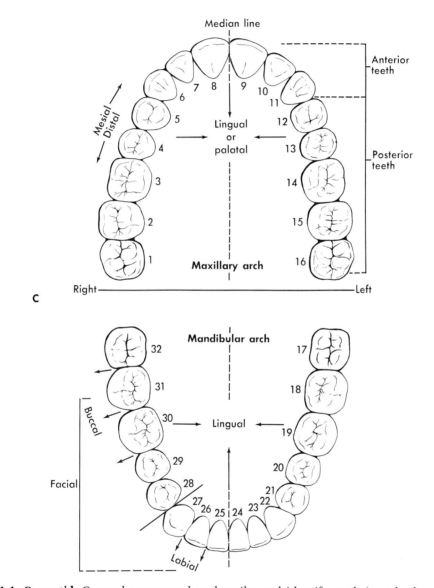

Fig. 1-1. C, cont'd. General terms used to describe and identify teeth (standard numbering system).

Classifications of cavities and restorations

Several terms are used to describe cavities, and at least three systems are used to identify or classify them.

G. V. Black formulated a commonly used system to describe types of cavities. The Black classification consists of five classes, to which a sixth is added (Fig. 1-2).

When a Class 2 situation includes Class 1 cavities, it is considered a Class 2 restoration.

Cavities may also be classified as follows:

Simple, involving only one surface of a tooth
Compound, involving two surfaces of a tooth when prepared
Complex, involving three or more surfaces of a tooth when prepared

A third classification, the one finding possibly the greatest practical utilization in clinical practice, is most specifically descriptive of the surfaces restored because it utilizes the initials of the surfaces treated. For example:

O—Occlusal surface
MO—Mesio-occlusal, or the mesial and occlusal surfaces
DO—Disto-occlusal, or the distal and occlusal surfaces
MOD—Mesio-occlusodistal, or the mesial, occlusal, and distal surfaces
B—Buccal surface
L—Labial surface or lingual surface (F for facial may be preferred. When used to identify a labial surface, L is confusing, thus the term *facial* is gaining preference.)
F—Facial (buccal or labial)
I—Incisal
DI—Distoincisal
MI—Mesioincisal
MID—Mesioincisodistal
DL—Distolingual
ML—Mesiolingual
MLD—Mesiolinguodistal
MF—Mesiofacial
DF—Distofacial
MFD—Mesiofaciodistal

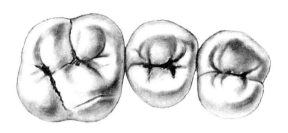

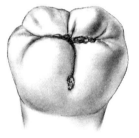

Class 1. Cavities beginning in structural defects of the teeth, such as in pits and fissures

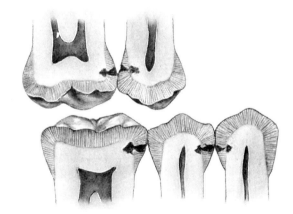

Class 2. Cavities in proximal surfaces of premolars and molars. (When a Class 2 situation includes Class 1 caries, it is considered a Class 2 lesion.)

Fig. 1-2. Black's classification of cavities. Class 6 is added.

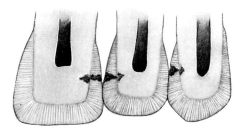

Class 3. Cavities in proximal surfaces of canines and incisors that do not involve removal of the incisal angle

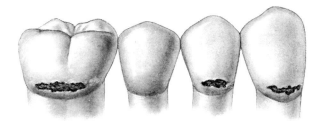

Class 5. Cavities in the gingival third of the labial, buccal, and lingual surfaces (excluding pit cavities)

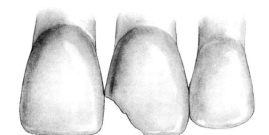

Class 4. Cavities in proximal surfaces of canines and incisors that require removal and restoration of the incisal angle

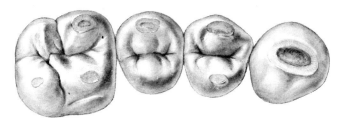

Class 6. Cavities on incisal edges and cusp tips (not included in Black's classification)

Fig. 1-2, cont'd. Black's classification of cavities. Class 6 is added.

Charting

TOOTH NUMBERING AND RADIOGRAPH MOUNTING

At its 1968 meeting the House of Delegates of the American Dental Association adopted the following system of numbering teeth and mounting radiographs.[1] The system adopted to designate permanent teeth assigns the maxillary right third molar the number 1. Each tooth of the maxillary arch is numbered in order to number 16, which is the maxillary left third molar. The mandibular left third molar is number 17 and the mandibular right third molar is number 32. Thus the teeth are numbered clockwise when viewed in the patient's open mouth from the front.

CHARTS

The proper method of mounting radiographs[1] is parallel with the approved numbering system. The upper right films are placed in the upper left side of the mount. The films are thus viewed as if from the front of the patient rather than viewed internally or as from within the patient's mouth.

Many popular types of charts resemble the one illustrated in Fig. 1-3. It has the advantage of being arranged in the same order as the human dentition viewed from the front. Also, radiographs mounted in the same order place chart and films parallel. Included in Fig. 1-3 is a system of charting borrowed largely from the armed forces. The items shown are solely for the purpose of illustration. Such a system is helpful in indicating quickly to the dentist or dental assistant exactly what type of treatment is to be performed.

Fig. 1-4, devised by Dr. Herbert Miller, has the teeth arranged as the mouth is viewed from the front and opened. In addition to being anatomically realistic, this chart has the advantage of providing proximal surfaces for the posterior teeth, and deciduous teeth are included.

Fig. 1-5 illustrates another type of chart and a second system of identifying teeth by numbers. The central incisors, for example, are all designated by the number 1, but teeth are identified as to quadrant by adding half boxes, such as ⎤1, maxillary left central incisor, or 6⎣, mandibular right first molar. This type of chart, unfortunately, lacks realism and does not afford the opportunity

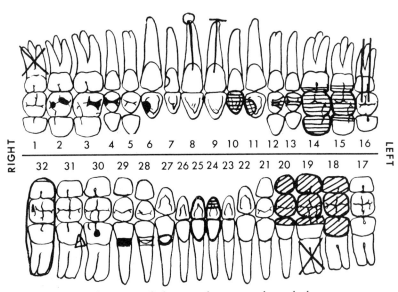

Fig. 1-3. A popular type of chart and suggested symbols to indicate various procedures.

1. Missing tooth
2. Occlusal amalgam
3. MO amalgam
4. MOD amalgam
6. DL amalgam
7. D silicate or plastic
8. Endodontic therapy indicated
9. Completed root canal treatment
10. Lingual gold
11. ML gold
12. DO gold
13. MOD gold
14. Three-quarter (4/5) crown
15. MOD overlay (gold)
16. To be removed
18. Full crown abutment
19. Gold-porcelain pontic (missing tooth)
20. Three-quarter (4/5) crown abutment (cross hatching may also be used to indicate splinted teeth)
24. Gold-porcelain (plastic) crown
25. Porcelain (plastic) crown
27. Labial silicate
28. Buccal gold
29. Buccal amalgam
30. Buccal pit amalgam
31. Mesial margin overhang
32. Impacted

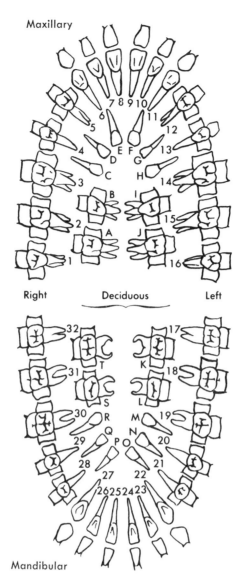

Fig. 1-4. Miller chart.

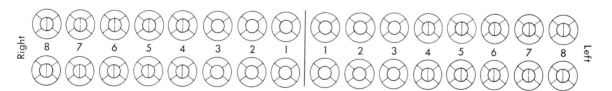

Fig. 1-5. Mechanical or geometric type of chart.

to chart the spectrum of conditions that the anatomical charts do.

Fig. 1-6 shows another example of mechanical outlines to represent the teeth but uses the standard numbering system. It is the type approved by the American Dental Association for the uniform claim form for insurance claims.

If charts provide no outlines for deciduous

teeth, it is suggested that the operative services be charted in the same manner as for permanent teeth and recorded by adding the letter "d" to the number used to identify the permanent tooth.

These charts represent only the dentition portion of a patient record and must, of course, be supplemented with other essential medical-dental information to form an adequate patient record and history.

Components of prepared cavities

Preparation of cavities results in the formation of various *walls, lines,* and *angles.* The following terms are used to describe a prepared cavity and its various components.

A *wall* is an enclosing side of a prepared cavity. It takes the name of the surface of the tooth toward which it is placed (Figs. 1-7 to 1-10). In an axial plane (long axis of the tooth) the internal wall is the *axial wall,* and in the horizontal plane it is the *pulpal wall.*

A *line angle* is formed where two walls meet (Figs. 1-11 to 1-15). At the place where three walls meet a *point angle* is formed (Figs. 1-16 to 1-18).

The *cavosurface angle* is the angle in a prepared cavity formed by the junction of the wall of the cavity with the uncut surface of the tooth (Figs. 1-14 and 1-19).

The term *margin,* although somewhat ambiguous, is commonly used to refer to the *cavosurface angle* of a prepared cavity and/or to designate the line of junction of the tooth surface and the restoration after the restorative material is placed. Margins of a wax pattern or gold casting are also examples of the use of this term to denote the edges that are to abut the cavosurface angle when placed in the prepared cavity.

The *dentinoenamel junction* is the junction of the dentin and the enamel as it appears in the walls of a prepared cavity.

The *enamel wall* is that portion of the wall that consists of enamel. It extends from the cavosurface margin or angle to the dentinoenamel junction.

The *dentin wall* is that portion of a wall that consists of dentin.

The peripheral extent of the cavosurface angle of a prepared cavity is termed the *outline* of the cavity.

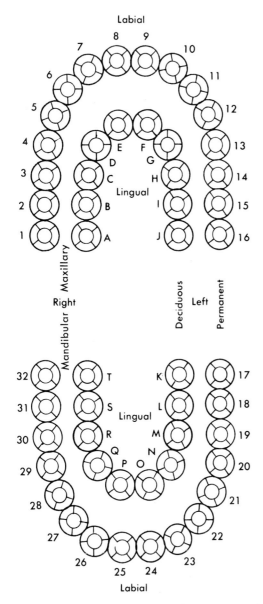

Fig. 1-6. Mechanical or geometric chart arranged anatomically.

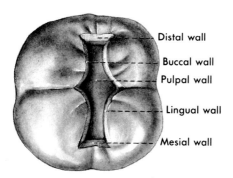

Distal wall
Buccal wall
Pulpal wall
Lingual wall
Mesial wall

Fig. 1-7. Walls of a prepared Class 1 occlusal cavity.

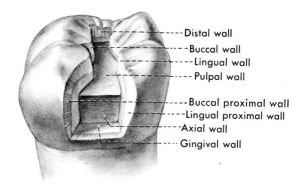

Distal wall
Buccal wall
Lingual wall
Pulpal wall
Buccal proximal wall
Lingual proximal wall
Axial wall
Gingival wall

Fig. 1-8. Cavity walls of a prepared Class 2 cavity.

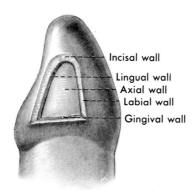

Incisal wall
Lingual wall
Axial wall
Labial wall
Gingival wall

Fig. 1-9. Walls of a Class 3 prepared cavity.

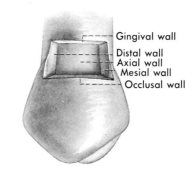

Gingival wall
Distal wall
Axial wall
Mesial wall
Occlusal wall

Fig. 1-10. Walls of a Class 5 prepared cavity.

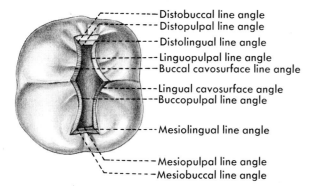

Distobuccal line angle
Distopulpal line angle
Distolingual line angle
Linguopulpal line angle
Buccal cavosurface line angle
Lingual cavosurface angle
Buccopulpal line angle
Mesiolingual line angle
Mesiopulpal line angle
Mesiobuccal line angle

Fig. 1-11. Line angles of a prepared Class 1 cavity.

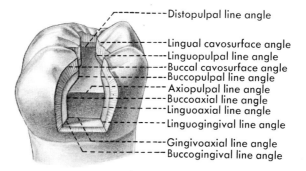

Distopulpal line angle
Lingual cavosurface angle
Linguopulpal line angle
Buccal cavosurface angle
Buccopulpal line angle
Axiopulpal line angle
Buccoaxial line angle
Linguoaxial line angle
Linguogingival line angle
Gingivoaxial line angle
Buccogingival line angle

Fig. 1-12. Line angles of a prepared Class 2 cavity.

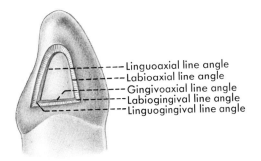

Fig. 1-13. Line angles of a prepared Class 3 cavity.

- - - Linguoaxial line angle
- - - Labioaxial line angle
- - - Gingivoaxial line angle
- - - Labiogingival line angle
- - - Linguogingival line angle

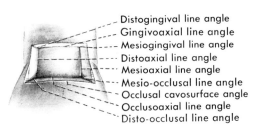

Fig. 1-14. Line angles of a Class 5 prepared cavity. Only one cavosurface angle is noted.

- - - Distogingival line angle
- - - Gingivoaxial line angle
- - - Mesiogingival line angle
- - - Distoaxial line angle
- - - Mesioaxial line angle
- - - Mesio-occlusal line angle
- - - Occlusal cavosurface angle
- - - Occlusoaxial line angle
- - - Disto-occlusal line angle

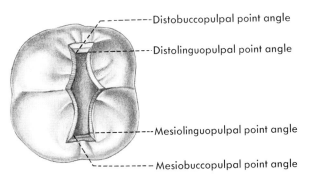

Fig. 1-15. Point angles of a prepared Class 1 cavity.

- - - Distobuccopulpal point angle
- - - Distolinguopulpal point angle
- - - Mesiolinguopulpal point angle
- - - Mesiobuccopulpal point angle

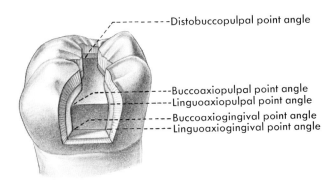

Fig. 1-16. Point angles of a prepared Class 2 cavity.

- - - Distobuccopulpal point angle
- - - Buccoaxiopulpal point angle
- - - Linguoaxiopulpal point angle
- - - Buccoaxiogingival point angle
- - - Linguoaxiogingival point angle

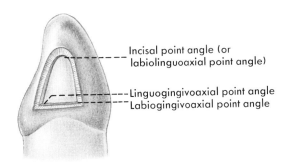

Fig. 1-17. Point angles of a prepared Class 3 cavity.

- - - Incisal point angle (or labiolinguoaxial point angle)
- - - Linguogingivoaxial point angle
- - - Labiogingivoaxial point angle

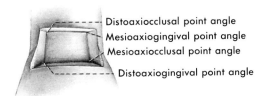

Fig. 1-18. Point angles of a Class 5 cavity preparation.

- - - Distoaxiocclusal point angle
- - - Mesioaxiogingival point angle
- - - Mesioaxiocclusal point angle
- - - Distoaxiogingival point angle

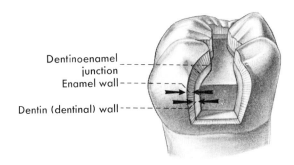

Fig. 1-19. Cross section of a prepared cavity showing enamel and dentin terms and cavosurface angle.

Dentinoenamel junction - - -
Enamel wall - - -
Dentin (dentinal) wall - - -

Treatment of cavosurface angles (margins)

Treatment of the cavosurface angle requires specific detail in cavity preparations, depending on a number of factors, such as length and direction of the enamel prisms, the particular restorative material being used, and the degree of anticipated stress on the area.

Examples of several types of margin finishes are illustrated in Figs. 1-20 and 1-21.

A *bevel*, in a cavity preparation, is the junction of the wall at an obtuse angle with the tooth surface. A cut or plane established in the line or plane of cleavage of enamel, as for gingival margins of amalgam and cohesive gold cavity preparations, is not considered a bevel. However, for practical purposes the term *bevel* is used to describe a cut or portion of a cavity preparation that cuts obliquely across the enamel at the cavosurface margin.

The terms *slight bevel, short bevel, long bevel,* and *full bevel* are used (Figs. 1-20 and 1-21).

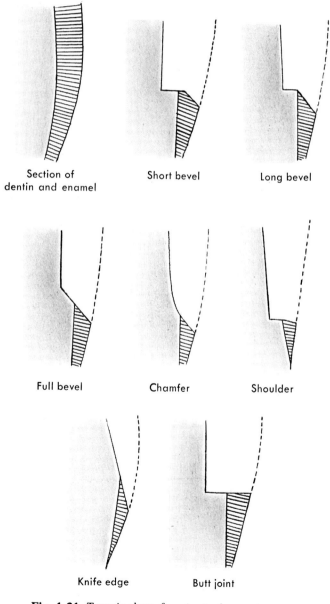

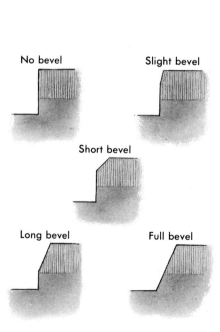

Fig. 1-20. Terminology for bevels on occlusal margins.

Fig. 1-21. Terminology for gingival margins.

Preparation for operative procedures

Prior to applying the principles of operative dentistry a thorough examination and diagnosis must be made of all aspects of the patient's oral cavity and the entire health picture. Detailed treatment planning must follow, and operative procedures are planned with consideration given to all the patient's needs and circumstances.

Certain aspects of the planned treatment program must normally precede operative procedures. For example, the patient's periodontal condition must be under control before operative procedures can be considered successful. The patient's occlusion should be analyzed, and any possible corrective measures must precede or be coordinated with operative treatment.

Basic concepts relative to tooth restoration

CONSERVATION OF TOOTH STRUCTURE

Conservation of tooth structure is of paramount importance in the preservation of esthetics and in the prevention of irritation to the dental pulp and supportive tissues.

Conservation of tooth structure is essential to the proper protection of the dental pulp. Not only is too deep a cavity preparation a hazard to the pulp, but the size of the area of the pulp affected must also be considered. For example, a full crown preparation will irritate all of the odontoblasts in the pulp chamber or within the coronal portion of the pulp. Of course, many factors can be considered relative to pulp irritation in dentistry, but deep and extensive preparations are critical factors that must always be considered.

ESTHETICS

No material is more esthetically beautiful than healthy, unmarred tooth enamel when it is supported by sound dentin. It is fortunate that techniques are available that allow conservative and esthetic treatment of carious lesions if detected and treated early in their development

CONTACTS AND CONTOURS

A thorough knowledge of dental anatomy is essential to understand the functions of the contours of a tooth crown. Contact areas and marginal ridges must be positioned correctly to minimize food impaction.

Contact areas should normally be restored to contours that were or are present in young teeth.

Axial contours will generally depend on the extent of gingival recession. The operator must continually observe conditions that contribute to the preservation of a healthy periodontium. For example, when a tooth receiving a gingival restoration exhibits gingival recession, in addition to consideration of occlusal correction the operator may observe the gingival contour of healthy teeth as an indication of the proper contour. Teeth with no gingival recession should generally be restored to their original contour (Fig. 1-22, *A*). If recession is present, the height of contour must always be moved apically to be placed in proper relation to the gingival tissue (Fig. 1-22, *B*).

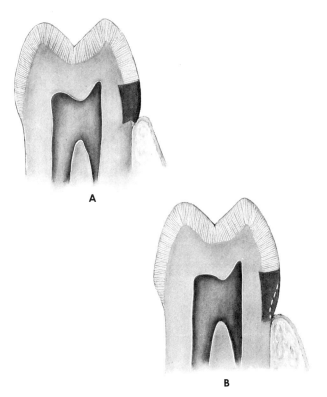

A

B

Fig. 1-22. Examples of placement of gingival contours. **A,** Desired buccal contour relative to normal gingiva. **B,** Proper contour relative to gingiva that has receded apically. Dotted line indicates the approximate original surface contour.

EXTENSION FOR PREVENTION

One of the objectives of operative dentistry is to prevent the recurrence of caries. Prepared cavity outlines must include deep developmental grooves on the occlusal surfaces of posterior teeth. Proximal margins should normally be extended at least slightly onto buccal (or labial) and lingual surfaces to an area where the operator can easily finish the margins and also where they can be easily cleaned by the patient. The hygienic condition of the mouth must be evaluated, and the possibility of a breakdown on tooth structure abuting the restoration considered; cavity outline is then designed accordingly.

Great judgment is demanded of the operator, for it is he or she who must design the restoration according to the factors mentioned, to which must be added the evaluation of whether or not the patient will respond to home care instruction.

Gingival extension of restorations has become somewhat controversial. Traditionally, margins are normally located slightly below the crest of the gingiva. However, every operator should carefully evaluate reasons for the location of the gingival margins. Erroneously, it has long been thought that the subgingival area is relatively immune to caries.

There are compelling reasons to keep gingival extension short of the soft tissues. Among these are conservation of tooth structure, better visual control, ease of finishing the restoration (fewer margin overhangs), and less gingival irritation. The "hiding" of gingival margins seems too often to be a means of hiding one's mistakes.

The procedures illustrated throughout this book are purposely conservative. Increased extension must be considered necessary only if required by an individual situation. The only reasons for locating margins subgingivally are (1) if essential to restore caries or other defects, (2) to cover highly sensitive dentition, or (3) if necessary for acceptable esthetics.

Cavity preparation

Several factors must be considered before a cavity is prepared to restore a defect within a tooth. *First*, the location of the lesion should be noted and the lesion classified according to Black's system. Thus the procedures and concepts to be followed are identified to assume that certain biomechanical principles are fulfilled.

Second, the extent of the lesion must be considered. Accordingly the operator must mentally outline the extent of the prepared cavity that will be necessary and, again, considering the possible biomechanical principles, elect a procedure to be executed for that particular restoration.

Third, and in combination with the two aforementioned factors, other requirements must be observed, such as additional areas to be restored in the same tooth, the depth of the lesion, the possible degree of occlusal stress, and esthetic factors.

In summary, after a diagnosis has been made, the following factors will normally have been evaluated in development of a treatment plan and will be reevaluated at the time the restorative procedure will begin, whether or not it is executed simultaneously with other procedures:

1. Location of the lesion or defect
2. Extent of the area to be restored
3. Other areas in the tooth to be restored
4. Depth of the lesion
5. Other procedures to be executed simultaneously
6. Degree of occlusal stress
7. Esthetic considerations

The above factors are not necessarily in order of priority but are offered as a basis for electing procedures and developing mental habits in the practice of restorative dentistry.

Experience of the operator is obviously another factor that will determine what procedures are elected in a treatment plan, assuming also that ability or degree of skill is also considered. An operator will tend to favor the use of materials with which he or she has the greatest familiarity and skill.

STEPS OF CAVITY PREPARATION

Preparing a tooth to receive any restorative material is an exacting process requiring specific attention to detail. Contrary to popular opinion, placing a restoration does not merely involve drilling a hole in the tooth and thumbing in some silver. Cavity preparation involves a definite process of thought and instrumentation to produce a lasting restoration that will not fail under any normal circumstance. G. V. Black has set forth a general sequence of cavity preparation that includes (1) outline form, (2) resistance form, (3) retention form, (4) convenience form, (5) caries removal, (6) smoothing cavity walls, and (7) cleaning the cavity preparation.

Cavity preparation is most efficiently executed if this order of procedure is followed with few exceptions; deviating from this sequence may mean unnecessary repetition of a step of the procedure already performed.

Outline form

Outline form circumscribes the area of the prepared cavity including (1) the area of the carious lesion, (2) the adjacent enamel defects such as pits and fissures, and (3) all undermined enamel that may be present owing to caries. All margins are placed (1) in areas least susceptible to caries, (2) where they can be finished, and (3) where they are easily reached by the patient by brushing or flossing. Access to caries, the type of restorative material to be used, and the functional requirements of the restoration also affect outline form.

Several factors that must be considered when establishing outline form are as follows:

1. *Access to the lesion or defect.* When a lesion cannot be reached without removal of a portion of the tooth adjacent to it, the means of approach to the lesion through the adjacent tooth structure is termed *access.* The tooth structure to be removed is outlined and space is created to allow adequate instrumentation and vision so that a lesion can be treated properly. Some aspects of access are further treated as convenience form.

2. *Extent of the lesion or defect.* The obvious objectives of restoration of any lesion or defect in a tooth are to restore and preserve form, function, and, when indicated, esthetics. To achieve these goals the cavity preparation must necessarily be extended to include the extent of the defect. Depending on the restorative material being utilized, it is normally necessary to extend the outline to include all *unsupported enamel.* Enamel that is not supported by normal, sound dentin is subject to fracture.

3. *Extent of the caries-susceptible tooth surface area.* The area of the tooth susceptible to further caries activity must be included in the restoration. This principles is called *extension for prevention.* Designing a proper outline to fulfill this requirement is frequently difficult because the benefits to be gained by a thorough program of prevention and the importance of the concept of conservation of *tooth structure* must be considered. Clinical judgment alone, therefore, must dictate the extent of outline form.

Extension for prevention normally requires that the outline form be such that the completed restoration is extended to a so-called self-cleansing area or enamel that is immune to caries by virtue of oral functional factors and /or good home care and preventive measures.

Areas of decalcification must necessarily be considered a possible indication for extension for prevention, as well as the inclusion of all defective or potentially defective developmental grooves and pits.

It has been traditionally taught that gingival extension is ideal when the gingival margin is placed below the crest of the gingiva. Conservative concepts augmented by effective prevention procedures as well as periodontal considerations have forced revision of this concept.

4. *Location and extent of developmental grooves.* Developmental grooves are normally included in outline form to avoid possible recurrence of caries and to establish smooth margins of the finished restoration. It is often preferable to polish out grooves rather than to cut them through the enamel.

5. *The restorative material to be used.* The individual properties of each material utilized to restore teeth demand certain design factors that must be incorporated into the creation of each cavity preparation. For example, relatively weak materials must depend on sound tooth structure to retain and support them—that is, the marginal strengths of such materials as cements, resins, and amalgam are such that the cavosurface margins must be prepared at an angle of approximately 90 degrees with the tooth surface. (There is evidence, however, that an acid-etched, 45-degree bevel provides better retention and strength.) Thus both enamel and the restorative material are provided maximum edge strength when abutted to each other.

Cohesive golds lend themselves to some degree to beveling (see the discussion of bevels on p. 11), provided that such bevels are not excessive and are not subjected to occlusal stress.

Cast gold restorations, because of their greater strength, allow extensive beveling and thus conservation of tooth structure.

The cavosurface angle therefore is an essential consideration in the establishment of outline form.

6. *Esthetic factors.* If a restoration is necessary in an area where it will be potentially visible when the patient smiles, a choice of materials is normally involved. If a lesion in an anterior tooth has not destroyed labial enamel, it may be possible to place cohesive gold from the lingual side of the tooth. Such a procedure demands its own outline form, especially to conserve labial and incisal enamel.

If, however, the operator is not capable of placing a cohesive gold restoration, or if the restoration extends labially, a restoration using a material of a compatible color may be necessary.

7. *Functional requirements of the restoration.* Occasionally, when a restoration may alter the contour of a tooth—for example, in restoring an open contact or improving occlusal function—the outline form must be altered to accommodate the desired objective.

Resistance form

Resistance form is the shape given to the preparation to prevent fracture of either the restorative material or tooth during insertion of the material or during function (for example, provision for adequate bulk of amalgam, surrounding walls at nearly right angles to the flat pulpal wall to withstand the forces of occlusion).

Retention form

Retention form is the shape of the internal aspects of a prepared cavity to prevent displacement of the restorative material (for example, nearly parallel opposing walls, retentive undercuts, grooves, dovetails, pins, and so forth).

Convenience form

Convenience form is that shape or form of the cavity that allows adequate vision, accessibility, and ease of instrumention during cavity preparation as well as insertion of the restorative material. This allows a large enough opening for instruments during preparation and access for placing the restorative material.

Convenience form also includes internal form created in a cavity preparation to facilitate the initiation of placement of the restorative material—for example, convenience points or pits to aid in the retention or stability of the first pieces of cohesive gold that are placed in a Class 3 compacted cohesive gold restoration.

Caries removal

At this stage the majority of decay may already have been removed owing to the extension of the cavity outline. However, there may remain a small amount of deeper decay that is removed at this time. (A suitable base or medication may be placed in the deepest areas to protect the pulp after the decay has been removed.)

Smoothing cavity walls

Cavity walls are smoothed by placing any refinements in the cavity that are necessary, such as elimination of unsupported enamel at the cavosurface angle or smoothing an irregular or jagged outline. This is to provide the best possible marginal seal and maximum strength to both the enamel and the restorative material.

Cleaning the cavity preparation

The final step in the preparation involves using an explorer, air, water spray, and cotton pellets to remove debris from the cavity preparation. A clean, dry cavity preparation is necessary before placing the restorative material.

REFERENCE

1. American Dental Association Transactions, 1968, p. 247.

CHAPTER 2

INSTRUMENTS

Modern instruments, when properly used, will easily produce the desired results the dentist requires. To successfully accomplish prescribed instrument manipulations in a precise fashion, the different types of instruments must be known as well as the function each performs.

The term *instrument* refers to a tool, device, or implement used for a specific purpose or type of work and is preferred in professional or scientific fields because delicate precision items are generally required to perform specific procedures.

Instruments for operative dentistry are classified into several categories. *Hand instruments* include a large group of instruments that are hand held when used. *Rotary instruments* are operated in a handpiece, which is in turn hand held. The term *cutting instrument* generally applies, unless otherwise specified, to a hand-held instrument used for operative dentistry during the process of preparing a cavity. However, burs and stones are also used to cut or reduce tooth structure.

There are many types of varieties of instruments on the market. It is important that the dentist be familiar with instrument terminology and formulas.

Hand instruments
CUTTING INSTRUMENTS

Cutting instruments are those instruments used to cut, plane, scrape, or cleave tooth structure during the preparation of a cavity to receive a restoration or other treatment. A trend exists to eliminate the use of cutting instruments by using the high-speed rotary instruments now available. Conservative, high-quality operative dentistry demands the use of hand instruments in most procedures.

Hand instruments are used to assist in cavity preparation and to insert or to finish the restorative material. They may be used in three ways (1) as explorers, (2) as gauges, and (3) as cutting and smoothing tools. The parts are the handle or shaft, the shank, and the blade. Hand instruments may be single- or double-ended (Fig. 2-1).

The *handle* of most dental instruments is octagonal in shape and slightly smaller than a pencil. It is used to hold the instrument and direct the action of the working surfaces. The *shank* is the tapered section of the instrument that connects the handle with the blade or the nib. The *blade* is the working end of a cutting instrument and normally has three cutting edges: one on the end and two on the sides. A *nib* is the working surface of an instrument used to insert, condense, and finish a restorative material. Hand cutting instruments are manufactured from one of two types of steel, either carbon or stainless steel. Carbon steel has the advantage of being harder and the cutting edge remains sharper, but it tends to rust and corrode.

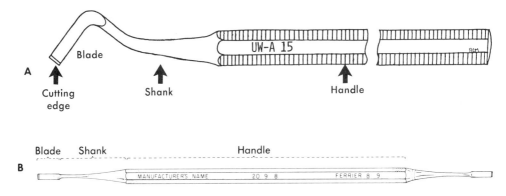

Fig. 2-1. A, Parts of cutting instruments. The rings on the shank to the right on the chisel, **B,** denote that the blade is contrabeveled. Black's formula is 20-9-8. The word *Ferrier* indicates the designer of the instrument or one who has arranged a set of instruments for operative procedures. The numbers 8 and 9 denote the order of instruments in such a set.

INSTRUMENT FORMULAS

A hand-cutting instrument is described by a series of numerals stamped on the side of the handle, which signify measurements in the decimal system. These formula names are made on the same principle as that used by the carpenter in identifying his chisels or augers; for example, ½-inch or 1-inch chisel, ¾-inch auger, and so forth. For the dentist, however, it is sufficient to describe the point of an instrument so that the particular instrument will be known on sight.

The numbers are placed in a definite sequence (Fig. 2-2):
1. The first numeral indicates the width of the blade in tenths of a millimeter.
2. The second numeral indicates the length of the blade in millimeters.

3. The third numeral designates the angle the blade forms with the long axis of the handle expressed in centigrades or ¹/₁₀₀ of a circle.
4. Certain instruments, such as gingival margin trimmers, are constructed with the cutting edge at an angle, other than a right angle, to the length of the blade. In such instances a fourth figure is placed in the formula designating the angle made by the cutting edge with the long axis of the handle. When this fourth figure is used, it is placed between the figures representing the blade width and the blade length (placed second). (See Figs. 2-3 and 2-4, dental instrument gauge.) *If only three numbers appear on the handle, the cutting edge is at right angles to the blade.*

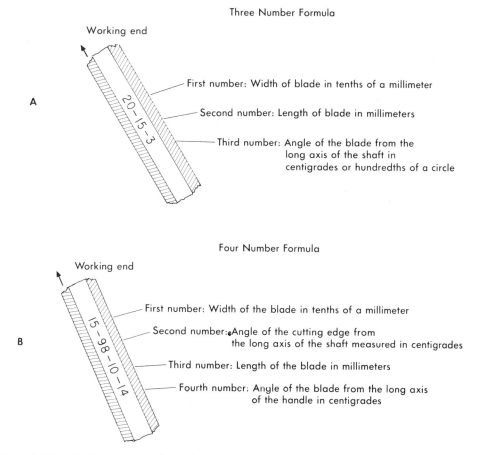

Three Number Formula

Working end

First number: Width of blade in tenths of a millimeter
Second number: Length of blade in millimeters
Third number: Angle of the blade from the long axis of the shaft in centigrades or hundredths of a circle

Four Number Formula

Working end

First number: Width of the blade in tenths of a millimeter
Second number: Angle of the cutting edge from the long axis of the shaft measured in centigrades
Third number: Length of the blade in millimeters
Fourth number: Angle of the blade from the long axis of the handle in centigrades

Fig. 2-2. Black's instrument formulas. **A,** Formula for three numbers. **B,** Formula for four numbers.

On the handle, in addition to the data usually included, other marks may be present to identify the placement of the working end or cutting edge. These marks may be inscribed rings on the base of the shank, dots on the handle adjacent to the working blade, or other distinguishing marks.

DENTAL INSTRUMENT GAUGE

A dental instrument gauge (Figs. 2-3 and 2-4) is used to measure the dimensions of hand instruments. The instrument formula can be related to an instrument by the following.

Measurements are made using the metric system. The length of the blade is found by using the right side of the ruler. The width of the blade is found by using the left side of the ruler inside the notch.

The angle of the blade is found by placing the handle parallel to the ruler, with the blade on the circle to the right of the zero line. Centigradation is now found parallel to the blade, indicating the angle with the handle. Figs. 2-3 and 2-4 show a gingival margin trimmer with a formula of 13-78-8-14.

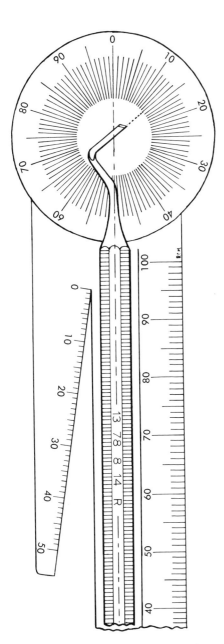

Fig. 2-3. Dental instrument gauge measuring the angle of the blade of a gingival margin trimmer.

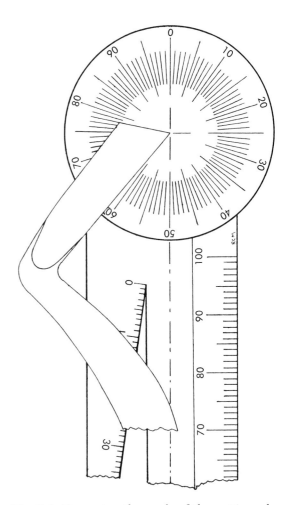

Fig. 2-4. Measuring the angle of the cutting edge.

INSTRUMENT BEVELS

Some instruments, such as enamel hatches and gingival margin trimmers, are designated right or left and may be marked with double rings or double dots on the shank. Such markings indicate that when the instrument is held away from the operator with the handle horizontal and the blade down, the cutting edge is on the right.

Wedelstaedt chisels (Fig. 2-8, *B*) have the bevel placed on the outside curve of the blade. Contra-bevel Wedelstaedt chisels (identified with rings on the shank) have their bevels on the inside curve (Fig. 2-8, *A*).

Bibevel hatchets are beveled on each side of the end of the blade. Other instruments are beveled on one side of the end of the blade only.

Newer designs of most cutting instruments have the sides of their working blades beveled. These designs facilitate the development of more conservative cavity preparations and allow use of the edge of the cutting blade in many situations.

CHISELS

Chisels are used to cleave enamel or plane cavity walls where they are accessible to straight or comparatively straight instruments. Their cutting edges are beveled on one side of the end of the blade, although newer designs also have the sides of the blade beveled.

Straight chisels

Straight chisels are just what the name describes (Fig. 2-5); they are commonly available as 10-10-0, 15-10-0, 20-10-0, or simply 10, 15, and 20, the important factor of a straight chisel being the width of its blade.

Fig. 2-5. Straight chisel.

Monangle chisels

Monangle chisels are those with one angle in the shank (Fig. 2-6).

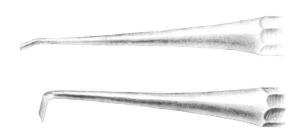

Fig. 2-6. Monangle chisels.

Binangle chisels

Binangle chisels have two bends in their shanks (Fig. 2-7) to place the cutting edge close to the long axis of the shaft as 10-6-6 and 15-8-6. They are used mainly for planing cavity walls of upper premolars and first molars.

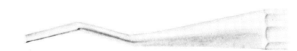

Fig. 2-7. Binangle chisel.

Wedelstaedt chisels

Wedelstaedt chisels have curved blades continuous with the shank, their formulas commonly being 10-10-3, 15-10-3, and 20-10-3 (Fig. 2-8). They are used mainly to plane Class 3 and 5 cavities with curved walls.

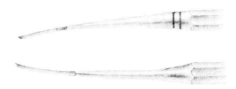

Fig. 2-8. Wedelstaedt chisels.

HOES

Hoes (Fig. 2-9) have their working blades at angles to their shanks. Their cutting action is developed either by thrusting the instrument in the direction of its cutting edge or dragging it much like a garden hoe. Their use is primarily to develop the internal form of cavities, although they are also used to plane enamel walls.

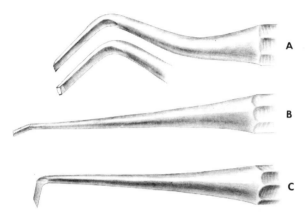

Fig. 2-9. Hoes. **A,** Binangle hoe, 20-10-16. **B,** Monangle hoe, 6½-2½-9. **C,** Another monangle hoe, 8-3-23.

HATCHETS

Hatchets generally have their cutting edges at various angles to the axis of the handle and the flat or broad sides of their blades parallel to the handles. Except for bibeveled hatchets they are paired and single beveled.

Enamel hatchets

Enamel hatchets are binangle (Fig. 2-10) and are used primarily to cleave and plane enamel and to plane proximal walls in Class 2 cavity preparations.

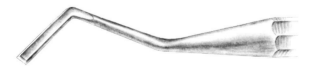

Fig. 2-10. Enamel hatchet.

Off-angle hatchets

Off-angle hatchets (Fig. 2-11) are similar to enamel hatchets (Fig. 2-10), but their working blades are rotated 12.5 centigrades on the blade axis. They are used for the same purposes as enamel hatchets but may also be used to plane cavity walls of lingual Class 5 preparations.

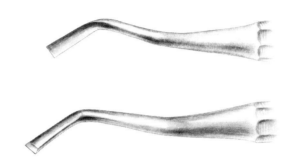

Fig. 2-11. Off-angle hatchets.

Jeffery hatchets

Jeffery hatchets (Fig. 2-12) are similar to off-angle hatchets (Fig. 2-11) but have their blades more nearly at right angles to the shaft. They are used in the preparation of maxillary anterior cavities from the lingual side of the teeth. These instruments have to be specially made for left-handed operators. Nos. 5 and 6 actually function as angle formers, and all three function as hoes.

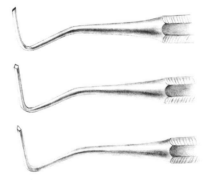

Fig. 2-12. Jeffery hatchets.

Bibevel hatchets

Fig. 2-13 shows a triple-angle bibevel hatchet. Another bibevel hatchet is monangle, 3-2-28 (not illustrated). Bibevel hatchets are used to develop internal or retention form in Class 3 cavity preparations.

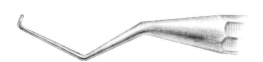

Fig. 2-13. Example of a bibevel hatchet, in this case a triple-angle or contra-angle bibevel hatchet.

GINGIVAL MARGIN TRIMMERS

Gingival margin trimmers have single beveled working blades, are binangled, and paired. Their working blades are curved toward their working edges, which are themselves at an angle from the axis of the blade (Fig. 2-14). These instruments may also be designated mesial and distal. Mesial margin trimmers have the point or acute angle of the blade (Fig. 2-14, *B*) nearest the shank, while distal margin trimmers (Fig. 2-14, *A*) have the point away from the shank.

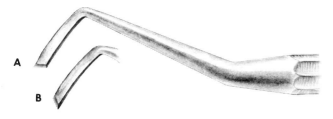

Fig. 2-14. Gingival margin trimmers. **A,** Distal gingival margin trimmer. **B,** Mesial gingival margin trimmer.

ANGLE FORMERS

Angle formers are similar to hoes, having their working blades at an angle to the axis of the shaft, but having their cutting edges at an angle to the axis of their blades rather than at right angles to them (Fig. 2-15, *A*). They are paired and are used to create retention form, mainly in Class 3 preparations, to place bevels in some preparations, and to accentuate line and point angles. Those with their working blades offset from the long axis of the shaft are termed *bayonet angle formers* (Fig. 2-15, *B*).

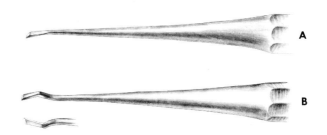

Fig. 2-15. Angle formers. **A,** Standard angle former. **B,** Bayonet angle former.

EXCAVATORS

The term *excavator* as used by G. V. Black included all cutting instruments. However, current usage of the term refers to those instruments, either spoon (Fig. 2-16, *A*) or discoid (Fig. 2-16, *B*), used primarily to remove carious dentin from a cavity. They are paired, usually binangled, and have the entire periphery of their working blades sharpened.

Spoon excavators generally have elongated, curved blades. *Discoid* excavators have disk-shaped working blades placed at a slight angle to their own shank adjacent to the instrument shank.

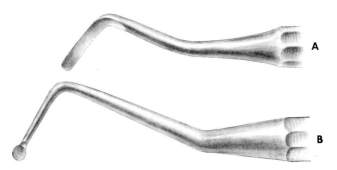

Fig. 2-16. Excavators. **A,** Spoon excavator. **B,** Discoid excavator.

CONDENSING INSTRUMENTS

Instruments used to pack or condense the restorative material into prepared cavities are referred to as *condensers;* the term *plugger* is now considered obsolete. The part of a condenser corresponding to the blade of a cutting instrument is the *nib,* the end of which is called the *face* of the condenser.

Designs of condensers are generally similar to those of cutting instruments and usually can be described by Black's formulas. They may be straight, monangle, binangle, bayonet, and so forth.

Nibs may be of various geometric designs: round, square, triangular, diamond, parallelogram, and so forth. Their ends may be smooth or serrated.

In addition to hand condensers, points are used in handpieces of various types powered by mechanical sources, such as air and electric motor.

CARVING INSTRUMENTS

Carvers (Fig. 2-17) are designed in various forms (square, discoid, cleoid, and so forth) to be used to form or shape plastic materials such as wax or amalgam. Many have elongated working blades of various shapes set at various angles to the shaft.

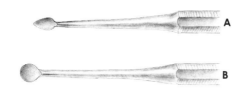

Fig. 2-17. A, Cleoid carver. **B,** Discoid carver.

INSTRUMENT GRASPS

Basically two grasps are used in handling instruments, and they can be varied with the task or the location of the tooth and cavity preparation.

Pen grasp (Fig. 2-18)

The pen grasp is the most commonly used grasp and is accomplished by positioning the hand as for writing. The instrument is held between the thumb and first two fingers, the last two fingers being used as rests or supports. This grasp offers the best control because the thumb and two fingers provide a tripod for the instrument, and this grasp should be used whenever possible because of the accuracy that is attained with its use.

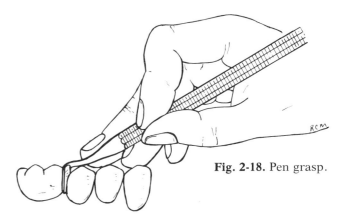

Fig. 2-18. Pen grasp.

Palm and thumb grasp (Fig. 2-19)

With the palm and thumb grasp the instrument handle rests in the palm and the cutting edge is directed by the four fingers and thumb. In most cases the thumb rests on tooth structure, usually the tooth adjacent to the one being prepared to support the movements. This grasp is most often used on the upper teeth because it is uncomfortable to use the pen grasp in some of these areas. It is seldom used when working on the lower arch, since it would be awkward to hold the instrument this way.

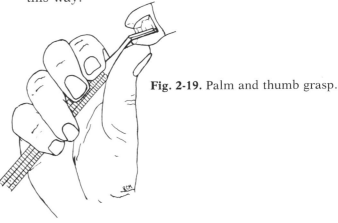

Fig. 2-19. Palm and thumb grasp.

INSTRUMENT STROKES

Dental hoes, hatchets, and chisels may be used to refine a cavity preparation in two ways. (1) The instrument can be used with a *cleaving stroke* (Fig. 2-20) to split off large irregular areas of enamel. Enamel tends to break or separate along a definite plane. If a sharp instrument is directed along this plane, with an adequate force, a separation of the enamel will occur. (The tooth fractures along a definite plane as opposed to being sliced.) (2) A dental instrument may be dragged across the tooth surface at right angles to the blade, *scraping stroke* (Fig. 2-20), thus removing small irregularities in the tooth structure and smoothing the surface.

A combination of these movements will be used when refining a cavity preparation. To use the hand instrument with greatest efficiency, it must be kept sharp. The instrument should be checked periodically during a procedure for any irregularities in the cutting edge and in sharpness.

Rotary instruments

Rotary cutting instruments have been beautifully discussed and classified by the Council on Materials and Devices of the American Dental Association.[1] Design standards of commonly used burs are established by the Council. Diamond rotary cutting instruments are much more difficult to classify. The American Dental Association classification of diamond points seem to be largely ignored by manufacturers; however, use of the classification is to be encouraged.

Rotary instruments are held in handpieces of various types powered by an electric motor or air or water turbines and either direct or belt driven. They may have *long shanks* (Fig. 2-21, *C*) for use in a straight handpiece, *short latch shanks* (Fig. 2-21, *B*) for use in a *latch* contra-angle, or *friction grip shanks* (Fig. 2-21, *A*) for use in an ultrahigh-speed handpiece.

Additional sizes of friction grip shanks include miniature and both longer (surgical) and shorter shanks.

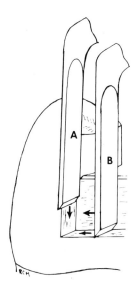

Fig. 2-20. Cleaving and scraping strokes. **A,** Cleaving stroke. **B,** Scraping stroke.

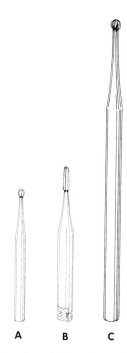

Fig. 2-21. The shanks of these burs illustrate those in common use. **A,** Friction grip. **B,** Latch. **C,** Straight handpiece.

BURS

Burs are rotary cutting instruments. They have three parts as illustrated in Fig. 2-22. The head of the bur has several cutting blades, usually 8 or 12, and may be shaped in a number of ways. Some of the basic bur designs are illustrated in Fig. 2-23. Burs are made with a steel shank, neck, and head, but sometimes the head is made of carbon steel (for additional hardness) and welded to the neck.

Each shape of bur comes in a series of different sizes designated by a specific number. The number indicates not only the size of the bur but also the shape. (As the number increases, so does the bur size.)

$^{1}/_{4}$-11	Round
$11^{1}/_{2}$-22	Wheel
$33^{1}/_{4}$-44	Inverted cone
$55^{1}/_{4}$-62	Straight fissure
$66^{1}/_{2}$-73	Tapered fissure

The burs listed above and their corresponding number series indicate the blades or flutings are straight. Numbers preceded by a 1, 5, 7, or 9 indicate various types of cutting edges.

0-99 series	Straight fluting or straight blades
100 series	Plain (spiral fluting, but not crosscut)
500 series	Crosscut (does not include tapered fissure bur)
700 series	Tapered fissure crosscut
900 series	End cutting

The standard classification of burs recognized by the American Dental Association* is:

$^{1}/_{2}$-11	Round
$11^{1}/_{2}$-16	Wheel
$33^{1}/_{2}$-40	Inverted cone
$55^{1}/_{2}$-62	Plain fissure
170-171	Tapered fissure noncrosscut
502-504	Round crosscut
556-563	Straight fissure crosscut
700-703	Tapered fissure crosscut
901-903	End and side cutting
957-959	End cutting

The letter "L" after a bur number, such as 169L, means the bur is longer than normal but retains the original shape.

---

*Guide to Dental Materials and Devices, ed. 6, Chicago, 1972, American Dental Association, contains a detailed classification of standards and specifications for types of burs in use today. For practical purposes, only the burs widely used are included here.

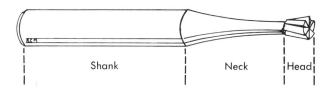

Fig. 2-22. Parts of a dental bur.

Examples of burs:
169L	Spiral fluting tapered fissure—long
556	Crosscut straight fissure
701	Crosscut tapered fissure

Flutings are indented spaces between the blades of the bur.

The term *crosscut* means the blades are notched.

Fig. 2-23 illustrates the types of dental burs common to restorative procedures. In some cases other sizes may be available in addition to those indicated.

Fig. 2-24 illustrates typical twelve-blade burs now available for various finishing procedures both of preparations and of restorations.

Fig. 2-25 illustrates typical shapes of diamond points. Many additional shapes are marketed and sizes vary greatly. Also their surface textures range from very coarse to very fine depending on the degree of abrasiveness desired. Some manufacturers coordinate sizes and shapes of diamond points with burs. This allows tooth reduction using diamond points and fine finishing of the same shape using burs.

ABRASIVE POINTS

Abrasive materials used for rotary instruments in operative dentistry include carborundum, Arkansas stone, and diamonds. The term *point* is frequently used to denote a small rotary instrument for intraoral use, such as "diamond point." These instruments defy rigid classification because of the endless variety of shapes and sizes manufactured.

FINISHING INSTRUMENTS

Rotary instruments used to finish and polish restorations include finishing burs, mounted stones, abrasive disks, rubber cups, and impregnated abrasive rubber disks and are illustrated throughout the text.

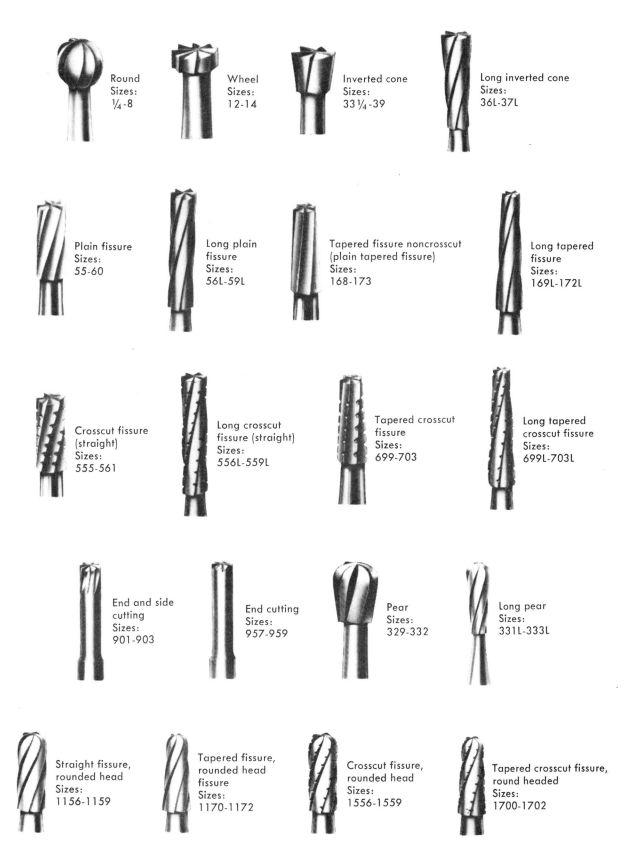

Fig. 2-23. Types of standard dental burs. (Courtesy Brasseler USA, Inc.)

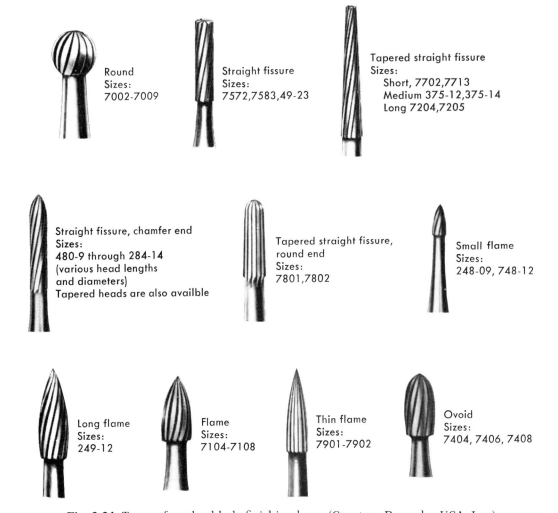

Round
Sizes:
7002-7009

Straight fissure
Sizes:
7572,7583,49-23

Tapered straight fissure
Sizes:
    Short, 7702,7713
    Medium 375-12,375-14
    Long 7204,7205

Straight fissure, chamfer end
Sizes:
480-9 through 284-14
(various head lengths
and diameters)
Tapered heads are also availble

**Tapered straight fissure,
round end**
Sizes:
7801,7802

Small flame
Sizes:
248-09, 748-12

Long flame
Sizes:
249-12

Flame
Sizes:
7104-7108

Thin flame
Sizes:
7901-7902

Ovoid
Sizes:
7404, 7406, 7408

Fig. 2-24. Types of twelve-blade finishing burs. (Courtesy Brasseler USA, Inc.)

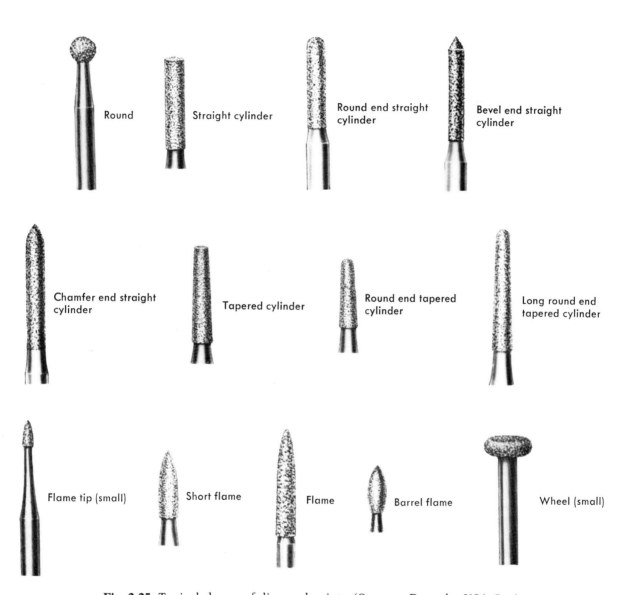

Fig. 2-25. Typical shapes of diamond points. (Courtesy Brasseler USA, Inc.)

Care of hand instruments

SHARPENING

Knowledge of the fundamental nature and uses of dental instruments and their maintenance is essential. A dull instrument in the hands of the best operator can accomplish very little.

There are several types of sharpening stones available for use with dental instruments. The most efficient are either the motor-driven rotary type or the oscillating type. Some of the motor-driven rotary stones on the market move too rapidly. Others move more slowly, but they move from side-to-side while rotating and have housings that restrict access to the stone.

A good rotary sharpener revolves at a slow speed, has a very fine circular stone, and has complete access to both sides of the stone. It should also have an accurate guiding plate to provide the correct bevel for sharpening instruments and a finger rest. The bevel should be cut by sighting visually.

For general purposes, dental instruments may be sharpened by movement back and forth on a good, flat Arkansas stone. The stone should be kept clean by frequent wiping with an alcohol sponge. For spoon excavators and cleoid-discoids, mounted Arkansas stones are available for use in the dental straight handpiece. Failing these, any fine stone can be used if cleaned beforehand.

The problem with sharpening any convex instrument (discoid-cleoid or spoon excavator—Fig. 2-26) is the gradual shortening or decrease in size and reduction of the tempered area. These instruments may be sharpened by applying the flat surface to the stone, but all too often sharpening the instrument in this way destroys the cutting efficiency of the instrument. The flat surface becomes unintentionally rounded, which does not produce a clean sharp cutting edge. Instead, the cutting edge remains somewhat rounded and dull.

The cutting edges of these instruments can be trued and sharpened by holding the flat surface nearly perpendicular but less than 90° to the moving stone and rotating the instrument so the full circumference of the cutting edge (Fig. 2-26) is eventually brought into contact with the stone. Care must be taken to use an even amount of pressure against the wheel and rotate the instrument in one uniform motion. Stalling at any one point will leave a flat area or facet on the blade.

A dull instrument:

1. Is less controllable
2. Takes more force to cut tooth structure
3. Takes more time to cut tooth structure
4. Produces a rough, irregular surface
5. Produces fatigue and strain on the operator

A sharp cutting instrument readily cuts tooth structure without digging into the wall of the tooth.

Hand cutting instruments such as hoes, hatchets, angle formers, gingival margin trimmers, straight chisels, binangle chisels, and Wedelstaedt chisels have one characteristic of the blade in common. They have cutting edges on three sides of the blade (Fig. 2-27). Each blade has *three cutting edges* all located on the same side of the instrument (Fig. 2-27). Each of these edges must be maintained by proper sharpening. Since the cutting edges on the side of the blade are angled more steeply and are not used as much, they usually do not require sharpening as often but nevertheless should be checked for wear or chips.

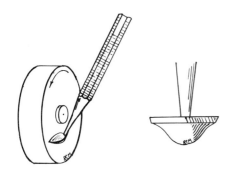

Fig. 2-26. Sharpening a cleoid instrument.

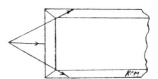

Fig. 2-27. Three bevels of a cutting blade.

Using the rotary stone sharpener

1 Check the instrument carefully before attempting to resharpen the cutting edge. Improper alignment of the cutting edge during sharpening can destroy the instrument.

2 Carefully orient the instrument on the instrument rest so that the proper angle of the cutting edge is restored. Fig. 2-28 illustrates the proper orientation of an angle former and a hoe.

3 Elevate or lower the instrument on the instrument rest so that a 45-degree cutting edge is produced (Fig. 2-29).

4 Use the side of the rotary stone (Fig. 2-30) to true the side cutting edges of the hand instrument. Orient the instrument while the machine is off to prevent accidentally nicking the instrument. NOTE: The sides of handcutting instruments are sharpened at a steeper angle than 45 degrees. The instrument must be rotated slightly (Fig. 2-31) to produce an acute angle (approximately 85 degrees).

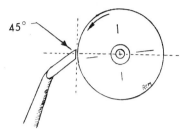

Fig. 2-29. Proper angle of a cutting blade to the sharpening stone.

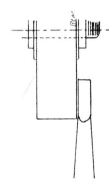

Fig. 2-30. Truing the side of a cutting blade.

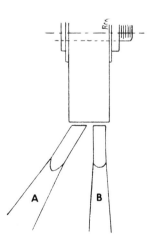

Fig. 2-28. Proper orientation of an angle former, **A,** and a hoe, **B,** to the sharpening stone.

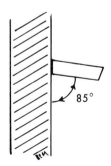

Fig. 2-31. Proper angle of the side of a cutting blade.

Arkansas stone

An Arkansas stone (must be kept cleaned and oiled) may be used to sharpen most hand instruments (Fig. 2-32). The instrument is held at its proper angle in the right hand while the stone is moved by the left hand. The instrument may, of course, be moved by the right hand, but a tendency exists to roll or move the instrument from its proper angle when this technique is used.

In many cases it is preferable for the dentist to have a sharpening instrument close to the operating area so that the instrument may be conveniently resharpened during a procedure.

When sharpening instruments, remember:

1. Use care; heat "blues" the instrument, an indication that the temper or hardness is lost.
2. Keep flat hand stones clean by wiping frequently with an alcohol sponge.
3. Never oil a rotary stone, as this will soften it in different places causing it to abrade more quickly and producing bumps on its surface. Oiling a rotary stone will also allow metal particles to clog the wheel and reduce its abrasiveness.
4. Make a short, definite bevel (approximately 45-degree angle) on hand cutting instruments. It will hold an edge longer than will a long, thin bevel (Fig. 2-33) and will cut just as well.

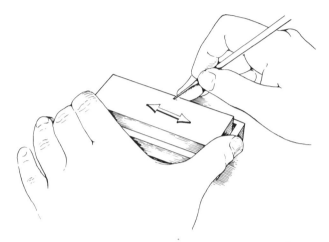

Fig. 2-32. Sharpening an instrument on an Arkansas stone. The instrument is held steady in the right hand as the stone is moved.

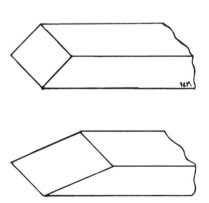

Fig. 2-33. Top, a 45-degree bevel (proper) and an instrument with too flat (sharp) a bevel, bottom.

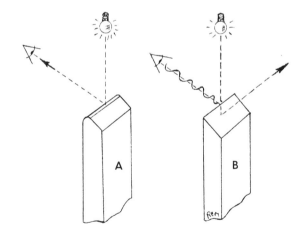

Fig. 2-34. Cutting blades with, **A**, a dull edge and, **B**, a sharp edge.

Detection of a dull cutting instrument

The following are indications of a dull cutting instrument:

1. Visibility of a reflection off the cutting edge (You will not see a reflection off the cutting edge of a sharp instrument [Fig. 2-34].)
2. Obvious irregularities in the cutting edge (Fig. 2-35)
3. Won't shave thumbnail
4. Won't cut tooth structure (If the cutting edge is dull, the instrument must be steeply inclined toward the surface being cut. This usually results in producing a rough or irregular surface by shattering the enamel prisms [Fig. 2-36].)

REFERENCE

1. Guide to dental materials and devices, ed. 6, Chicago, 1972, American Dental Association.

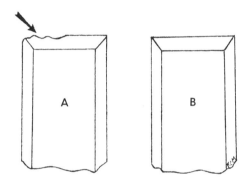

Fig. 2-35. A, Irregularities on the cutting edge. **B,** A sharp straight cutting edge.

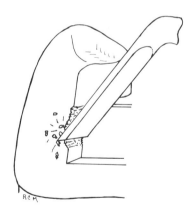

Fig. 2-36. A dull cutting edge is difficult to control and can shatter enamel prisms.

CHAPTER 3

OPERATING FIELDS

While executing operative procedures, specific areas of the dental arch are commonly isolated to enhance access for instrumentation and visibility. Proper isolation will control moisture, maintain a clean surgical field when needed, and protect the patient from harsh chemicals or mechanical trauma.

The area to be isolated may be only a single tooth as for endodontic procedures, or it may include an entire arch as for extensive restorative treatment. The extent of isolation is dependent on the particular requirements of the operation. There are numerous methods for isolating teeth; the method used is dictated by the extent of the area to be isolated, the type of operation to be performed, and the length of time the area is to remain isolated.

Mouth mirror and suction

The use of a mouth mirror to retract adjacent soft tissue in combination with high volume suc-

tion is helpful for controlling moisture and providing moderately clear vision in localized areas of the mouth for short durations. This method is useful when preparing teeth for crown or bridge restorations. It allows checking occlusal relationships as needed with a minimum of difficulty.

Cotton rolls

Cotton rolls are available in a wide variety of lengths and diameters and may be used in conjunction with a saliva ejector to absorb excess moisture. They have a disadvantage of not improving access or visibility to a great extent because of the close proximity to the teeth. Cotton roll isolation may be used during impression procedures for cast gold restorations or application of topical fluoride. Cotton rolls are placed in the vestibule where moisture control is desired. They may be used for varying lengths of time depending on how fast they become saturated. Wet cot-

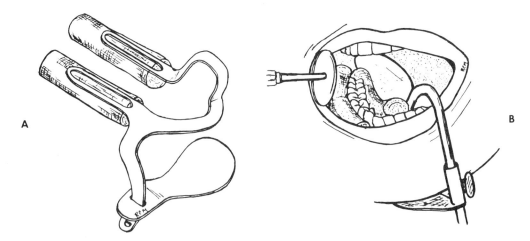

Fig. 3-1. A, Cotton rolls in place on a typical cotton roll holder. **B,** Cotton rolls in place on either side of mandibular posterior teeth with Svedopter in place to retract and protect the tongue.

ton rolls may be exchanged for dry ones from time to time as needed. Slightly better visibility and access may be obtained in the lower arch by using a cotton roll holder (Fig. 3-1, *A*). This device forces the cotton rolls deeper into the buccal and lingual vestibule and holds the tongue and cheek slightly farther away from the teeth. An alternative to the use of cotton rolls to retract and protect the tongue is the use of a Svedopter (Fig. 3-1, *B*).

Rubber dam

A rubber dam is a thin sheet of latex or rubber that may be purchased in a variety of sizes (6 inches by 6 inches, 5 inches by 6 inches, and 5 inches by 5 inches being the most common sizes) and several thicknesses (thin, 0.006 inch; medium, 0.008 inch; heavy, 0.010 inch; extra heavy, 0.012 inch; and special extra heavy, 0.014 inch). A rubber dam is used to obtain an operating field that is dry and antiseptic and to retract the surrounding soft tissues (gingiva, tongue, lips, and cheek). A rubber dam also protects the soft tissues from rotating instruments and medications or drugs that may be injurious or distasteful; it also protects the patient from swallowing tooth debris or accidentally aspirating foreign bodies. When properly applied, the resultant dry field and soft tissue retraction provide the dentist with a better view of the operating area. All restorative services are completed more efficiently and are of better quality when performed using a rubber dam. With a little experience, a rubber dam can be placed in one to three minutes.

Even if considerable time is devoted to application of a good dam, the reasons cited not only justify but demand its use.

The only reason for not using a rubber dam is lack of interest or lack of ability on the part of the operator, except for occasional situations in which it may be impossible to place adequate clamps or retainers. The operator who consistently places superb restorations will seldom operate without the use of a rubber dam if it is possible to use one.

If the dentist is positive concerning the use of the rubber dam, patients frequently volunteer comments on the advantages of having it used. They normally feel more secure during operative procedures with a dam in place. The frequently heard excuse for not using a dam, "patients don't like it," is a misconception. What patients really do not like is the awkwardness of the inept operator who has never learned to use it with ease.

MATERIALS

As indicated previously, rubber dam material is available in thicknesses ranging from thin to special extra heavy. The heaviest thicknesses are decidedly preferable. Extra heavy (or special extra heavy) rubber may have a somewhat more awkward feel to those not familiar with it, but contrary to the opinion of many it is actually easier to place. It is much tougher and may be passed through contacts without tearing as frequently as lighter grades. It also resists catching rotary instruments (burs, finishing disks, and so forth), is more effective for tissue retraction, and is less likely to leak.

The material is supplied in rolls or precut in sizes 6 inches square and 5 inches by 6 inches; the smaller size is used for isolating anterior teeth and on children. Rubber dam is supplied in dark and light colors. The dark color is generally preferred because it contrasts with the teeth and reflects less light. A green-colored rubber has recently been placed on the market.

APPLICATION

The first step in applying a rubber dam is to look at the patient's teeth in the quadrant to be isolated. To prevent unnecessary bunching or stretching of the dam, it is necessary to note the number of teeth, size of teeth, curvature of the arch, location of missing teeth, teeth that may be in buccoversion or linguoversion, height of the gingiva, and location and size of any diastemas or edentulous areas. These observations are necessary so that one may correctly locate and punch the holes in the dam.

Templates or rubber stamps are also available that may be used to help those inexperienced in the location of holes in the rubber dam. An experienced operator will vary the arrangement according to individual conditions in each case.

Basic rules for punching rubber dam

1 The rubber dam is punched differently for each specific operation; therefore keep in mind the tooth requiring the restoration.

2 Select the correct size of rubber dam for the operation, 6 inches by 6 inches for posterior and 5 inches by 6 inches for anterior applications.

3 Make the key punch in the correct position, using the rubber dam punch patterns as a guide. This hole will serve as a guide for positioning the remaining holes on the dam. A pattern for punching rubber dam is shown in Fig. 3-2.

Fig. 3-3 shows several patterns for segments of the dental arch and location of the key punch.

4 Consider the following when punching the remaining holes:

a. The correct size hole for each tooth should be included in the rubber dam (Fig. 3-4).
   (1) Smallest hole: upper lateral, lower incisors
   (2) Second hole: upper central incisor, upper and lower cuspids and premolars

(3) Third and fourth holes: large premolars and molars
(4) Largest hole: exceptionally large molars and tooth to be clamped

b. The spacing and position of the teeth (labioversion, linguoversion, bridge connectors, splinted teeth, diastema, edentulous areas, and so forth) should be considered.

c. The shape of the arch—punching the curve of the arch too flat or straight (Fig. 3-5) will result in folds and stretching of the rubber dam labially, and punching the dam with too

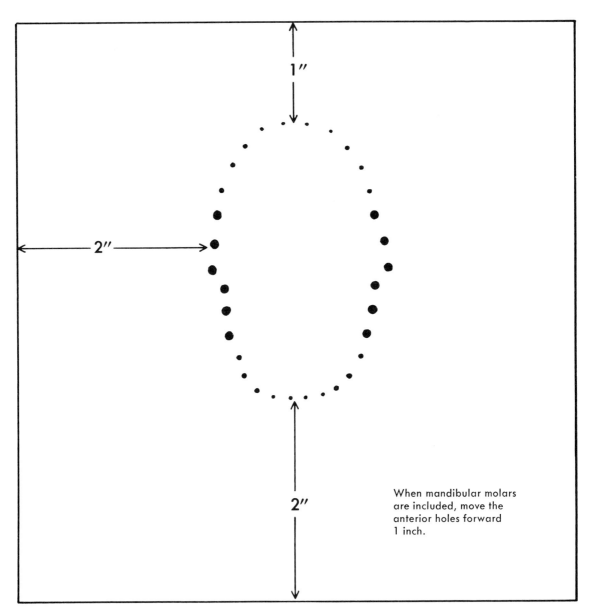

1″

2″

2″

When mandibular molars are included, move the anterior holes forward 1 inch.

Fig. 3-2. Template or guide to aid in the arrangement of holes using 6-inch rubber dam material.

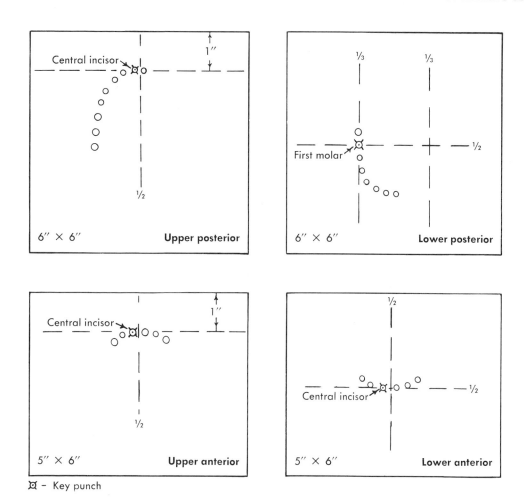

Ⅺ – Key punch

Fig. 3-3. Various patterns of hole arrangements for segments of the dental arch.

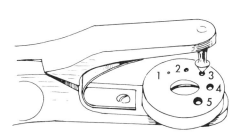

1. Smallest incisors
2. Upper central incisors, canines, and premolars
3 and 4. Large premolars and molars
5. Large molars and clamps

Fig. 3-4. Suggested relative sizes of holes to be punched for a rubber dam.

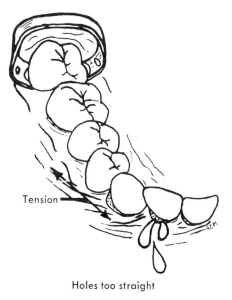

Holes too straight

Fig. 3-5. Result of punching the holes in too straight a line.

much curvature (Fig. 3-6) will result in folds and stretching lingually. In either case there will be increased difficulty in sealing the dam around the teeth.

d. The holes are generally punched in the configuration of a curve or arc slightly smaller than the arch of teeth (Fig. 3-7) on which the dam is to be placed. Particular care must be taken, however, to observe the size of the interproximal papillae. In cases of high, full papillae the holes should be spaced farther apart (Fig. 3-8).

e. In general, 3.5 mm. of rubber should be left between holes—not between centers. Holes for lower anterior teeth are punched slightly closer. Holes too close together will allow leakage around the teeth owing to excessive stretching of the rubber dam (Fig. 3-9). If the holes are too far apart, the rubber bunches up between the teeth (Fig. 3-10).

f. When convenient, include two teeth distal to the tooth to be operated on and one tooth beyond the midline. This provides for increased access and visibility in the working area and better lay of the dam.

g. For Class 5 restorations, the hole for the tooth to be operated on is punched 1 mm. buccally or labially, at the same time allowing 1 mm. extra rubber between adjacent teeth (Fig. 3-11).

h. When punching posterior dams, the hole for the incisors should be located near the midline of the dam.

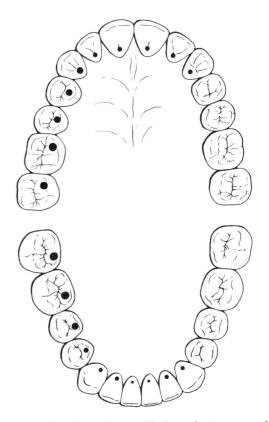

Fig. 3-7. Usual positions of holes relative to teeth.

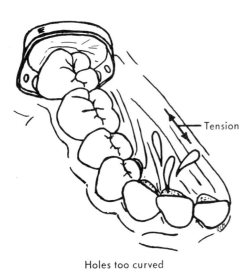

Holes too curved

Fig. 3-6. Result of punching the holes in too tight a curve.

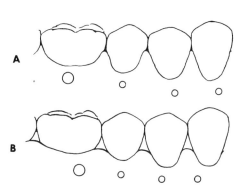

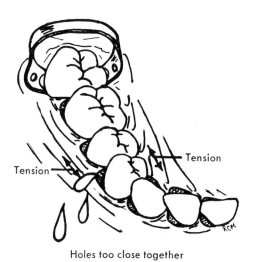

Holes too close together

Fig. 3-8. Examples of how the spacing between holes must be considered relative to the height and fullness of the interdental papillae. **A,** High papillae, full gingival tissues. **B,** Smaller papillae.

Fig. 3-9. Holes punched too close together may leave space between the dam and the teeth.

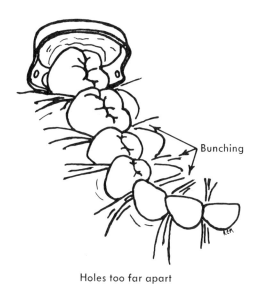

Holes too far apart

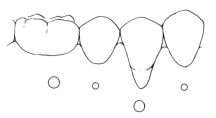

Fig. 3-10. Bunching of the rubber because the holes are punched too far apart.

Fig. 3-11. Relative location and size of a hole for a mandibular first premolar when an extensive Class 5 lesion is to be treated.

TECHNIQUES FOR STABILIZING THE DAM

Techniques to hold the dam in place on the most posterior tooth during the dam application include use of (1) clamps, (2) ligatures, (3) interproximal retention (including reliance on the dam itself, floss, strips of rubber dam, or segments of rubber bands), and (4) compound.

Clamps (retainers)

Clamps of various types (tungsten steel is preferred) are used generally for stabilizing the distal aspect of the dam and for gingival retraction. Use of a clamp to retain the distal aspect of the dam is frequently unnecessary but is usually essential on short teeth such as in younger patients. *It must be emphasized that clamps should be avoided when control of the dam is possible without them because they may be uncomfortable to the patient and may injure gingival tissues if not well controlled.*

A variety of clamps should be kept available, and the operator should never hesitate to modify a clamp to improve its function for a given situation. New clamps should always be inspected to be certain the edges that will engage the tooth are smooth. If they are sharp or rough, they must be smoothed and polished with an abrasive rubber wheel.

The use of clamps with or without wings is a matter of personal preference; however, we usually prefer wingless clamps. Those with wings can generally be improved by cutting off the anterior tabs.

The list at the right should be helpful as a guide to the uses of various clamps. The list is a compilation of popular clamps. Those followed by an asterisk (*) are especially useful. Fig. 3-12 shows at a glance which clamps may be selected for most cases.

POPULAR CLAMPS
Premolars and anteriors

MANUFACTURER	NUMBER	GENERAL FUNCTION AND ADVANTAGES
		Anterior teeth and premolars
SSW	212*	Gingival retraction; must be stabilized with compound (Figs. 3-50, 3-65, and 3-66)
	27	Usually best when altered; can accommodate some third molars
Ivory	00*	Mandibular incisors and small premolars
	0	Mandibular incisors and small premolars
	2*	Premolars; may be altered for gingival retraction on molars
	S1, S2, S3	Gingival retraction; must be stabilized with compound
		Molars
SSW	1A* and 2A*	Deciduous molars
	26	General molar use, especially lowers
	30* and 31*	Gingival retraction; an additional pair should have wings reduced to facilitate placement of the SSW No. 212 clamp on an adjacent tooth
Ivory	4*	Gingival retraction, maxillary molars
	7	Mandibular molars when space limited
	7B	Large molars
	8	Gingival retraction, maxillary molars, larger than No. 4
	W8A*	Partially erupted molars, deciduous molars, small third molars
	10 and 10A*	Maxillary left molars
	11 and 11A*	Maxillary right molars
	14 and 14A*	Partially erupted molars
	16	Gingival retraction; must be modified (Fig. 3-56)
	27*	Large molars; has unusually large bow permitting distal access

A properly placed clamp should engage the tooth on four points (Fig. 3-13). A two- or three-point contact allows the clamp to rock or tilt unduly, engaging and damaging soft tissues.

Ligatures

The use of ligatures to stabilize the rubber dam is usually not necessary. However, ligatures are occasionally helpful on some types of teeth, such as deciduous molars. Use of a heavy-gauge dam will generally preclude the nuisance and damage created by using ligatures.

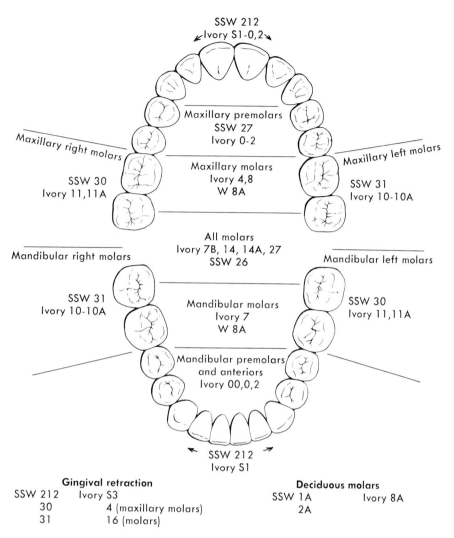

Fig. 3-12. Chart of suggested clamps.

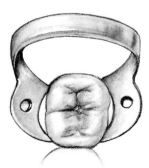

Fig. 3-13. A clamp should firmly engage four points on the tooth to prevent rocking or shifting.

Interproximal retention

Often a dam terminated forward of the last tooth in the arch will remain in place with nothing used to retain it. This is especially true with most anterior dams and those extended as far as the mesial aspect of the first molar, except in youngsters.

Suggested means of wedging the dam between teeth when necessary are (1) dental floss, doubled or tripled if necessary (Fig. 3-14, *A*), (2) use of a strip of rubber dam material about an inch in length and about 4 to 5 mm. wide stretched and inserted between the teeth (Fig. 3-14, *B*), or (3) small-sized rubber band material.

Modeling compound

Compound can frequently be used to retain the distal aspect of the dam on the last tooth in the arch (Fig. 3-15).

FACE PADS (NAPKINS)

Flannel or absorbent paper napkins are used between the rubber dam and face to provide for patient comfort and prevent chafing the skin. They are available ready-made or can be inexpensively made from flannel. Fig. 3-16 and 3-17 illustrate two patterns that may be used to make napkins.

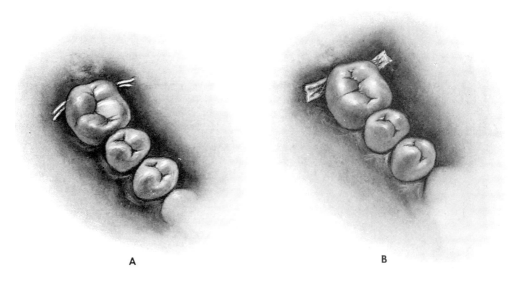

Fig. 3-14. Interproximal retention. **A,** With dental floss. **B,** With a small strip of rubber dam material.

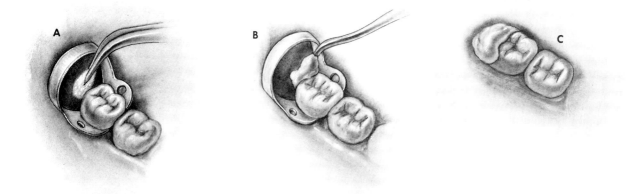

Fig. 3-15. Method of placing modeling compound to retain rubber dam on a posterior tooth to allow removal of the clamp. **A,** The tooth is painted with cavity varnish. **B,** Warm compound is placed with a large plastic instrument. **C,** The clamp is removed.

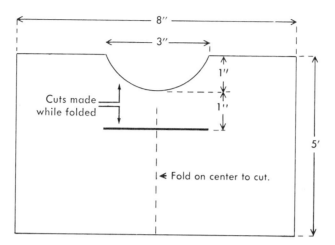

Fig. 3-16. Suggested outline for cutting flannel napkins. (1) Cut a piece of flannel 5 inches by 8 inches. (2) Fold in the middle as indicated by dotted line. (3) Cut out top crescent. (4) Make a straight 3-inch (1½ inches when folded) cut indicated by heavy dark line. This opening goes over the mouth.

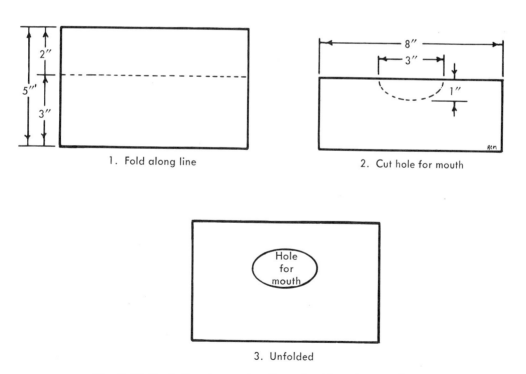

1. Fold along line

2. Cut hole for mouth

3. Unfolded

Fig. 3-17. Variation for cutting flannel rubber dam napkins.

RUBBER DAM HOLDERS

A rubber dam holder stretches the otherwise limp rubber dam taut to provide a clear view of the patient's mouth. There are several types available, each has advantages and disadvantages.

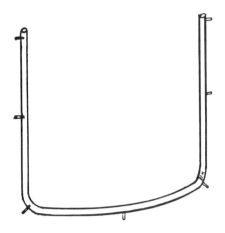

Fig. 3-18. Young rubber dam frame.

Young frame (Fig. 3-18)

The Young frame (Fig. 3-18) does not provide the degree of lip and cheek retraction desired for operating on posterior teeth. It has the sometimes distinct advantage of not unduly disturbing a glamorous hairdo, as well as being quickly and easily placed. It is most practical when used to isolate anterior teeth in adults (Fig. 3-19), for endodontic treatment, and for work on children (Fig. 3-20). Another advantage is that the upper border of the dam may be extended above the patient's nose, thereby protecting the patient from breathing dust from the operative field. The frame can be placed under the rubber, where it is out of the operating area and does not reflect light to create an irritating glare.

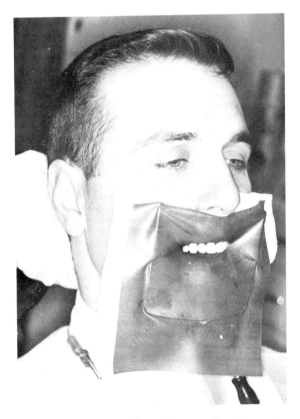

Fig. 3-19. Anterior rubber dam application using a Young rubber dam frame. Note that the frame is behind the dam. This protects the frame from being bumped or caught and eliminates chrome glare.

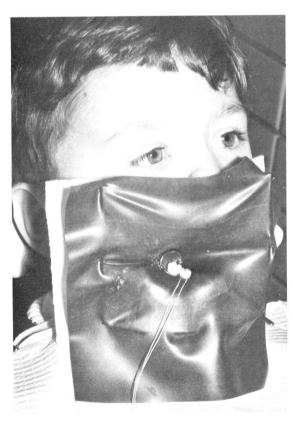

Fig. 3-20. Rubber dam on a child, using a Young rubber dam frame.

Woodbury holder

The Woodbury (Cleve-Dent) holder provides three clips on each side and two straps around the head (Fig. 3-21). It provides an excellent operating field since it firmly retracts the cheeks. However, too much tension over a long period of time can be unduly fatiguing to the patient.

Wizard (Cleve-Dent) holder

The Wizard (Cleve-Dent) holder (Fig. 3-22) provides two clamps on each side. It can be greatly improved by making a strap from ⅝-inch elastic (Fig. 3-23) to stabilize it on the patient's head.

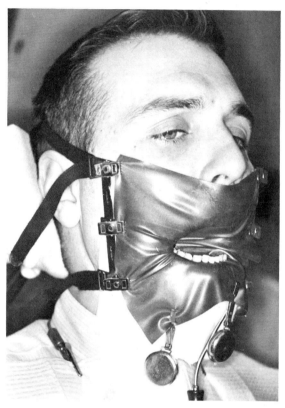

Fig. 3-21. Woodbury (Cleve-Dent) rubber dam holder.

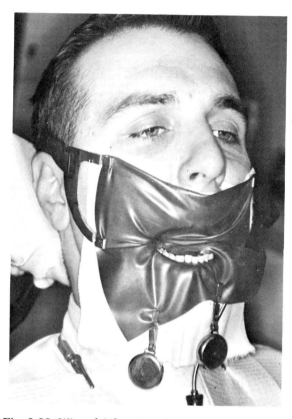

Fig. 3-22. Wizard (Cleve-Dent) Rubber dam holder.

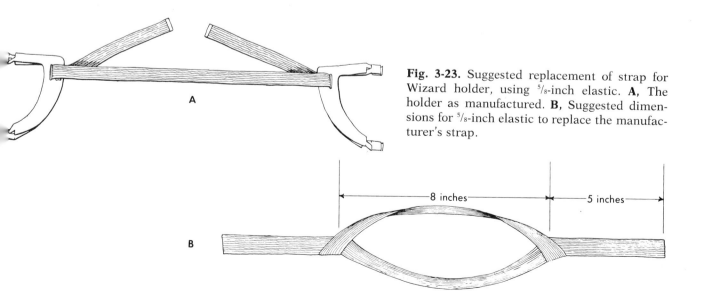

Fig. 3-23. Suggested replacement of strap for Wizard holder, using ⅝-inch elastic. **A,** The holder as manufactured. **B,** Suggested dimensions for ⅝-inch elastic to replace the manufacturer's strap.

8 inches

5 inches

PLACEMENT OF RUBBER DAM

Following are the usual routines for isolating the mandibular right quadrant for operative procedures. The functions of the dental assistant are not specifically noted since operators differ on what assistance they desire. The assistant should, of course, pass instruments as appropriate and help by holding the dam out of the operator's view as it is placed.

Three general approaches used in placing the dam are as follows:

1. Placement of the clamp, after which the dam is placed over it (Figs. 3-27 to 3-31)
2. Placement of the dam over the bow of the clamp prior to placing the clamp on the tooth (Figs. 3-32 to 3-34)
3. Placement of the clamp after the dam is already on the teeth, thereby allowing each septum to be tilted and stretched to slip it through the contact (Figs. 3-37 and 3-38)

It is often helpful to punch a hole in the upper left-hand corner of the dam as a guide to avoid confusion during placement.

Combinations of these various approaches will be used by most operators as conditions vary.

The following series of steps and illustrations includes the various alternatives listed. Not shown is the method of placing the dam on the wings of certain Ivory clamps as illustrated in the manufacturer's catalog.

1 Pass a ligature through the contacts where the dam is to be placed (Fig. 3-24). Use of the ligature should acquaint the operator with rough areas that may be difficult to pass. It may be advisable to reduce sharp edges with strips or disks. It may be helpful, on occassion, to rough out the cavity preparations prior to placing the dam to avoid the frustration of tearing the dam with a sharp interproximal edge.

2 Lightly lubricate the patient's lips to protect them against irritation (Fig. 3-25).

3 When possible, punch the rubber (extra heavy) to include two teeth distal to the one being restored and the canine on the opposite side of the mouth. It is important that enough teeth be included to provide an adequate field free from the space restriction often created when the dam includes too few teeth.

4 Place a small amount of tincture of green soap (shaving cream or other water-soluble materials may be sparingly used) over the holes to facilitate passage through the contacts (Fig. 3-26).

5 Place a clamp over the second molar, gently against the gingiva. Carefully release the clamp (Fig. 3-27). The clamp should now be against the gingiva *below* the height of contour (Fig. 3-28) not on the height of contour or above it as in Fig. 3-29.

6 Slip the dam over the clamp (Figs. 3-30 and 3-31). If the rubber slips easily onto the teeth, place it over each succeeding tooth in the arch beginning with the molars. The assistant should dry the teeth as the dam is slipped over them while also holding the edges of the dam out of the operator's visual field.

In some cases it is difficult to slip the dam over a previously placed clamp, such as when the bow is in close proximity to the mandibular ramus. An alternate method is that of grasping the clamp with forceps and then slipping the clamp bow

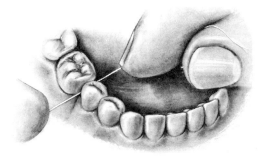

Fig. 3-24. Check contacts with floss.

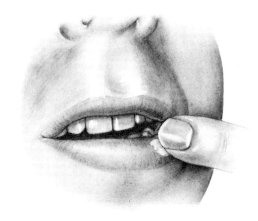

Fig. 3-25. Lubricate lips with protective ointment.

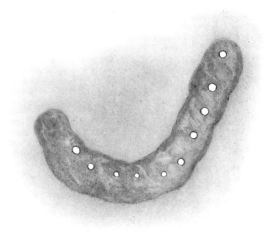

Fig. 3-26. Lubricant placed on punched rubber.

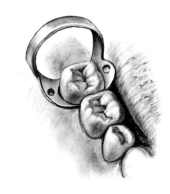

Fig. 3-27. Molar clamp in place.

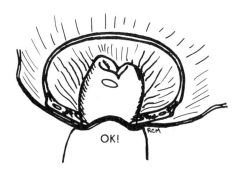

Fig. 3-28. Molar clamp in correct position.

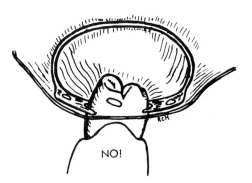

Fig. 3-29. Molar clamp too high on tooth.

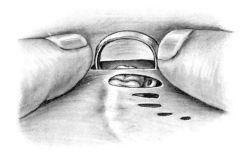

Fig. 3-30. Slip the dam over the clamp bow.

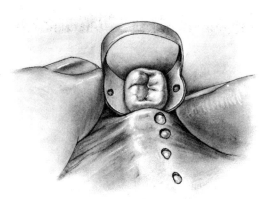

Fig. 3-31. Snap the dam under the clamp jaw.

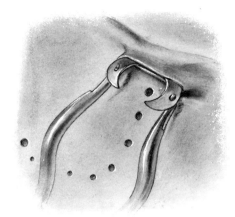

Fig. 3-32. Alternate method: Place the clamp bow through the last molar hole.

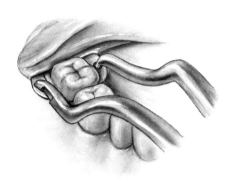

Fig. 3-33. Alternate method: Second step, place the clamp on the molar.

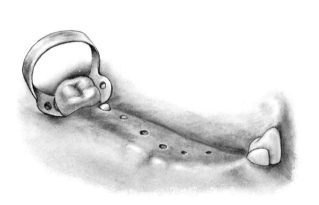

Fig. 3-34. Dam secured by clamp and on opposite canine.

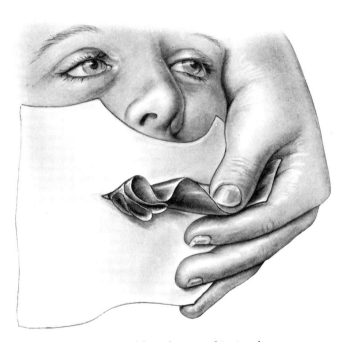

Fig. 3-35. Rubber dam napkin in place.

through the hole (Fig. 3-32), then placing it on the tooth with one hand while holding the dam out of the way with the other (Fig. 3-33).

7 If the rubber does not easily pass between the teeth, place it over the left canine and lateral incisor (Fig. 3-34).

8 Slip a napkin over the rubber and spread it over the face (Fig. 3-35).

9 Attach the rubber dam holder and adjust it so that the rubber is under gentle tension (Figs. 3-21 and 3-22). A Young frame is often helpful in controlling the dam during preliminary adjustment

prior to placing a strap-type holder. Should tight contacts cause difficulty in placing the dam, stretch the rubber over the contact areas (Fig. 3-36) and start an edge of rubber between the teeth.

10 An alternate step is shown in Fig. 3-37. It is often easier to slip the dam through the contacts as shown, stretching the septal rubber and tipping it parallel with the contact areas, after which the clamp is placed if needed.

11 Use of waxed floss (Fig. 3-38) to carry the dam through the contact is helpful if skillfully used. However, it may cut holes or tear the rub-

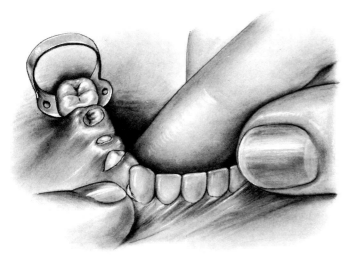

Fig. 3-36. Slip the rubber septa through the contacts.

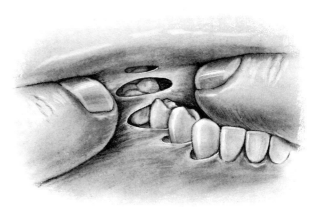

Fig. 3-37. Stretching the septal rubber to facilitate passage through contacts.

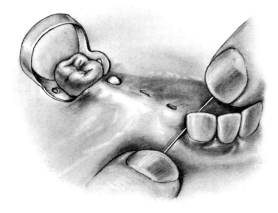

Fig. 3-38. Waxed floss used to guide the rubber through the contacts.

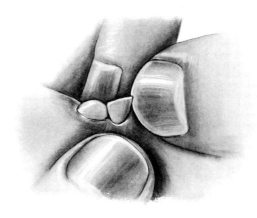

Fig. 3-39. Use of a thumb nail to open a contact slightly.

ber, especially lighter gauges. When used, it should start one edge of the rubber between the teeth and carry it through. Never force a bulk of rubber with waxed floss or allow it to snap through since such clumsy action may injure the gingiva.

12 Separation with a thumbnail will sometimes allow the rubber to slip through (Fig. 3-39).

13 If the contact is particularly difficult, a blunt instrument such as a plastic instrument can be inserted through the rubber and under the contact (Fig. 3-40). Careful but firm forcing of the instru-

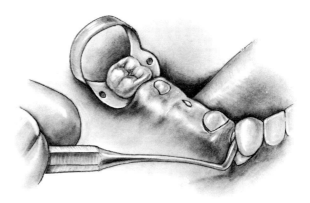

Fig. 3-40. Use of an instrument to lift upward under the contacts to facilitate passage of a rubber septum.

ment upward should open the contact to allow the rubber to pass through.

14 Adapt a saliva ejector tip to accommodate the patient and slip it between the rubber and the napkin distal to the canine on the side not being operated. Some operators prefer inserting the saliva ejector through a hole in the rubber in the lingual area (Fig. 3-41), either by punching a hole with the rubber dam punch when the tooth holes are punched or by cutting a hole with scissors after the dam is placed. Many patients do not re-

quire the saliva ejector. Also, placement of a hole in the lingual area of the dam can be a nuisance. Disposable ejector tips are excellent since they are adjustable and afford maximum control. At no time should the ejector be placed in a manner that might allow it to impinge on the floor of the mouth.

15 After the dam has been slipped through all the contacts, use an instrument to turn the edge of the dam gingivally while having the assistant dry the area with air (Fig. 3-42). When the dam is not easily turned under with an instrument, pass floss around each tooth and push it gingivally (Fig. 3-43). Dry with air and gently remove the floss.

16 Place weights if needed to hold the lower part of the rubber down. Sometimes the rubber can be attached to the napkin using the weight clips, thereby creating slight tension to hold the rubber out of the operating field.

17 Place a protective coating of *cocoa butter,* lacquer, or varnish over silicate restorations to prevent dehydration.

Occasionally, especially with very short molars, when the clamp is placed first and the dam slipped over it, an adequate seal may not result. When this occurs, the assistant should retract the dam outward and gingivally to retain it on the tooth. The operator then retracts the dam similarly on the other side while lifting the clamp slightly off the tooth. The dam is then relaxed slightly and the clamp replaced to its desired position. This should allow the dam to seal around the tooth.

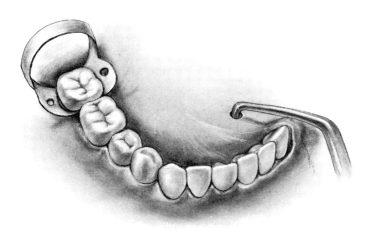

Fig. 3-41. Saliva ejector in place.

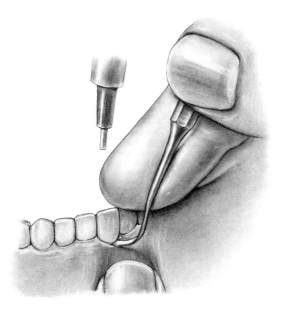

Fig. 3-42. Tipping the edge of the rubber dam under a stream of air to seal the dam.

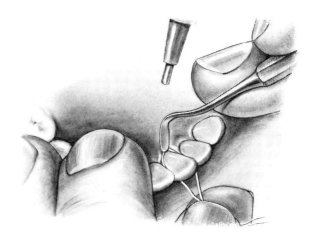

Fig. 3-43. Use of floss looped around a tooth to turn in the edge of the rubber as air dries the field.

PROBLEMS

Following are several errors that may be observed in rubber dam placement. Clinical experience using the accompanying suggestions should make rubber dam placement an easily executed routine procedure.

Spaces between the teeth and the dam

When spaces remain between the teeth and the rubber after the dam has been placed, the holes have been punched too close together. (See Fig. 3-9.) A properly placed dam will uniformly cover the interdental papillae. If the rubber dam retainer is not arranged properly, the dam may be pulled askew, which can also create open spaces between the teeth and the rubber. Proper balanced tension on the holder should correct this problem.

Rubber dam is bunched up between the teeth

A rough appearing rubber dam application may be the result of poor application of the rubber dam holder. If, however, the rubber remains bunched up between the teeth (see Fig. 3-10) after tension of the holder is made, the holes have been punched too far apart.

Tight rubber in the lingual area, loose in buccal area

If the rubber is too taut in the lingual area and loose in the buccal area, the holes have been punched in too tight an arch. (See Fig. 3-6.)

Rubber bunched up in lingual area

If the rubber is bunched up in the lingual area but taut in the buccal or labial area, the holes have been punched in too straight a line. (See Fig. 3-5.)

Rubber dam not located properly on the face

A properly arranged rubber dam will be located with its upper margin passing just below the patient's nose (Fig. 3-44). It should be smooth, adequately retract the lips and cheeks, and be comfortable for the patient. The elastic strap should be located in a stable position on the back of the patient's head.

If the dam is placed too low, it will slip below the patient's upper lip (Fig. 3-45), thereby not properly retracting the lip from the field of operation. The holes have been punched too close to the edge of the dam.

If the rubber lays across the patient's nose (Fig. 3-46), the patient may not be able to breathe comfortably. An exception may be when a Young-type frame is used and the rubber is held taut enough not to be drawn down over the patient's nostrils. (See Fig. 3-20.) Punching the holes too near the center of the dam causes the dam to be placed in too high a position. This problem may be quickly solved, usually, by simply folding down the upper margin of the rubber until it is below the patient's nose. (See Fig. 3-22.)

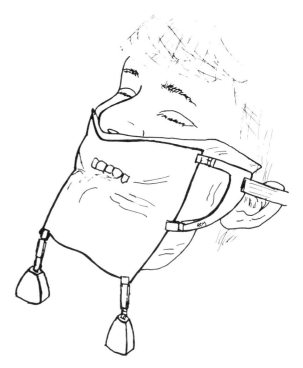

Fig. 3-44. Proper location of a rubber dam on a patient's face.

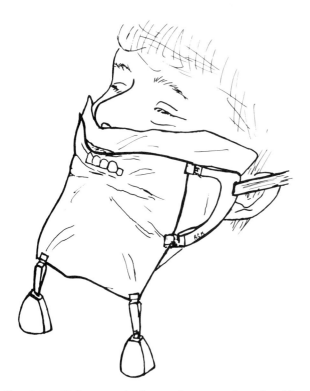

Fig. 3-45. Holes punched too close to edge of rubber causing the dam to slip under the patient's lip.

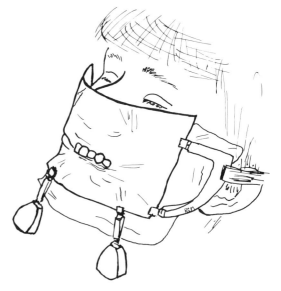

Fig. 3-46. Holes punched too far from the edge of rubber causing the dam to cover the patient's nose.

REMOVAL

While the teeth are still dry, it is excellent practice to *apply a fluoride solution or gel.* The gel, especially, will usually lubricate the rubber so that it may easily slip up over the teeth without cutting the septa. An eyedropper may be used to inject the gel around the teeth. If contacts are tight, however, the following standard procedure should be employed.

If ceramic restorations are present in the operative field, extreme care must be exercised to protect them from etching by acidulated fluoride gels. It is suggested that the operator test the fluoride preparation he uses on glass to note its effect.

1 Apply fluoride (Fig. 3-47) and wait two minutes.

2 Remove separators, compound, or other materials used to stabilize the dam. Cut ligatures with a gold knife (Fig. 3-48).

3 Stretch the rubber septa outward and cut with crown and bridge shears (Fig. 3-49). Remove clamps.

4 Remove the saliva ejector.

5 Remove the holder.

6 Remove the rubber and napkin. Wipe the patient's face.

7 Rinse the mouth with warm water.

8 Thoroughly examine the mouth to be certain it is free of rubber and other material incident to the operation. Also examine the rubber removed to further ensure that no tags or bands of rubber are unaccounted for.

9 Massage the gingival areas where clamps were placed.

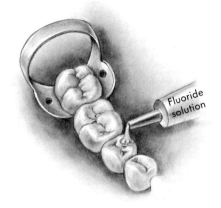

Fig. 3-47. Application of fluoride solution to moisten teeth to facilitate dam removal.

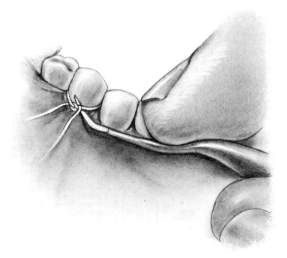

Fig. 3-48. Cutting a ligature with a gold knife.

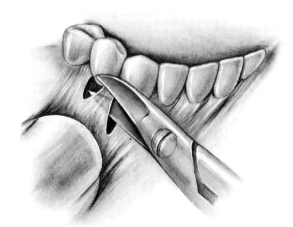

Fig. 3-49. Cutting rubber septum to facilitate easy dam removal.

GINGIVAL RETRACTION FOR CLASS 5 CAVITIES

Gingival retraction is usually essential to the proper restoration of lesions in the gingival third of any tooth. The most easily controlled retraction for most cases is attained using the Ferrier No. 212 clamp. It functions best on anterior teeth and premolars. Some teeth may require the use of a clamp of the Schultz type (Ivory No. S1, S2, or S3) as placed on the premolar in Figs. 3-80 and 3-81.

It is essential, whatever type of gingival retraction employed, that it be adequate to expose the entire involved area to view. An additional area of sound tooth structure must also be exposed for adequate operating room and to ensure adequate extension of the restoration. The clamp should protect the gingival tissues and, when stabilized with compound, serve as a finger rest and distribute operating forces to several teeth.

As it comes from the manufacturer, the lingual jaw of the S. S. White No. 212 clamp usually needs to be altered to properly accommodate most cases. Fig. 3-50 shows a clamp as manufactured (dotted lines) and the desired change. This is accomplished by removing the temper from the lingual jaw by heating it in a pinpoint flame until red. Two pairs of pliers are then used to bend the lingual jaw upward, one holding the clamp at the base of the jaw.

Caution should be used if it is even deemed desirable to bend the buccal jaw downward, since to do so may tend to seriously restrict the operating area. Fig. 3-51 illustrates the effect of this jaw when bent downward. The gingival margin is much less accessible than when the proper relationship is used as shown in Fig. 3-52. The notches may also be deepened to accommodate the clamp forceps. Also, the ends of the jaws that contact the tooth may be deepened slightly to ensure better tooth contact so that the rubber will not creep under them after it is placed (Fig. 3-53).

It is suggested that several No. 212 clamps that have been altered be kept on hand to serve a variety of situations. For example, one may have its labial jaw narrowed to accommodate crowded anteriors (Fig. 3-54). Another should have all its temper removed so that it may be quickly altered to an unusual situation. Such a clamp can then be quickly formed to accommodate an abnormal requirement. All points that contact tooth structure should be polished with a rubber wheel to avoid scratching the tooth surface (Fig. 3-55).

Gingival retraction on molars can often be accomplished with the No. 212 clamp. However, clamps such as the S. S. White Nos. 30 and 31 are also useful. An Ivory No. 16 is frequently to be preferred; however, it must be altered to function well (Fig. 3-56).

Another suggestion is removal of the chrome finish by sandblasting or heating the clamp carefully in a flame to blue the metal. Glare from a mirrorlike surface is most annoying and contributes to operator fatigue.

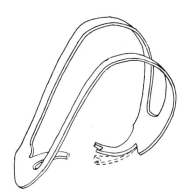

Fig. 3-50. A No. 212 clamp indicating the desired modification prior to use.

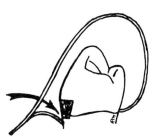

Fig. 3-51. Effect of improperly tipping the facial jaw downward on a No. 212 clamp.

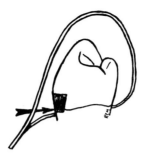

Fig. 3-52. Access provided by a properly modified No. 212 clamp.

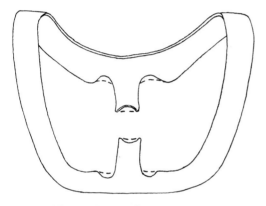

Fig. 3-53. Additional modifications suggested for the No. 212 clamp to improve its function.

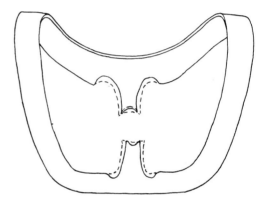

Fig. 3-54. Narrowed jaws of a No. 212 clamp to facilitate placement on small and possibly crowded lower incisors.

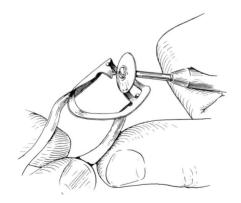

Fig. 3-55. Polishing a No. 212 clamp using a rubber wheel to eliminate sharp edges.

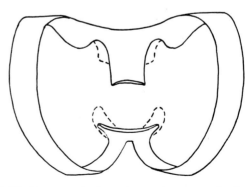

Fig. 3-56. Suggested alteration to improve the function of the Ivory No. 16 clamp.

Placement of SSW No. 212 clamp

1 Explore the gingival sulcus on the buccal (labial) aspect with a blunt instrument to determine the level of the gingival attachment relative to the area to be restored (Fig. 3-57).

2 The hole punched for the tooth to be operated on may be placed somewhat buccally and an additional 1 mm. of space allowed between the holes for adjacent teeth (Fig. 3-58). If the gingiva is greatly receded, the hole should be quite large to accommodate the circumference of the area to which it is applied (Fig. 3-11).

3 Place the rubber dam, including at least two teeth if possible, distal to the tooth to be operated on. If it is essential to use a clamp on a tooth ad-

jacent to the one to be operated on, the clamp should be substantially reduced so that it will not interfere with the buccal bow of the No. 212 clamp (Figs. 3-59 and 3-60).

4 Keep the teeth *dry* and paint the teeth on which compound will be placed with varnish to ensure that the compound will not loosen during the operation.

COMMENT: *It must be emphasized that seldom is a clamp on the adjacent tooth necessary as shown in Fig. 3-59. Its use is to be avoided if possible.*

5 Grasp the No. 212 clamp with the rubber dam forceps and place it over the tooth while stretching the rubber outward away from the tooth to provide a clear view of the area to be isolated and

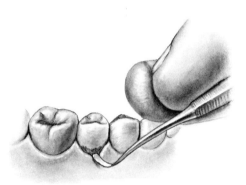

Fig. 3-57. Using a plastic instrument to explore the area of a carious lesion.

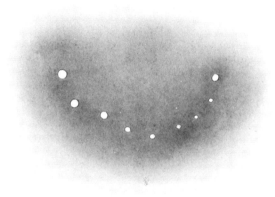

Fig. 3-58. Holes punched for a Class 5 rubber dam.

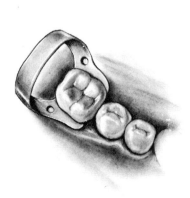

Fig. 3-59. Modified molar clamp in place.

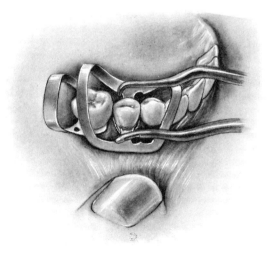

Fig. 3-60. Placing the No. 212 clamp over the modified molar clamp.

to avoid placing the jaw of the clamp over the rubber (Fig. 3-60). Place the clamp gently against the gingiva and release it while holding the buccal (labial) jaw firmly with the thumb or forefinger to prevent it from creeping while it is stabilized (Fig. 3-61). While moving the clamp gingivally with the forceps, the lingual jaw should be held against the tooth to ensure that it will not be placed over the margin of the dam. Also, it is sometimes helpful to have the assistant retract the dam slightly on the lingual side to avoid placing the clamp jaw on its margin. If, after the clamp has been released from the forceps, it is found that the buccal jaw should be placed farther apically, it can be moved (if not blocked by the cavity shoulder) by placing

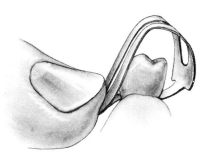

Fig. 3-61. Use of the thumb or finger to control the position of a No. 212 clamp while stabilizing compound is applied.

a blunt instrument such as an amalgam condenser on the clamp jaw, next to the tooth, and forcing it firmly apically to the desired position (Fig. 3-62).

Some operators may prefer to support the clamp with the thumb or finger on the lingual side. However, using the buccal (labial) clamp jaw as a fulcrum, pressing on the outer aspect of the clamp affords complete control against the lingual jaw slipping gingivally.

COMMENT: *Although a great deal of concern is commonly expressed about encroaching on the gingival attachment and thereby possibly damaging it, it is also essential to the protection of the attachment that the restoration of the tooth be done properly. This sometimes requires bold retraction to gain absolute control of the defective area of the tooth. Also, it must be emphasized that control of the No. 212 clamp can usually be maintained by keeping a thumb or finger on the buccal (labial) clamp jaw. The buccal jaw serves as a fulcrum, and the lingual jaw can thus be prevented from encroaching on the gingiva (Figs. 3-60 and 3-61). If this cannot be done, the thumb should be kept on the buccal jaw and the index finger held under the lingual side of the clamp while it is stabilized with compound.*

6 Still holding the buccal side of the clamp with the thumb or forefinger, slowly warm the end of a stick of red compound until it softens slightly (do not overheat) and place it around one bow of the clamp (Fig. 3-63). Twist the softened

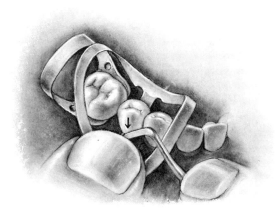

Fig. 3-62. Use of an instrument as an aid to force the facial jaw gingivally.

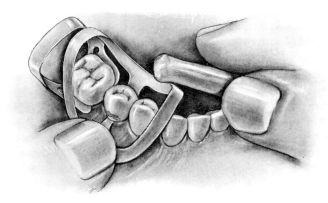

Fig. 3-63. Place warm compound under one bow.

compound off the stick and, with slightly moistened fingers, mold the soft compound around the teeth and bow, forcing it into the embrasures to lock it (Fig. 3-64). While this is done, the assistant should blow a stream of cold air over it. Care should be taken not to place a bulk of compound on the outside of the clamp in a manner that might tend to restrict the field of operation.

7 Repeat the procedure for the other bow, still holding the clamp with the thumb or forefinger (Fig. 3-65). It is permissible, and sometimes desirable, to block the entire lingual area with compound (Fig. 3-66) to block a group of teeth together more rigidly.

8 If any of the interdental papillae are not covered by the dam, it should be adjusted to cover them.

9 Free the patient's lip if it is locked under the clamp bow.

If it is found desirable to place the clamp farther apically after it has been stabilized, this can usually be done without removing it. Heat a large plastic instrument or wax spatula and soften the compound around the clamp while holding the buccal side with the thumb or forefinger. Use ample time to allow the heat to penetrate the compound. Then use a blunt instrument to firmly force the buccal jaw apically, or make the movement with the forceps if preferred. This technique is difficult, however, if a large amount of compound has been used.

Some operators prefer placing compound on the teeth prior to placing the clamp. When this procedure is followed, the compound is softened and placed on the teeth, the clamp is placed, and the compound is molded into place and chilled.

Another alternative is to place the softened compound on the bows of the clamp prior to its placement on the teeth.

The key to successful placement of a stable No. 212 clamp is the adhesion of the compound to the teeth while the compound supports the clamp. To assure this the teeth must be dry where the compound is to attach.

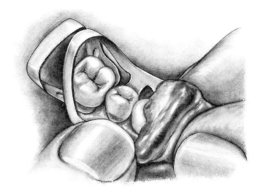

Fig. 3-64. Press the compound around the bow and into embrasures.

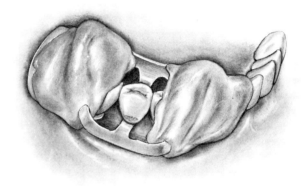

Fig. 3-65. Compound placed on both bows.

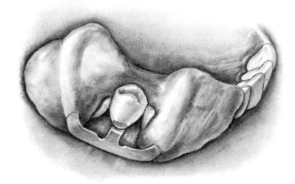

Fig. 3-66. Lingual area blocked out by compound to facilitate stability.

Removal of SSW No. 212 clamp

Removal of the SSW No. 212 clamp is most easily managed by placing an instrument that will hook under the buccal bow (Fig. 3-67) next to the clamp jaw. Markley suggests an altered crochet hook (Fig. 3-68). Force the buccal jaw buccally off the tooth and rotate it occlusally to break the clamp loose. Do not remove a clamp by this method if it is not stabilized by compound.

Forceps can, of course, be used if the bows are free of compound, but the clamp can slip off the forceps when attempting to loosen it from the compound, thereby marring the restoration.

If the operator wishes to use the forceps on a No. 212 clamp when proper positioning of the forceps on the clamp is blocked by compound, the ends of the forceps may be warmed and pushed into the compound.

Periodontal dressing

Occasionally the gingival tissue will necessarily be traumatized during the restorative procedure. In such cases it is excellent practice to place a small periodontal pack. The teeth can be dried and varnished (Fig. 3-69, A), and the dressing can be placed (Fig. 3-69, B). The patient is instructed that it will probably fall away in a few hours, but in case it does not it should be removed in forty-eight hours.

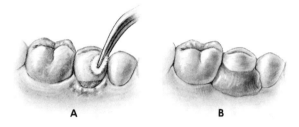

Fig. 3-69. Placement of a periodontal dressing. **A,** Varnish the teeth. **B,** Periodontal dressing pressed in place.

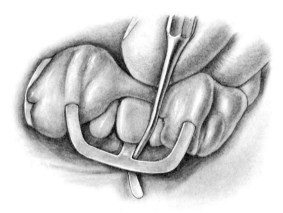

Fig. 3-67. Use of a plastic instrument to remove a No. 212 clamp.

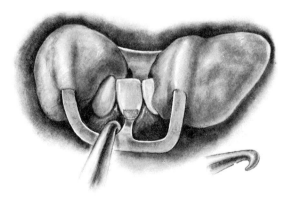

Fig. 3-68. Use of a button hook to remove a No. 212 clamp.

GINGIVAL RETRACTION ON ABUTMENT TEETH OF FIXED PROSTHESES

Obtaining gingival retraction on a tooth serving as an abutment for a fixed bridge (Fig. 3-70) can be accomplished by the following method, which has the advantage of sealing the dam so that it will not leak.

1 Punch the rubber to isolate the field of teeth desired, plus a hole for the pontic. The septum between the abutment tooth and the pontic hole should be extra wide (Fig. 3-71).

2 Place the dam on the teeth and the napkin and holder as usual (Fig. 3-72).

3 Thread floss through the pontic hole and the abutment tooth hole (Figs. 3-73 and 3-74).

4 Using a floss threader (Fig. 3-75), thread the ends of the floss through the abutment tooth hole, under the solder joint, and lingually through the abutment tooth hole. Frequently the floss can be simply threaded under the solder joint without using an instrument. (A floss threader can be made from a sickle explorer. Heat the explorer in flame until it is red. It can then be easily formed into an effective floss threader.)

5 Varnish the teeth to aid retention of the modeling compound (Fig. 3-76).

6 Place an SSW No. 212 clamp over the tooth, holding the buccal jaw down in place with the thumb or forefinger while the clamp is stabilized with modeling compound. The compound should be blocked well behind (lingual) the tooth to be operated on, but the floss must be kept free (Fig. 3-77). Chill thoroughly with air.

7 The floss may now be drawn firmly to the lingual side to place tension on the papilla under the solder joint. The amount of tension desired is established, and the floss is secured to the compound with an additional dab of modeling compound (Fig. 3-78).

If the amount of tension on the papillae should need to be changed, the floss may be released and the adjustment made. This technique should provide ample retraction in most cases to completely expose the distal margin of the abutment if desired.

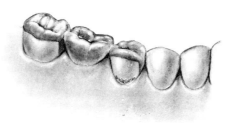

Fig. 3-70. Fixed bridge with Class 5 cavity in one abutment tooth.

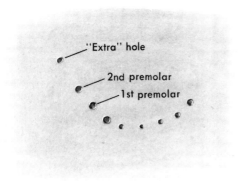

Fig. 3-71. Configuration of holes in the rubber.

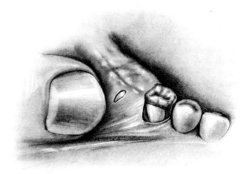

Fig. 3-72. Dam slipped over anterior teeth and the anterior abutment tooth.

OPERATING FIELDS **59**

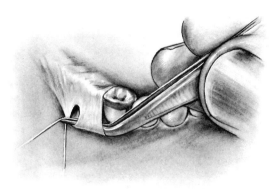

Fig. 3-73. Cotton forceps used to draw floss under septum.

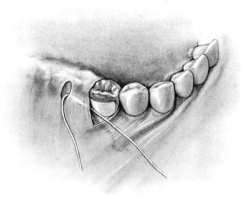

Fig. 3-74. Floss under septum.

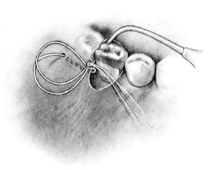

Fig. 3-75. Floss threader used to reach under the connector and thread the floss through toward the lingual area.

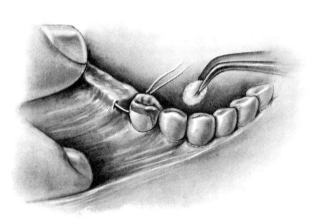

Fig. 3-76. Floss around the septum and under the connector.

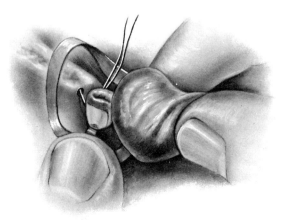

Fig. 3-77. No. 212 clamp placed and stabilized on one end.

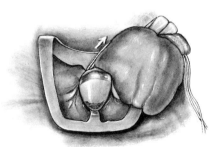

Fig. 3-78. Floss drawn taut to pull the rubber under the connector and secured with a dab of compound.

Multiple abutments

A method of retracting the gingiva adjacent to a bridge pontic on both abutment teeth is shown in Figs. 3-79 to 3-81. Two holes are punched as shown in Fig. 3-79. An Ivory Schultz clamp is placed on the premolar (Figs. 3-80 and 3-81). The distal floss is drawn under the solder joint, under the lingual jaw of the molar clamp, and around the distal surface to secure it to the compound. This can help to place more pressure on the gingiva (Fig. 3-78).

Use of wire hooks instead of floss threader

Another method of drawing the rubber under the solder joint to facilitate gingival retraction follows.

1 Punch the dam as indicated, but *do not* punch a hole for the pontic, and place the dam, napkin, holder, and saliva ejector.

2 Ball the end of a piece of 21-gauge gold wire and bend it to create a hook on each end as shown in Fig. 3-82. About ¹/₂ inch in length is desirable. Slip the hook through the lingual portion of the abutment tooth hole, under the solder joint (Fig. 3-83).

3 Place and stabilize the No. 212 clamp.

4 Engage as much rubber on the buccal side as indicated.

5 Loop floss into the lingual hook of the wire (Fig. 3-83), pull it to the lingual side, and "tack" the floss to the compound (Fig. 3-84). If the procedure is carefully done, the hook will not punch through the rubber.

Several additional methods of placing a dam adjacent to pontics include (1) insertion of a stick, wood wedge, or pipe cleaner through the abutment hole and under the solder joint, (2) insertion of a cotton ball saturated with cavity varnish under the solder joint, or (3) two beads (or other objects) tied together under the solder joint.

Also, two holes may be punched about 5 or 6 mm. apart in a buccolingual line about 5 mm. distal to the abutment tooth. The dam is placed and floss is threaded (using a ligature needle or wire) through the abutment hole, under the solder joint, and back through the two other holes under the pontic. The floss is then tied tightly to draw the dam around the solder joint.

Other methods include cutting the dam between the abutments and punching four or more holes to allow the dam to be sewn together under the pontic.

The methods mentioned in the preceding three paragraphs, for the most part, are awkward and provide generally less than satisfactory control of saliva and soft tissue.

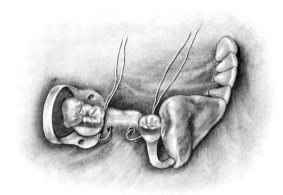

Fig. 3-80. Clamps in place on abutment teeth and floss threaded under the bridge connectors.

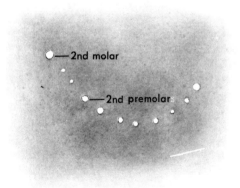

Fig. 3-79. Holes punched for both abutments of a three-unit fixed bridge.

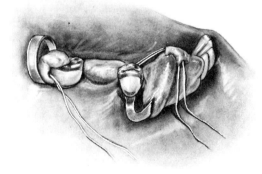

Fig. 3-81. Floss drawn tight under the bridge connectors and secured by compound.

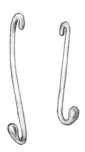

Fig. 3-82. Wire hooks used to engage the compound instead of punching an extra hole and threading floss under the connector.

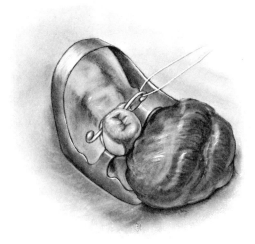

Fig. 3-83. Hook ready to engage the rubber on one end and held by floss on the lingual end.

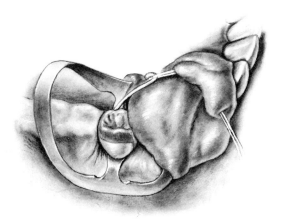

Fig. 3-84. Floss and hook drawn taut and secured to the compound.

Separators

Separators used in conjunction with a rubber dam have the primary purpose of slightly separating two teeth to facilitate the placement of proximal restorations. A secondary function is gingival retraction. In situations where teeth are already without contact, placement of a separator can occasionally retract the papilla, although separating tension is not necessary in such cases.

Probably the most popular separator is the type designed by W. I. Ferrier.* It is easily stabilized with modeling compound and does not tend to twist or move. It is available in several sizes. The No. 1 size is also available as modified by Alex Jeffery, making it somewhat smaller and more versatile. Most of the separators as supplied can be improved by thinning the jaws slightly where they engage the teeth and by removing some of the bulk from the bows.

PLACEMENT OF FERRIER SEPARATOR

1 Select the separator to be used. The No. 1 will accommodate most anterior teeth and occasionally the distal side of canines.

2 With the jaws of the separator closed, place it between the teeth to be separated. If the jaws do not lightly engage the teeth, extend them until they do, while keeping the rubber from being pinched between the jaws and the tooth.

3 Cautiously move the separator gingivally until both labial and lingual jaws are clear of the operative area and in gentle contact with the teeth. At the same time the rubber dam should be retracted slightly (Fig. 3-85).

---

*Now manufactured by Almore International Inc., 1095 S.W. 5th, Beaverton, Oregon

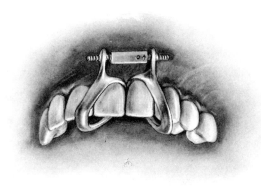

Fig. 3-85. Ferrier separator.

4 Warm the end of a stick compound, place the softened compound under one bow, and mold it onto the teeth to stabilize the separator. Chill with air.

5 Repeat for the other bow (Fig. 3-86). Sufficient compound should be used to prevent the clamp from rocking or moving gingivally during the operative procedure.

6 With the separator wrench, very slowly open the jaws of the separator until slight separation is observed.

> COMMENT: *Always remain alert to the possibility of increased separation after separating tension is applied to the teeth, especially in young people. When more than normal force is necessary to obtain separation, it must be very cautiously and slowly applied. Never attempt separation with this instrument without stabilizing it with compound since it readily moves apically as it is tightened.*

Removal of the separator is accomplished simply by backing the jaws together as indicated. If much pressure has been applied to the teeth, it must be released very slowly to avoid pain. If the possibility exists of scratching the restoration with the separator, it can be spread somewhat with rubber dam clamp forceps as it is removed.

TRUE SEPARATOR

The separator designed by Harry True is preferred by many operators because of its capability of providing unimpeded access from one side (Fig. 3-87). It must be firmly secured with compound (Fig. 3-88) and closely watched to be certain it does not move gingivally as separating tension is applied.

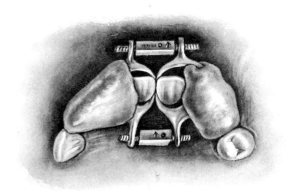

Fig. 3-86. Ferrier separator stabilized by compound.

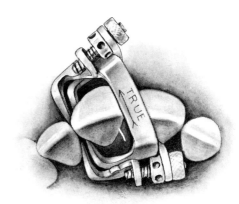

Fig. 3-87. True separator.

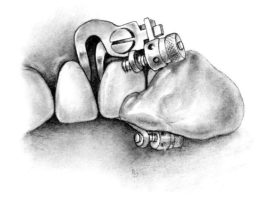

Fig. 3-88. True separator stabilized by compound.

Miscellaneous suggestions

As with all operative procedures, variations prohibit description of all circumstances. Following are a few suggestions that may prove helpful.

TORN RUBBER DAM

If the dam is torn in the course of operating, it need not be removed, but an additional one can be placed over it. It is possible to do this occasionally without removing some types of clamps, unless they are stablized with compound.

PROTECTION OF SEPTAL RUBBER

Wood wedges may prove helpful when using a bur interproximally (Fig. 3-89) to avoid tearing the rubber dam or injuring the gingiva. The operator may cut into the wood while preparing the cavity with no fear of catching the dam or injuring the gingiva.

REDUCING THE HEIGHT OF THE INTERDENTAL PAPILLA

Occasionally a resistant high papilla may partly obscure an operative area. A pellet or two of cotton (or a wood wedge), slowly but firmly wedged between the teeth for a few minutes, can assist the rubber dam in retraction of interproximal soft tissue (Fig. 3-90). It should then be removed before the cavity preparation is performed.

Clamps may also be used to reduce the height of gingival papillae effectively. For example, use an Ivory No. 0 or 00 on premolars to increase tension on the dam.

PATIENT UNABLE TO BREATHE

On rare occasions a patient is reluctant to submit to rubber dam placement because of a feeling that the ability to breathe may be impaired. Whether this problem is real or imagined, the patient may be relieved by using Young's frame for anterior cases. This usually leaves the corners of the mouth free of obstruction. A hole may be cut through the dam in the area toward the palate to facilitate passage of air. It may be fairly large and should be placed high to keep the saliva contained.

GAGGING

Although patients susceptible to gagging may object to placement of the rubber dam, it can be successfully placed if the operator is firm regarding its necessity and is deft and quick in placing it. The dam, once in place, eliminates gagging and makes the patient more comfortable. This is a great asset since gagging can remain a problem throughout the procedure if the dam is not used.

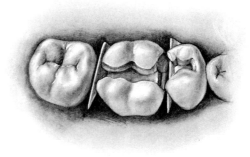

Fig. 3-89. Wood wedges cover the rubber septa between teeth to protect the rubber during operative procedures.

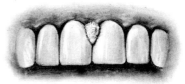

Fig. 3-90. Insertion of cotton pellet between teeth to hasten gingival retraction.

PLASTIC INSTRUMENT USED AS SHIELD

A relatively large plastic instrument can be used to protect the rubber when preparing gingival cavities and finishing restorations close to the rubber dam. The instrument is easily held by the left hand with the dam retracted while cutting is accomplished with a bur or using an abrasive disk or stone (Fig. 3-91).

SINGLE TOOTH DAMS

Too often when placing a simple restoration such as a simple occlusal restoration on a molar, placement of a dam may seem unnecessarily burdensome. Control of such a circumstance can, however, be quickly gained simply by placing a dam on the one tooth (Fig. 3-92). Unless gingival protection, as required for Class 2 and Class 5 cavities, is indicated, time need not be wasted isolating additional teeth.

CATCHING THE DAM WITH ROTARY INSTRUMENTS

While using finishing disks on proximal restorations or cavities, it is easy to prevent the dam from wrapping up on the disk by forcing the dam gingivally with the fingers. Use of extra heavy rubber reduces the problem, and holding the dam taut while using disks makes it difficult to catch. Some operators recommend using petroleum jelly to lubricate the dam, but it is messy and really not needed.

PROTECTION OF SILICATE AND GOLD RESTORATIONS

Subjecting silicate restorations to a dry environment will damage them. As soon as the dam is placed, they should immediately be protected with a coat of lacquer, petroleum jelly, or cocoa butter.

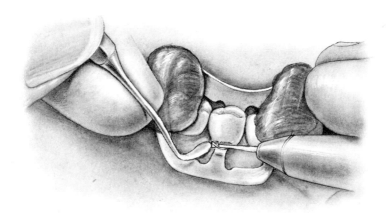

Fig. 3-91. Use of a plastic instrument to shield the rubber while preparing a Class 5 cavity.

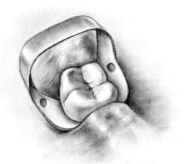

Fig. 3-92. A single tooth rubber dam application.

When amalgam is being placed in proximity to existing gold restorations, the gold should be painted with some sort of varnish to protect it from mercury contamination.

Chair operating positions for dental procedures

When working on a patient in a dental chair, the object of positioning the patient is to allow the dentist to work more comfortably for longer periods of time and with minimal fatigue. Likewise, if the patient is kept reasonably comfortable, he or she will be more relaxed and be able to tolerate longer appointments. The net result is a more efficient operation. When considering the position to operate on a patient, a number of interrelated factors must be kept in mind (1) visibility of the operating area, (2) access to the operating area, (3) areas of activity, and (4) body mechanics.

VISIBILITY OF THE OPERATING AREA

The operator may use either direct vision when viewing an operation or indirect vision using a mouth mirror. If the operator and the patient are suitably positioned and the lighting is adequate, the operator may easily see and operate, using direct vision, most of the facial, lingual, and occlusal surfaces of teeth, the proximal surfaces of anterior teeth, often the proximal surfaces of premolars, and occasionally the proximal surfaces of molars.

Direct vision is most desirable since one less instrument (mouth mirror) is usually required in the operating area. Sometimes a mouth mirror is used to retract soft tissues (cheek or tongue) away from the operating area. In addition, when a mouth mirror is used for indirect viewing, it must be kept clean to provide good visibility. This may require frequent interruption since water spray and debris, which collect on the mirror, must be removed. If direct vision can be used without imposing prolonged strain on either the operator's or the patient's body, then it may be used.

Almost invariably, the line of sight and direction of the external light source should coincide. The position of the light should be adjusted overhead so the direction of the beam closely coincides with the operator's line of sight. This allows the light to illuminate most clearly the operating area. If the operator is using a mouth mirror for indirect vision, this position of the operating light will allow light to simultaneously illuminate the area viewed in the mouth mirror (Fig. 3-93).

The operating light should also be adjusted to the proper distance from the patient's mouth to focus the most intense beam where it is needed.

An increased number of dentists have found the use of fiber optics beneficial in transmitting a high-intensity light beam into the mouth. Currently there are many companies that produce fiber optic handpieces and accessories for intraoral illumination (Fig. 3-94).

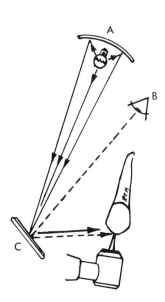

Fig. 3-93. Beam of the overhead light, *A*, should closely coincide with the line of sight, *B*, to simultaneously illuminate the area viewed in the mouth mirror, *C*.

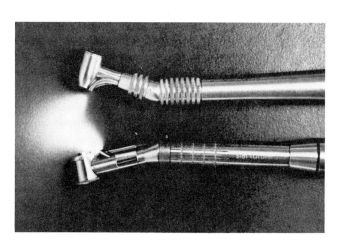

Fig. 3-94. Fiber optic handpieces.

ACCESS TO THE OPERATING AREA

The focus of the dentist's attention is on one area of the patient's mouth. The operator's light, vision, and instruments all converge on this one area. If any one of these is compromised, the result of the operation will likewise suffer. Earlier in this chapter we discussed the proper grasp of hand instruments. The type of hand instrument (this includes rotary cutting instruments as well as chisels, hoes, and so on) and the way these instruments are held and manipulated will determine the degree of access the operator has to the operating area. Each has been designed to perform in a specific manner when applied from a certain direction. If the access to the tooth being restored is limited, this will usually dictate how the external light source is to be adjusted and the line of sight to the tooth. If the opposite is true, that is, if the line of sight or light is restricted, then the access may be varied to allow the best visibility.

AREAS OF ACTIVITY

In the past the style of operating on a patient was with the dentist either standing or seated on a high stool with the assistant often standing behind the dentist. The patient in this scene was usually sitting upright or slightly reclining.

The concept of modern dentistry is one in which the dentist and assistant are comfortably seated near the head of the patient. The patient is lying back horizontally or reclining at approximately a 45-degree angle and the center of attention is the patient's mouth. If the dentist is right-handed, he or she will usually be seated to the right of the patient's right shoulder. The assistant will be located at the patient's left. Instruments and materials are passed from the assistant to the dentist over the patient's bib (never across the patient's eyes). If the dentist is left-handed, he or she is seated to the patient's left, and the assistant is seated to the patient's right.

Imagine looking down on the dental chair from above the patient. The patient's mouth represents the center of the face of a clock with twelve o'clock being the location of the patient's head and six o'clock the patient's feet (Fig. 3-95). A right-handed dentist would operate in an area between eight o'clock and twelve o'clock, and the assistant would work in an area between one o'clock and four o'clock. Instruments would be passed between four o'clock and eight o'clock, and the area between twelve o'clock and one o'clock would have very little activity since this area represents the area over the patient's eyes. The mirror image would be true for a left-handed dentist.

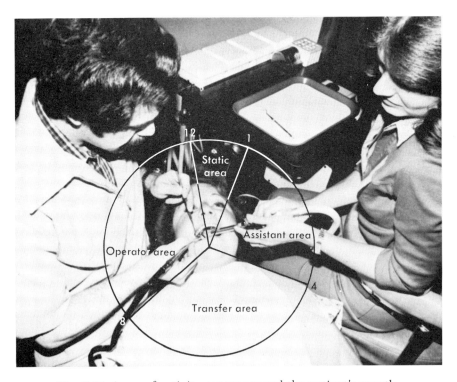

Fig. 3-95. Areas of activity center around the patient's mouth.

BODY MECHANICS

The dentist and assistant must always be positioned in relation to the patient in such a way that neither they nor the patient must assume a stressful body position. This is especially true for the dentist and assistant since a good deal of time is spent each day working on patients, whereas a patient will usually have to endure a slightly awkward position, at most, for the duration of the dental appointment. Oftentimes the dentist's attention to details of restoring teeth will limit concern for the physiological welfare of his or her body. The dentist becomes lost in work and forgets that the neck is bent, the shoulders and back are twisted, he or she is nose to nose with the patient, and so forth.

Merely sitting while operating does not eliminate the stress on muscles, ligaments, and joints. Many dentists suffer from back problems even though they practice sit-down dentistry. The dentist's posture affects the distribution of weight and pull on the joints, thus proper posture is the key in minimizing the complications of low back pain, bursitis, and neuritis.

There are several things the dentist may do to ensure proper posture for himself or herself and comfort for the patient.

1 The patient may be tilted back in the chair to the point where the maxilla is perpendicular to the floor. To ensure comfort, patients should not be tilted back farther than the point at which their back is horizontal since they may feel like they are standing on their head (Fig. 3-96).

2 The patient may be tilted forward to a position where the mandible is parallel to the floor or anywhere between this position and the first position (Fig. 3-97).

3 The patient's head may lie on either the right or left ear, if necessary, so that the dentist may have better visibility or access.

4 The patient's head should be at chest level or slightly lower and over the dentist's lap (Fig. 3-98).

5 For esthetic reasons, the dentist should not be so close as to touch noses with the patient when operating. The normal focus distance from eye to object should be about 12 to 16 inches.

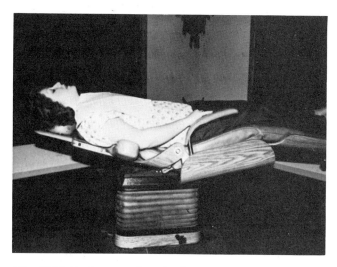

Fig. 3-96. Patient can be tilted so maxillary arch is perpendicular to the floor.

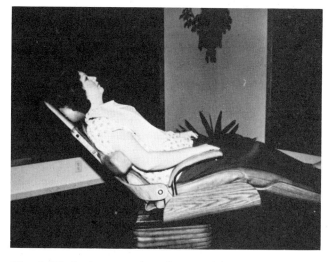

Fig. 3-97. Patient can be tilted so mandibular arch is parallel to the floor.

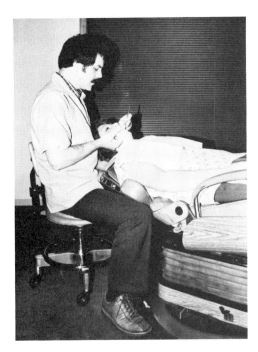

Fig. 3-98. Proper elevation of patient's head and mouth relative to the dentist's seated position.

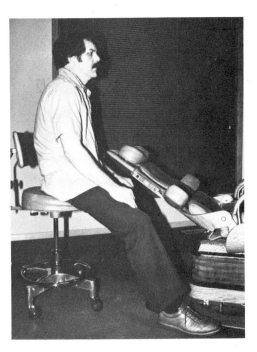

Fig. 3-99. Operator should not be perched on the edge of the chair when operating.

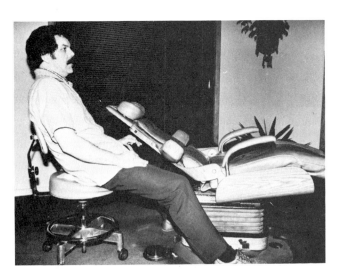

Fig. 3-100. Operator should not slouch in the chair when operating.

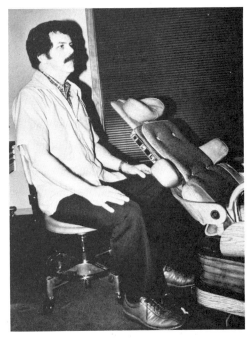

Fig. 3-101. Operator should have good posture with his back against the backrest of the chair.

6 Ideally, the patient's mouth should be at the dentist's elbow level or slightly higher, and the dentist's elbows should be close to the sides to minimize arm fatigue (Fig. 3-98).

7 The dentist should neither be perched on the edge of the chair (Fig. 3-99) nor slouching (Fig. 3-100). The dentist's back should be straight and against the backrest of the chair (Fig. 3-101).

8 The dentist's chair should be low enough to allow the knee level to be slightly higher than the hips (Fig. 3-101).

9 The dentist's shoulders should be parallel to the floor (Fig. 3-101).

10 The dentist's feet should be flat on the floor (Fig. 3-101).

11 The dentist may sit behind the patient or, if right-handed, to the patient's right or if left-handed, to the patient's left (Fig. 3-95).

12 The operating light should be adjusted the proper distance from the patient's mouth to focus the most intense light where it is needed. This distance may vary from 2½ to 3½ feet from the light. This distance can be checked by shining the light on a nearby surface and noting the distance at which the spot of light is brightest and focused (Figs. 3-102 and 3-103).

13 The position of the light should be adjusted overhead so the direction of its beam closely coincides with the line of sight of the dentist. This allows the light to most clearly illuminate the operating area. If the dentist is using a mouth mirror for indirect vision, this position of the operating light will allow light to simultaneously illuminate the area viewed in the mouth mirror (Figs. 3-93 and 3-104).

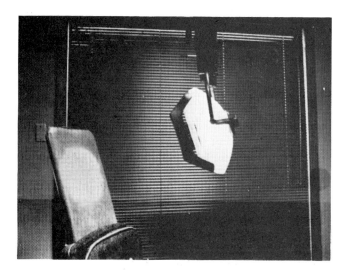

Fig. 3-102. Light is too close. Beam is diffused on the surface and not focused.

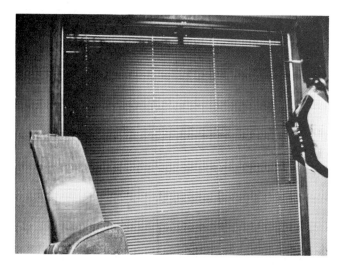

Fig. 3-103. Light is at the proper distance. Beam is intense and focused.

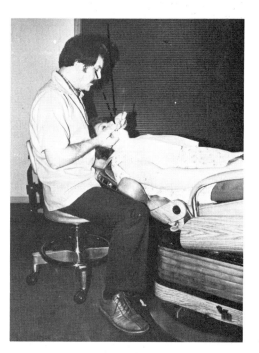

Fig. 3-104. Overhead light should be adjusted so its beam (solid line) closely coincides with the line of sight (dotted line) of the dentist.

INITIAL PATIENT POSITION

Before seating a patient, the base of the chair (Fig. 3-105, *A*) should be lowered (or raised) to a comfortable height with the back upright (Fig. 3-105, *B*). The operating light (Fig. 3-105, *C*) should be swung out of the way and the arm of the chair (Fig. 3-105, *D*) raised or moved to the side for easier access.

When the dentist is ready to work on the patient, the entire chair is tilted until the back of the chair is at the appropriate level. The patient is moved toward the head of the chair and the dentist's side of the chair.

SUGGESTED OPERATING POSITIONS

The following describes positioning for the operator and the patient for operations in each quadrant of the mouth:

Maxillary right posterior tooth (The patient's back is elevated approximately 30 degrees from the horizontal.)

Buccal—The dentist should sit at the ten o'clock position using direct vision with the patient's head rotated away from the dentist.

Occlusal—The dentist should sit at the eleven o'clock position using indirect vision with the patient's head rotated slightly away from the dentist and the chin tipped upward as much as possible.

Lingual—The dentist may use either direct or indirect vision while sitting in the ten o'clock position with the patient's head rotated toward the dentist.

Maxillary left posterior tooth (The patient's back is slightly elevated from the horizontal.)

Buccal—The dentist should sit in the eleven o'clock position with the patient's head rotated as much as possible toward the dentist so direct vision may be used.

Occlusal—Indirect vision from the eleven o'clock position should be used and the patient should rotate the head slightly toward the dentist.

Lingual—The dentist may use direct vision from the ten o'clock position if the patient will tip his or her chin up and rotate the head away from the dentist.

Mandibular right posterior tooth (The patient's back is elevated at about a 40-degree angle with the horizontal.)

Buccal—Direct vision is possible if the dentist is seated in the nine o'clock position and the patient's head is rotated slightly away from the dentist.

Occlusal—In the eleven o'clock position direct vision can be used by moving the patient's head slightly toward the dentist or straight ahead.

Lingual—The dentist may operate on the lingual surfaces using direct vision from the eleven o'clock position with the patient's head rotated toward the dentist.

Mandibular left posterior tooth (The patient's back is horizontal.)

Buccal—The patient's head should be rotated toward the dentist while he or she is seated in the eleven o'clock position using direct vision.

Occlusal—If the dentist is seated at the eleven o'clock position, direct vision may be used to operate on the occlusal surface if the patient rotates the head slightly toward the dentist.

Lingual—direct vision can be used from the ten o'clock position if the patient's head is rotated slightly away from the dentist.

Maxillary anterior tooth (The patient's back is slightly elevated above the horizontal.)

Labial—The dentist will use direct vision from the eleven o'clock position.

Lingual—The dentist may use indirect vision from the eleven o'clock position.

Mandibular anterior tooth (The patient's back is elevated at about a 40-degree angle above the horizontal.)

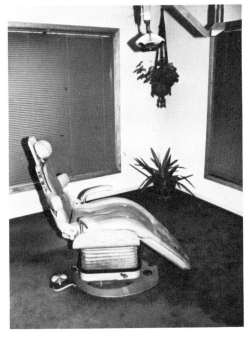

Fig. 3-105. Dental chair is positioned for easy patient seating.

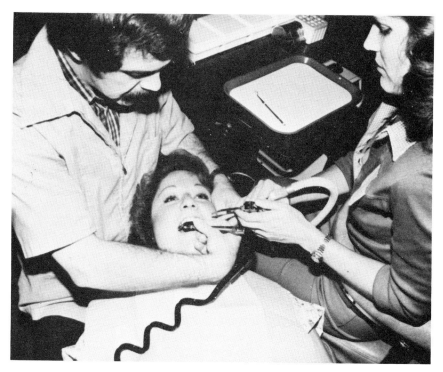

Fig. 3-106. Poor operating position owing to strained position of dentist's right wrist and elbow.

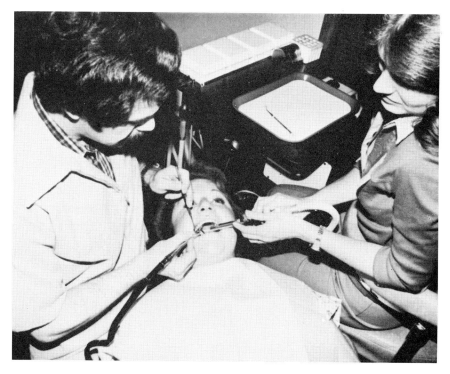

Fig. 3-107. Correct position for operating the same area as in Fig. 3-106. Wrist is in line with the forearm and elbows are close to the dentist's sides.

Labial—The dentist will use direct vision from the ten or eleven o'clock position.

Lingual—The dentist may use either direct or indirect vision from the ten or eleven o'clock position.

It should be kept in mind that these are only guides for operating on a tooth. The dentist may vary the position of the patient's head to improve access and visibility. The patient can be asked to tip the head forward or backward or turn the head to lay more on the left or right ear. The dentist should not become a contortionist by operating in an awkward and stressful manner. The dentist's position and /or the patient's position may be changed to achieve a more comfortable position while maintaining equally good access and visibility. For example, if the dentist finds he or she is working with good visibility and access but the wrist is severely bent and the shoulder is sore because the elbow is not close by the side (Fig. 3-106), the dentist may roll the chair around and reposition the patient so the elbow is closer to the side and the wrist is not severely bent (Fig. 3-107).

It is less fatiguing to the operator to place the patient in a convenient position during operating procedures. Patients can generally tolerate inconvenient posture better than the dentist.

CHAPTER 4

DENTAL CARIES

Dental caries is the second most common reason for patient's losing teeth; periodontal disease is the primary cause. Oftentimes, the detection of decay is quite easy when the patient has neglected proper home care and gross tooth breakdown occurs. At other times, scrupulous attention to radiographs and careful tactile and visual examination with an explorer and mouth mirror may be necessary to detect decayed areas.

The actual process of tooth decay has long been debated, but there is general agreement that there is progressive decalcification of the inorganic structures with concurrent bacterial invasion and disintegration of the organic matrix of the enamel, dentin, and cementum. It can be safely said that the presence of acidogenic microorganisms and a suitable carbohydrate substrate in dental plaque are essential for development of a carious lesion. Initial caries that has penetrated into dentin demonstrates a form peculiar to the type of tooth surface on which it occurs (Fig. 4-1).

Pit and fissure caries

The path of decay diverges from the pit or fissure toward the dentinoenamel junction (DEJ) (Fig. 4-1). The path in dentin then converges toward the pulp. The general appearance is that of two cones with their bases back to back at the DEJ (Fig. 4-2). Once the decay reaches the DEJ, it spreads rapidly in a lateral direction and undermines the enamel.

Smooth surface caries

There is penetration of the enamel forming a conical shape with the base at the cavosurface and the apex at the DEJ (Figs. 4-1 and 4-2). Once the decay reaches the DEJ, it spreads laterally and then converges inward, again forming a cone with the base at the DEJ and the apex toward the pulp.

The presence of decay necessitates immediate removal of the infected tooth structure and restoration of the tooth's original form; otherwise there will be continued destruction of the dental tissue, pain, and loss of function.

Caries detection

Before examining a patient for dental caries, the dentist must have at hand a good set of bite-wing radiographs, a sharp explorer for probing, a mouth mirror, and an air syringe or gauze sponge to dry the teeth for inspection.

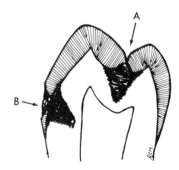

Fig. 4-1. Cross section of progressive development of dental caries in enamel and dentin when initiated in a fissure, *A*, and on a smooth surface, *B*.

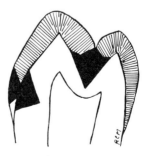

Fig. 4-2. Schematic drawing of Fig. 4-1 illustrating "cones" of decay.

PITS AND FISSURES

Deep enamel fissures are predisposing to caries. They afford retentive areas for caries-producing agents. Caries rapidly penetrates the floor of fissures since the enamel is very thin there. Carious enamel usually appears as a brown or black line. Visual confirmation of the discolored pits or fissures is not conclusive since these areas may not be decayed and yet be darkly stained. A radiolucent area can often be seen on a radiograph if the lesion is of moderate size and the radiograph is clear. Tactile probing should be done to confirm the presence of decay. The tip of a sharp G-3 explorer will stick or catch if a lesion is present.

SMOOTH SURFACES

Carious enamel in smooth surfaces appears chalky white or opaque and usually rough. Often times, pieces of enamel will break loose when probing because of the fragile nature of the enamel. Interproximally it is possible to detect decay by a cone-shaped radiolucent area just below the proximal contact. Large interproximal lesions are readily detected by mirror and explorer examination. A G-2 explorer allows reaching interproximally gingival to the contact area, and by slightly rotating the probe tip toward the suspicious area it is often possible to catch it on the decay.

DENTINAL CARIES

Distinguishing sound dentin from carious dentin is often complicated by deep staining of adjacent healthy dentin. Carious dentin may also be confused with the slightly darker reparative or secondary dentin formation, particularly when decay approaches the pulp chamber. Proper identification of decayed and normal dentin often requires noting a combination of several factors, any one or all of which may be noticed on investigation of a suspicious area:

1. Radiographic appearance
2. Color and texture
3. Feel with explorer or spoon excavator
4. Sound elicited when scraping
5. Odor

Carious dentin can appear in a range of colors from light yellow to brown or black. Normal dentin is a light yellow or cream color and has a smooth hard consistency when explored. Decayed dentin is usually rougher than normal dentin and has a soft leatherlike feel when scraped with a spoon excavator. A sharp G-3 explorer will often

sink or stick into carious dentin and will produce a dull sound when dragged over the surface. Healthy dentin produces a sharp ring under similar treatment. Radiographically, carious dentin is radiolucent, whereas normal dentin is relatively radiopaque. Normal dentin is odorless; decay has a foul odor when being cut or ground. There are several chemical indicators that selectively stain carious dentin, but they are seldom used clinically.

Secondary dentin may be distinguished from carious dentin primarily by its hardness and location. Secondary dentin feels smooth and hard like normal dentin but differs from normal dentin in that it is usually light brown in color. Secondary dentin is deposited within the pulp chamber in response to pulpal irritation; therefore knowledge of the normal pulpal anatomy of the tooth will help distinguish it from caries.

Caries removal

Incipient pit fissure, and smooth surface caries are usually removed when establishing the outline form for a restoration. When the decay is more extensive, it tends to spread laterally along the dentinoenamel junction. The resulting undermined enamel must be included when establishing the outline of the cavity preparation (Fig. 4-3).

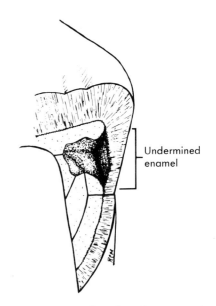

Fig. 4-3. Proximal box of a Class 2 preparation showing enamel wall undermined after caries is removed.

Early removal of undermined enamel allows easier access and visibility to the deeper regions of decay, thus avoiding the possibility of leaving unwanted decay in the finished restoration. In general, the principles of obtaining the outline, resistance, retention, and convenience forms should be met before removing the deeper decay; this minimizes the risk of pulp exposure at an early stage of cavity preparation.

The cavity preparation is not to be extended beyond normal depth to include deep decay. Instead, deep decay is left until the preparation is completed. It is then removed with a spoon excavator or large round bur in the slow-speed contr-angle. What remains is a subsurface (subpulpal, subaxial) wall that may be slightly irregular (Fig. 4-4).

The area is then filled with an insulating base and built up with crown and bridge cement if necessary to restore ideal cavity form (Fig. 4-5).

SEQUENCE OF DEEP DECAY REMOVAL

Figs. 4-6 to 4-19 illustrate a tooth with radiographic evidence of mesioproximal decay as well as deep buccal and occlusal decay.

1 The G-3 explorer is used to probe the involvement of the occlusal pits and fissures (Fig. 4-6).

2 Preparation is being rinsed with water spray (Fig. 4-7) after initial outline form was established at normal axial and pulpal depth using a fissure bur in the high-speed handpiece. The mesiobuccal cusp disintegrated during this procedure since it was completely undermined by decay. The cavity outline is extended so that a clean (decay-free) DEJ is obtained around the perimeter of the preparation.

3 On reexamination of the preparation more undermined enamel was discovered (Fig. 4-8). This is removed and the preparation is checked again.

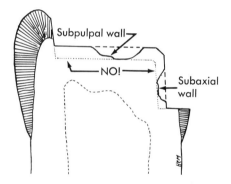

Fig. 4-4. Pulpal and axial walls should be prepared to ideal depth in dentin. Deeper caries is removed leaving a subpulpal or subaxial wall.

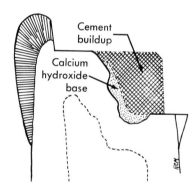

Fig. 4-5. Calcium hydroxide base is placed over dentin areas closest to the pulp. A copal varnish may be placed over remaining dentinal walls and, if necessary, a cement buildup can be placed.

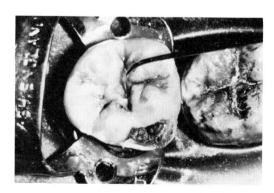

Fig. 4-6. Evaluate extent of carious involvement.

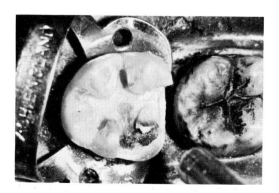

Fig. 4-7. Initial outline form.

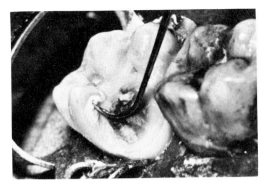

Fig. 4-8. Undermined enamel remains, which must be included in the modified outline.

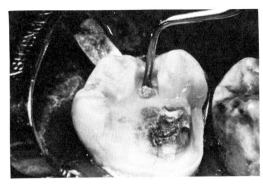

Fig. 4-9. Removal of remaining carious material.

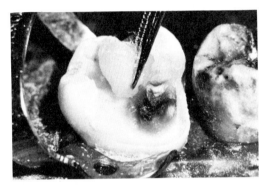

Fig. 4-10. Moistening the cavity aids in detection of remaining carious material.

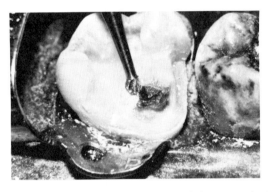

Fig. 4-11. Removal of larger areas of decay with slow-speed round bur.

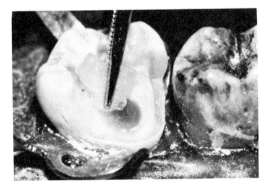

Fig. 4-12. Remoistening cavity.

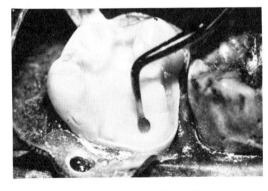

Fig. 4-13. Final check to assure that all carious material has been removed.

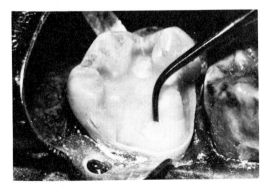

Fig. 4-14. Placement of cavity base.

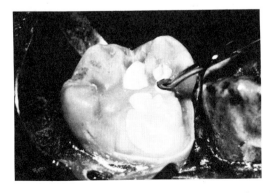

Fig. 4-15. Removal of cavity base from enamel walls.

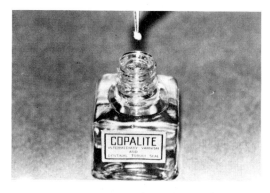

Fig. 4-16. Cavity liner (varnish).

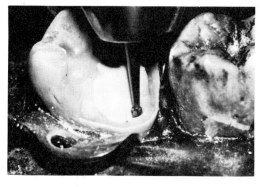

Fig. 4-17. Placing a small depression with a high-speed round bur to act as an index for twist drill.

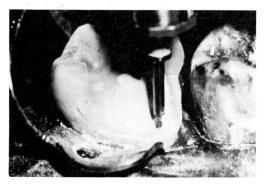

Fig. 4-18. Twist drill in slow-speed handpiece used to place pin hole.

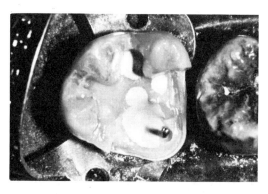

Fig. 4-19. Completed preparation with auxilliary pin retention.

4 The cavity walls have been planed with burs and hand instruments to the desired form. Only deep decay remains. A spoon excavator may be used to scoop out small areas of deep decay leaving a subpulpal wall (Fig. 4-9).

5 Moisten the preparation often. This softens any remaining decay, making it easier to detect and remove (Fig. 4-10).

6 A large round bur in the slow-speed contra-angle handpiece is used to remove larger areas of decay (Fig. 4-11). Proceed from the periphery of the decayed area and work inward, following the clean dentin and leaving the deepest decay until last.

7 More decay has been removed and the preparation is again being moistened (Fig. 4-12).

8 The last bit of decay may be removed with either the round bur or spoon excavator. At this point a sharp spoon excavator is being used to test for complete decay removal. Decay removal is complete when the area sounds and feels like normal caries-free dentin (Fig. 4-13).

Figs. 4-14 through 4-16 illustrate placement of a cavity base and cavity liner. A threaded pin has been added to supplement retention of an amalgam filling material (Figs. 4-17 to 4-19).

CHAPTER 5

TREATMENT OF DENTAL CARIES

Treatment of dental lesions

INITIAL OR SHALLOW CARIES

Lesions that are incipient and those that have not penetrated deeply into dentin (Fig. 5-1) will normally be eliminated by the procedures outlined throughout this atlas.

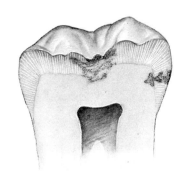

Fig. 5-1. Shallow carious lesions.

MODERATELY EXTENSIVE CARIES

Lesions that have penetrated comparatively deeply into dentin but have not encroached on the dental pulp (Fig. 5-2) are normally managed by operative procedures described to prepare the cavity, *after* which the remaining carious material is removed either with a round bur using a slow speed and light pressure or preferably with an excavator.

If the depth of the lesion is well away from the pulp, it is doubtful that a cement base is of value, in which case the dentin should be well coated with cavity varnish and the restoration inserted. However, if any doubt exists about possible pulp irritation, a cement base should be placed consisting of either a thin layer of quick-setting zinc oxide and eugenol or zinc phosphate cement for metallic restorative materials.

DEEPLY EXTENSIVE CARIES

Caries that radiographically is demonstrated to have penetrated half or more of the distance from the enamel to the pulp should always receive special treatment in addition to the placement of the external restorative material. As a general rule, radiographs do not demonstrate the full extent of the carious penetration, and it must be assumed that the depth of damage is greater than that seen on the film.

The following outline of treatment is suggested.

No history of pain

1 Test tooth vitality. If the tooth is not vital, endodontic therapy may be elected, if indicated, or the tooth may be removed. If it is vital, proceed with the following treatment.

2 Anesthetize the area and place a rubber dam.

3 With a No. 171 bur or diamond point quickly open the peripheral walls to sound dentin.

4 If no pulp exposure is expected and no history of pulpitis is present:

    a. Remove all caries with an excavator.

    b. Place retentive pins, if indicated, in sound dentin.

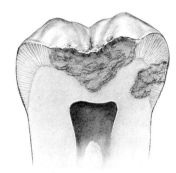

Fig. 5-2. Moderately extensive caries.

c. Place a protective layer of zinc oxide and eugenol and/or zinc phosphate cement over the area near the pulp. Zinc phosphate cement should be preceded by a thorough coat of varnish.

5 Place the restorative material. Pin-retained silver amalgam is recommended as a foundation for cast restorations in such cases.

With a history of pain

When a tooth has a history of pain, it should be evaluated very carefully before arriving at a treatment plan. Always to be considered, of course, is the possibility of occlusal trauma. In a case of deep caries, however, the assumption must be made that the pulp is irritated when pain is present, and the possible extent of pulpal pathology must be considered.

If pain is experienced from heat but relieved by cold, the pulp is probably irreversibly dying or devital and endodontic therapy is indicated. Such a tooth will frequently be acutely sensitive to percussion, making the diagnosis and treatment plan definite.

If the tooth has experienced symptoms of hyperemia and pain has not been severe, corticosteroid treatment may be elected as the treatment of choice to reduce the pulpal inflammation before proceeding to the final restoration.[1]

ARMAMENTARIUM

No. 171 bur (diamond point)
Excavator
Metimyd
Zinc oxide and eugenol

1 Place a rubber dam.

2 With a No. 171 bur or diamond point remove the carious dentin to sound tooth structure in the peripheral walls.

3 With a sharp round bur cautiously remove the bulk of the carious dentin.

4 Use a sharp excavator to remove the remainder of the carious tissue.

5 With a cotton pellet wet the floor of the cavity with Metimyd* or a solution of prednisolone in para-monochlorophenol (PMC) for two or three minutes.

6 Place a layer of zinc oxide and eugenol over the pulpal area.

7 If the proximal area is involved or the tooth is otherwise extensively involved, margin integrity must be established to positively contain the treatment. This may be accomplished by one of the following alternatives, elected according to the case.

a. Place a band (copper or steel).
b. Place an aluminum shell crown if the occlusal surface is reduced.
c. Cover the treatment with a very plastic mix of amalgam.

CARIOUS PULP EXPOSURES

Clinically, many exposed pulps are treated successfully by the average practitioner, much of the literature notwithstanding. The following procedures are included to afford the operative dentist a choice of treatment. They all have wide successful use. Perhaps as research continues, more clear-cut diagnostic methods and thinking will evolve. It may be true that many pulps survive in spite of what is done to them rather than because of what is done for them. This remark is not intended to reflect on what is offered here but, rather, on some of the drugs and procedures used in past years.

To afford a reasonable chance for a successful exposed pulp treatment the following factors should be present:

1. The pulp must be vital.
2. The tooth should be asymptomatic. (A history of pain, depending on its cause and severity, indicates a poorer prognosis.)
3. The exposure should be made in a dry environment and with sharp, sterile instruments.
4. The pulp must not be unduly abused during the procedure.
5. The size of the exposure should be small.
6. The patient should be in good health.

Indirect pulp capping

Indirect pulp capping is a procedure wherein after removal of the superficial carious material a layer of carious dentin is left over the suspected exposed pulp, over which are placed the materials that should enable the pulp to build secondary dentin. The procedure may be executed without anesthesia or the rubber dam; however, if the vital pulp should be encroached upon, the operator will wish both had been utilized.

The procedure is executed in two treatments as follows.

*Schering Corp., Bloomfield, N.J.

First treatment (Fig. 5-3)

1 Open the carious lesion with a No. 171 bur or a diamond point and establish the periphery of the lesion in sound tooth structure or at least strong enamel (Fig. 5-3, *C*).

2 With a sharp excavator remove the outer layer of carious dentin. This can usually be peeled out quickly, exposing a sizable area of sound dentin surrounding the site of the suspected exposure. If a pulp exposure is anticipated, leave a layer of carious dentin in place over the pulp.

In removing the carious tissue avoid pressure in a pulpal direction. Start the removal of the caries as far from the center of the tooth as possible.

3 Place a layer of calcium hydroxide over the pulpal area of the lesion.

4 Place a layer of zinc oxide and eugenol over the calcium hydroxide.

5 If inadequate tooth structure remains to contain the dressing by itself (one or more missing peripheral walls), place a band or an aluminum shell crown if the occlusal surface is reduced adequately. A layer of amalgam may be used instead to ensure that the dressing and an absolute seal will be maintained.

Second treatment
(after a two-month interval)

1 Place a rubber dam.

2 Remove the entire dressing and remaining caries (Fig. 5-3, *D*).

3 If no exposure is found, place a thin layer of calcium hydroxide and a thin layer of zinc oxide and eugenol. If an exposure is found, proceed as outlined under direct pulp capping.

4 Proceed with the restorative steps as appropriate (Fig. 5-3, *E*).

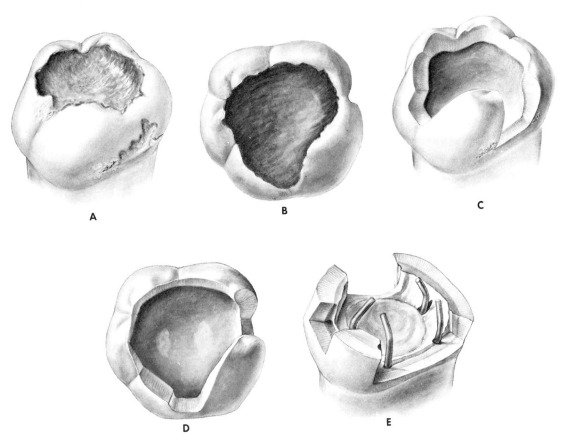

Fig. 5-3. Extreme caries destruction. **A** and **B,** Before removal of carious tissues. **C,** Sufficient enamel removed to facilitate removal of carious material. **D,** As such a tooth should appear after the first treatment of an indirect pulp capping procedure. **E,** Preparation to receive an amalgam foundation (pin and cement base).

Direct pulp capping
Calcium hydroxide

Probably the most widely used methods of pulp capping currently being taught utilize calcium hydroxide.

1 Control bleeding by pressing gently with a sterile cotton pellet. If bleeding cannot be thus controlled, use a 1% solution of epinephrine. Commercially prepared pellets containing epinephrine are excellent for this purpose. Do not use hydrogen peroxide.

2 Lack of bleeding or excessive bleeding renders the prognosis less than desirable, and other treatment may be indicated. The pulp should be made to bleed so that an evaluation may be made.

3 Place a thin layer of calcium hydroxide over the exposure.

4 Place a small quantity of quick-setting zinc oxide and eugenol over the calcium hydroxide.

5 Place a layer of zinc phosphate cement.

6 Proceed with the final restoration.

Pulpotomy

For pulps of young permanent teeth severely exposed a pulpotomy should be considered. Pulpotomy is the surgical amputation of the dental pulp coronal to the dentoenamel junction. It is performed in combination with the preliminary steps outlined in the foregoing procedures as follows.

1 With a round bur (No. 5 or 6) open the coronal portion of the pulp around its entire periphery.

2 Remove the pulp to the root canals with a sharp discoid excavator.

3 The cavity can be cleaned and bleeding controlled with an anesthetic solution containing a vasoconstrictor or cotton pellets containing epinephrine.

4 Place a layer of calcium hydroxide over the "stump" of each canal.

5 Place a thin layer of zinc oxide and eugenol.

6 The bulk of the crown can be restored with amalgam if desired, or zinc phosphate cement can be used to build up the bulk of the volume. Pins are also recommended for cross splinting[2] since such involved cases frequently leave the sides of the tooth vulnerable to splitting.

A *formocresol pulpotomy procedure* is recommended for primary teeth.

Pulpectomy

Endodontic therapy is an essential aspect of operative dentistry, but it is a field of dental practice too extensive to warrant inclusion here.

PULPALLY INVOLVED PRIMARY TEETH

The following procedures, taught by Charles "Pop" Sweet,[3] are highly successful for treating involved pulps in primary teeth.

ARMAMENTARIUM

No. 171 bur
Large round burs
Band material
Thymol
Calcium hydroxide
Quick-setting zinc oxide and eugenol

Pulp not exposed

1 Anesthetize the quadrant.

2 Place a rubber dam, including the canine.

3 Remove unsupported enamel. Establish peripheral walls in sound dentin.

4 If peripheral walls are destroyed, place a band.

5 Excavate the carious dentin using a large round bur (Nos. 6 to 10).

6 If no exposure is found, paint the dentin with liquefied thymol to desensitize. Wipe the excess out with cotton.

7 Place a layer of calcium hydroxide.

8 Place a layer of quick-setting zinc oxide and eugenol.

9 Place the amalgam or steel crown restoration.

Pulp exposed

Contraindications to pulpotomy are as follows:
1. Early root resorption
2. Presence of pus
3. Sensitivity to percussion
4. History of unprovoked toothache
5. Poor physical health (rheumatic fever and so forth)
6. Abnormal pulpal hemorrhage (or lack of it)

If the pulp is vital and the preceding contraindications are not present, the following pulpotomy procedures are recommended. The first is accomplished in two appointments.

ARMAMENTARIUM

No. 171 bur
Large round burs
Anesthetic solution
Buckley's formocresol
Zinc oxide and eugenol
Quick-setting zinc oxide and eugenol

First appointment

1 Anesthetize the quadrant.

2 Place a rubber dam. Wash the field with alcohol.

3 Open the tooth with suitable burs. Remove the caries at the gingival seat.

4 With a clean, frest bur (Nos. 6 to 9) remove the bulbous portion of the pulp, running the bur *counterclockwise* and with light pressure. Sever the pulp flush with the entrance to the root canal.

5 Control hemorrhage with sterile anesthetic solution containing epinephrine. Epinephrine-impregnated cotton pellets may be used.

Do not disturb the blood clot while cleaning the cavity. Never use hydrogen peroxide on an exposed pulp since it may create emboli in the remaining filaments of the pulp.

6 Place pellets of cotton moistened with Buckley's formocresol over the stumps of the pulp.

7 Seal the cavity for three to five days with zinc oxide and eugenol.

Second appointment

1 Anesthetize the quadrant.
2 Place a rubber dam.
3 Remove the previously placed treatment.
4 Remove all stain and debris from the cavity with clean instruments.
5 Place a creamy mix of zinc oxide and eugenol and formocresol (half and half). Press the paste into place with a cotton pellet.
6 Place a layer of quick-setting zinc oxide and eugenol and a layer of zinc phosphate cement if desired.
7 Fill the remaining crown as appropriate.

Single appointment procedure

A single appointment procedure, presumed less successful for severe cases, varies from the preceding outline only in that in step 6 of the first appointment the formocresol is left on the root canals for five minutes, and then the procedure outlined for the second appointment is completed.

REFERENCES

1. Fry, A. E., Neely, A. R., Ruhlman, D. C., and Phatak, N. K.: Topical use of corticosteroids for the relief of pain sensitivity of dentin and pulp. Clinical observations, J. Oral Ther. **2**:88, 1965.
2. Markley, M. R.: Pin retained and reinforced restorations and foundations, Dent. Clin. North Am., pp. 229-244, March, 1967.
3. Sweet, C.: Latest in pulpal therapy. Lecture to the Multnomah County Dental Society, Portland, Ore., April 18, 1967.

CHAPTER 6

DENTAL AMALGAM

M. Traveau is credited with advocating the first form of dental amalgam-silver-mercury paste in 1826 in Paris, France. It was presented by the Crawcour brothers to the dental profession in America in 1833 as "Royal Mineral Succedaneum," as a substitute for gold. The ensuing chaos in organized dentistry of the time is known historically as the "Amalgam War."

Dr. J. Foster Flagg and Dr. G. V. Black studied amalgam, and the research of Black led to the development of the formula in 1896 that has been closely adhered to until recent years.

Since amalgam is the most widely used single restorative material in dentistry, its overwhelming importance cannot be ignored. It is relatively easy to use, a fact that perhaps invites its use in many unwarranted circumstances and widespread abuse. Restorative dentists must continually reevaluate the indications of the various restorative procedures relative to their individual ability to perform and practice within the limitations of the physical properties of the materials employed.

Indications

Amalgam is indicated for relatively small restorations if the material will not be subjected to excessive stress and where it is supported and contained by sound tooth structure. It must not be expected, therefore, that it can be consistently relied on to serve for extended periods of time when a relatively large portion of the occlusal surface to be restored will be subjected to heavy masticatory forces. Normal indications for the use of amalgam include the following:

1. Restoration of proximal cavities, defective pits and fissures, gingival third lesions of posterior teeth, the distal surfaces of canines, and other areas where its placement will not result in diminished esthetic results
2. Repair of defective restorations
3. As a temporary protective covering over pulp treatments
4. To build bases or foundations, often with pins, to retain cast restorations
5. For general use in deciduous teeth in preference to gold

The following factors should be considered when amalgam is to be used:
1. Size of the area to be restored
2. Other materials in the tooth or adjacent teeth
3. Economic factors
4. Esthetic result

Contraindications

Precautions to be observed in using amalgam have been noted in the discussion of indications. However, consideration must also be given to its relatively low tensile strength, which contributes to marginal deterioration. The following are contraindications:

1. Extensive restorations, which are subject to excessive stress, preclude the use of amalgam.
2. If the restoration would be unduly displayed, there is a poor esthetic result.

Composition and properties

Amalgam is defined as an alloy, one of the constituents of which is mercury.[1] Silver alloys used for dental purposes are primarily silver and tin, to which are added copper and zinc. The alloy, mixed with mercury, produces the dental amalgam.

1. Silver, by itself, unites with mercury with difficulty. It increases expansion, retards setting time, enhances strength, decreases flow, and resists tarnish.
2. Copper unites with mercury with some difficulty, reduces setting time, increases expansion, increases strength and hardness, reduces flow, and tarnishes readily.
3. Tin is included in silver alloys for dental purposes because it unites readily with mercury, retards setting time, improves plasticity of the material, reduces expansion, and increases flow. In increased percentages it increases shrinkage.
4. Zinc combines readily with mercury, causes expansion, increases setting time, increases flow, lends plasticity, and inhibits oxidation.[5] It also seems to decrease porosity.[6]

The percentage of mercury in a completed amalgam restoration should generally be about 50%,[3,7,8] but less is better, provided the restoration is properly condensed.

More than fifty alloys are marketed that meet American Dental Association Specification No. 1 for dental amalgam alloy.* Additionally, silver alloys formulated without zinc are in use.

Extensive research has been done on amalgam throughout the period of time it has been used. This has resulted in extensive improvements, especially in recent years.

Newer alloy systems

Recent years have seen the introduction of alloy systems that utilize a strengthening material of silver-copper eutectic based on the principle of dispersion strengthening of alloys, a principle used successfully in developing exotic metals in the space program.† The formula contains 70% silver, 16% tin, 13% copper, and 1% zinc (or nonzinc).

Dispersalloy is an alloy system that is a mixture of conventional filings and silver-copper dispersant particles in a spherical form. Its physical properties demonstrate a high compressive strength and low creep, whereas clinical trials show it has a lower incidence of marginal fracture as compared to conventional and spherical alloys.*

Mercury

Mercury that is used for dental restorative procedures must meet certain acceptable criteria. The American Dental Association Specification No. 6[2] sets the standard of purity, labeling, and packaging.

Labeling of mercury for dental purposes should state that it meets American Dental Association Specification No. 6, or if the mercury is obtained from a chemical house, it should be labeled "U.S.P." (United States Pharmacopeia), "A.C.S." (American Chemical Society), or "Analytical Grade." Mercury sold as "pure," "redistilled," or "triple distilled" may not be pure or in any way meet dental standards.[2]

Mercury hygiene

A high level of concern about mercury in our general environment has developed in recent years. Prudent mercury hygiene is essential to good practice.

Rupp and Paffenburger[9] have compiled the following summary of recommended mercury hygiene for dental offices:

Store mercury in unbreakable, tightly sealed containers;
Confine any inadvertant spills to an easily cleaned tray or similar work space;
Design the dental offices with seamless flooring that extends two inches up each wall;
Coat the cavity surfaces with a varnish or a base;
Salvage all amalgam scrap and keep it in a tightly covered container;
Work in well-ventilated spaces;
Eliminate the indiscriminate use of mercury-containing solutions;
Avoid heating mercury or amalgam;
Use water spray and [high-volume] suction when . . . [removing old] amalgam [restorations],

*Guide to dental materials, ed. 8, Chicago, 1978, American Dental Association.
†Dispersalloy, American Silver & Mercury Producers, El Cajon, Calif.

*Guide to dental materials, ed. 8, Chicago, 1978, American Dental Association.

Use conventional dental amalgam compacting procedures, manual and mechanical, but should not use ultrasonic amalgam condensers.*

They further concluded that their review of the literature did not indicate a significant hazard to patients in the use of amalgam, and that risks to dental personnel, although normally low, must not be ignored and have been shown to be of unacceptable levels in some offices.

Alloys
FORMS IN WHICH SUPPLIED

Alloys for dental use are available in a variety of forms: in bulk, such as filings (powder), in tablets (pellets), or in capsules. Tablets and capsules contain measured amounts to facilitate accuracy and efficiency clinically and to prevent mercury contamination of the operatory.

Tablets

Tablets are produced by compressing a measured amount of alloy filings into a pellet. The pellet quickly breaks up into loose filings during trituration.

Capsules

Because of their potential uniformity and efficiency, disposable capsules are convenient to use. They should contain accurately measured amounts of alloy and mercury. Capsules aid in avoiding operatory contamination by mercury. Such capsules vary in construction, some brands being more convenient than others, but they provide a means of introducing the mercury into an alloy and contain a mixing pestle. To mix, the mercury is released and the capsule is activated in a mechanical amalgamator for the time specified by the manufacturer.

STORAGE

Alloys are generally considered to possess very long shelf life. However, they should not be stored in an area subject to heat.[2] Normal room temperatures should not affect them.

PARTICLE SIZE

The *particle size* of traditional alloys is generally classified medium, fine, or ultra-fine. Recent re-

search has revealed much evidence in support of the clinical superiority of fine particle size[8,10,11] in preference to ultra-fine.[5] High-quality alloys also have controlled particle sizes, the mesh or particle sizes being restricted to certain micron ranges.

SPHERICAL ALLOYS

One of the newer particle forms for dental alloys, introduced in recent years, is spherical owing to the manufacturing technique. It presents some different manipulative characteristics—requiring larger-sized condensers for the same condensing force as filings, for example. In fact, it flows so readily under condensing force that it requires an especially well-formed and well-placed matrix to produce adequate contact areas when it is used to restore proximal surfaces. Operators accustomed to relying on condensing pressure to expand the matrix laterally to create proximal contact with the adjacent tooth may experience difficulties with this form of alloy.

Clinical properties

Various physical and working properties of silver alloys are controlled by the manufacturer. These include the setting time, plasticity, strength, creep, dimensional change, corosion and tarnish, and tensile strength.

SETTING TIME

Fast-setting alloys must be rapidly condensed, otherwise the strength of the restoration will be reduced[12] and marginal adaptation will be inadequate.

PLASTICITY

Plasticity of the freshly mixed amalgam relates to the technique employed to condense it in the prepared cavity. Low plasticity requires greater condensing force to achieve good adaptation to cavity walls and margins.

STRENGTH

Relative to setting time and to the need for rapid condensation, fast-setting alloys achieve strength more rapidly if they are managed properly. Amalgam nears its final strength about twenty-four hours after placement.

The amount of mercury remaining in the matrix of the completed restoration, in the reactant products, relates to its strength. Strength does not diminish appreciably unless the mercury content is

---

*Rupp, N. W., and Paffenburger, G. C.: Significance to health of mercury used in dental practice; a review, J. Am. Dent. Assoc. **82**:1401, 1971.

more than approximately 52% of the final restoration.[8]

CREEP

Creep or flow correlates rather closely to clinical marginal breakdown. Creep is the percentage of flow under pressure at mouth temperature.[13]

DIMENSIONAL CHANGE

Researchers using isotope tests do not seem to demonstrate a difference in leakage patterns between expanding and contracting amalgams.[8] It is logical to achieve slight expansion of the material to support margins.

Excessive expansion, caused by inclusion of moisture in the material during manipulation, is of great clinical significance. Expansion as great as 5% may occur, resulting in postoperative pain, cracked teeth, extrusion of the amalgam from the prepared cavity, decreased strength, and increased corrosion. Protection of the amalgam from moisture during manipulation and condensation procedures is obviously mandatory if acceptable results are to be achieved.

There is no effect on the dimensional change induced by moisture after the amalgam is placed in a prepared cavity. Moisture is a factor entering into the corrosion of the surface, especially if the amalgam is left unpolished. Researchers identify the corrosion of amalgam on its interface with the prepared cavity as a factor toward improving the marginal seal.[8,12]

CORROSION AND TARNISH

Deterioration of the surface of an amalgam restoration depends on the quality of technique during placement (proper trituration, adequate condensation, proper alloy-mercury ratio, freedom from moisture, and smooth surface) and the quality of the oral environment and personal oral hygiene as well as the type of alloy used. Polishing reduces corrosion, and the selection of a good alloy is essential to avoid corrosion.

TENSILE STRENGTH

Chipping or loss of material at the margin of amalgam may be a result of any or all of several factors. Cavity preparation is a major factor if the enamel is not adequately planed and a butt joint (90 degrees) created.

Tensile strength of amalgam is reduced if the final mercury content is too high[14] (more than about 52%), possibly because of inadequate condensation. Ultra-fine–cut alloys have been shown to produce low tensile strength[13]; the fine-cut alloys are superior.

Alloy-mercury ratios

Of critical importance to an amalgam restoration is the percentage of mercury remaining after amalgam is condensed and finished.

Eames[7] has popularized the concept of trituration of the alloy and mercury in the same percentage as that desired in the finished restoration, or a ratio of about 1:1. Although such a concept may seem desirable, it creates some critical demands on several technical steps. Dispensing, trituration, and time of condensation are all of critical importance, and condensation must be skillfully accomplished to achieve proper results.

Sweeney and Burns[15] have shown that proportion is not a critical factor provided that proper condensation procedures are observed.

Because "dry," or low-ratio, mixes require longer trituration time, proper plasticity may not be achieved. The result may be more porosity and poorer physical properties in the final restoration.

Trituration

Trituration is the making of amalgam by mixing silver alloy with mercury.

Hand trituration is the making of amalgam using a hand mortar and pestle.

Mechanical trituration is the making of amalgam by means of a powered mechanical device. Mechanical trituration has the advantage of producing a more uniform consistency of amalgam time after time.

Adequate trituration requires that the alloy particles be coated with mercury. It is essential that this coating be thoroughly achieved so that a continuous matrix can be created surrounding the particles in the completed restoration.

Overtrituration will produce contraction of the completed amalgam. Undertrituration will cause the following:
1. Inadequate wetting of the alloy particles
2. Decreased strength
3. Increased expansion
4. Corrosion
5. Generally poorer clinical behavior

It is essential to determine the best trituration time for each size of mix to be made. Trituration times may vary from one amalgamator to the next since trituration intensities often vary.

REFERENCES

1. Boucher, C. O., editor: Current clinical dental terminology, ed. 2, St. Louis, 1974, The C. V. Mosby Co.
2. Guide to dental materials and devices, ed. 6, Chicago, 1972, American Dental Association.
3. Phillips, R. W., Swartz, M. L., and Norman, R. D.: Materials for the practicing dentist, St. Louis, 1969, The C. V. Mosby Co.
4. Suprinick, H.: Relating reactions in silver-mercury and tin-mercury to properties of amalgam alloys, J. Dent. Res. **50:**944, 1971.
5. Skinner, E. W., and Phillips, R. W.: The science of dental materials, ed. 6, Philadelphia, 1967, W. B. Saunders Co.
6. Weikel, M. M. (American Silver and Mercury Producers): Personal communication, July 18, 1972.
7. Eames, W. B.: Preparation and condensation of amalgam with a low mercury-allow ratio, J. Am. Dent. Assoc. **58:**78, 1959.
8. Mahler, D. B.: Physical properties and manipulation of amalgam, Dent. Clin. North Am., pp. 213-228, March, 1967.
9. Rupp, N. W., and Paffenburger, G. C.: Significance to health of mercury used in dental practice. A review, J. Am. Dent. Assoc. **82:**1401, 1971.
10. Mitchem, J. C., and Mahler, D. B.: Influence of alloy type on marginal adaptation and final residual mercury, J. Am. Dent. Assoc. **78:**96, 1969.
11. Mitchem, J. C., and Mahler, D. B.: The adaptation of amalgam, J. Am. Dent. Assoc. **76:**787, 1968.
12. Phillips, R. W.: Research on dental amalgam and its application in practice, J. Am. Dent. Assoc. **54:**309, 1957.
13. Mahler, D. B., Terkla, L. G., Van Eysden, Jan, and Risbeck, M. H.: Marginal fractures vs. mechanical properties of amalgam, J. Dent. Res. **49:**1452, 1970.
14. Nadel, R., Phillips, R. W., and Swartz, M. L.: Clinical investigation on the relation of mercury to the amalgam restoration (II), J. Am. Dent. Assoc. **63:**488, 1961.
15. Sweeney, W. T., and Burns, C. L.: Effect of mercury alloy ratio on the physical properties of amalgam, J. Am. Dent. Assoc. **60:**374, 1961.
16. Jacobson, F. L. (Seattle, Washington): Study club demonstrations.

CHAPTER 7

CAVITY PREPARATIONS FOR AMALGAM

Amalgam restorative procedures

As a restorative material silver amalgam is used for a variety of purposes. In addition to the situations for which it is normally indicated it may be used as a temporary material over pulp treatments, for repairs of defective restorations, as a stable base under cast restorations, and, with pins, to rebuild the foundation structure upon which cast restorations or porcelain jacket crowns can be placed.

Its selection as the material of choice for operative procedures is generally based on (1) the size of the area to be restored, (2) materials used in adjacent areas of the tooth or adjacent teeth, (3) economic factors, and (4) whether or not it will be esthetically acceptable.

Amalgam finds its greatest success when used to restore areas that are not extensive or subjected to unusual stress. Its edge strength is not great, and unless adequately supported by sound tooth structure and properly prepared cavosurface margins, it is subject to failure.

The necessity of using hand instruments in amalgam preparations is sometimes questioned, the opinion being that with high-speed techniques all margins may be adequately planed with rotary instruments. Although this may be true in some circumstances, superior resistance form is created only when hand instruments are properly used. It is dangerous to the adjacent tooth in most in-stances to attempt to prepare the proximal part of Class 2 cavities with rotary instruments only. Inevitably, the operator who avoids the use of hand instruments in preparing Class 2 cavities does four undesirable things. He or she must (1) remove too much tooth structure by over extending the outline, (2) leave unsupported enamel on the proximal cavosurface margins, (3) leave rough gingival margins with unsupported enamel prisms, and (4) damage the adjacent tooth. Orthodontists also complain if bands are damaged. A thorough and conservative cavity preparation that ensures the greatest longevity of the restoration is far more important than saving the few seconds required to properly use the hand instruments indicated.

Although the preceding is true when placing single restorations, simultaneous restoration of several adjacent teeth occasionally presents opportunities to vary the techniques illustrated. Obviously, the care taken to protect an adjacent tooth surface may be overlooked if it is to receive a restoration. Also, when preparing two adjacent proximal cavities, a better opportunity presents itself to plane the proximal walls using a straight fissure bur. Skillfully performed, this may be adequately accomplished without overextending proximal margins. However, to form ideal resistance form in the gingival wall and to plane the gingival margins, hand instruments must be used.

Cavity preparations

The designs of prepared cavities to contain and retain silver amalgam result from the following physical properties of the material:

1. Low edge strength
2. Flow or distortion when subjected to stress
3. A tendency to extrude from the cavity when adequate retention is not created (Dimensional change expansion occurs from moisture contamination.[1])
4. Low tensile strength
5. High conductivity

The physical characteristics of the material dictate basic characteristics of cavity design. Virtually all writers indicate the following common ideals:

1. Cavosurface angles must be at or approach 90 degrees.
2. Cavities must be prepared so that the remaining tooth structure will support the amalgam.
3. Cavities should be prepared conservatively.
4. Deep cavities require insulation to protect the pulp.
5. Retentive factor is essential.
6. Adequate bulk for strength must be considered.

It is interesting to note that of all attributable causes for failure of amalgam restorations, the major factor has been identified as improper cavity preparation.[2,3]

INTERPRETATIONS OF FUNDAMENTALS

Many of the various basic fundamentals of cavity design are interpreted differently by educators. Variations in methods of fulfilling basic principles may be confusing, even perplexing to some, but differences in philosophy are important to progress in any endeavor. It is paramount, however, that the basic objectives of conservation be adhered to and that one never be guilty of rationalizing to justify poor technique.

BULK FOR STRENGTH

The principle of providing adequate bulk of amalgam to ensure strength does not mean that the preparation should be large in extent, but refers only to the depth (thickness) of the material to be subjected to stress. Cavity preparations, therefore, must have sufficient depth, the periphery of the material being contained by walls. Where the material is not contained by an outer wall, as in a Class 2 restoration, pulpal depth must be sufficient to provide adequate bulk (thickness) to contribute resistance to fractures and displacement.

When cusps are overlayed, the amalgam must be thick enough, and adequately supported, to resist fracture under stress.

Thus cavities should never be widened buccolingually to provide bulk for strength.

CLASS 1 AMALGAM CAVITY PREPARATIONS

Detected early, pit and fissure cavities can be easily treated. When pits or grooves are sufficiently deep in young patients to be deemed susceptible to caries, they should be restored. Such a procedure is termed *prophylactic odontomy* and must be considered conservative preventive dentistry in every respect. This does not, of course, justify use of the procedure in all teeth simply because pits and fissures happen to be present. Judgment on the part of the operator is essential. Recontouring defective grooves using twelve-blade burs is also recommended if they are not defective to the dentinoenamel junction.

The outline form may be established by the use of one bur, a straight (Nos. 55 or 56) or tapered fissure bur (Nos. 169L, 170, or 171) bur, as advocated by some writers, or, as advocated by Black[4] and others, the area to be restored may be penetrated or opened by using a No. $\frac{1}{2}$ round bur or, as taught by Markley,[5] a No. 330 bur, and then extended by using other burs or the No. 330 bur. Strickland[6] advocates a No. 245 bur for the entire preparation. *The principles of cavity outline and internal wall alignment remain the same regardless of which bur is used. However, the orientation of each bur is modified as it is used to prepare the cavity so the proper internal form is produced.*

If a round bur is utilized, the enamel may be undermined by removing carious material, after which a No. 34 bur is used to further break away enamel to approach outline form and/or achieve access to the dentin.

It must be emphasized that, according to circumstances, an operator may wish to use all these concepts at one time or another. For example, a tooth extensively involved by caries on its occlusal surface will obviously not require opening with a No. $\frac{1}{2}$ or No. 330 bur. A round bur may be indicated to quickly remove the bulk of the caries and undermined enamel.

Occlusal cavities

Cavity preparation

ARMAMENTARIUM

No. 170, 329, or 330 bur

Mandibular molar (Figs. 7-1 to 7-5)

1 Enter the distal pit using a No. 170, 329, or 330 bur and extend the cut distally only to the beginning of the distal marginal ridge, then buccolingually only far enough to remove any deep fis-

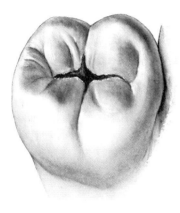

Fig. 7-1. Occlusal caries, lower right second molar.

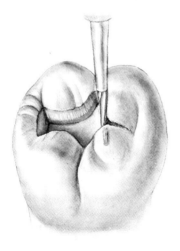

Fig. 7-2. Distal wall established.

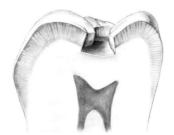

Fig. 7-4. Buccolingual cross section of preparation.

sures (Fig. 7-2). While establishing the *distal wall*, the angle of the bur must be such that the distal marginal ridge is not weakened. This usually requires that the distopulpal line angle be obtuse (Fig. 7-5).

Establish the pulpal wall at a depth to remove a small amount of dentin. If caries exists to a depth beyond that at which the pulpal wall is normally placed, prepare the cavity as illustrated here and manage the carious area as described in Chapter 4.

2 Extend the cut mesially into the central pit (Fig. 7-2) and then laterally into the buccal and lingual grooves. As the cavity walls are established, use a brushlike motion in removing the tooth structure. The enamel is thus planed and sufficient tooth structure removed to facilitate proper placement of the restorative material. The distal portions of the buccal and lingual walls should be slightly undercut (Fig. 7-4). It is not necessary to undercut the walls in the narrow portions (isthmus) of the preparation if the cusps are relatively flat. If the cusp height is relatively steep where the cavosurface margin is established, it

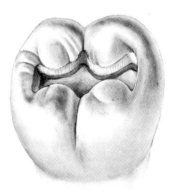

Fig. 7-3. Completed cavity preparation.

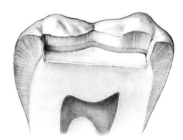

Fig. 7-5. Mesiodistal cross section of preparation.

should be undercut accordingly (Fig. 7-6). The walls should be established in a manner that will maintain the bulk of amalgam at the margins in the completed restoration.

The pulpal wall of the cavity will be relatively flat, and it should be smooth and continuous as the preparation is made.

COMMENT: *Amalgam cavosurface margins are, because of lack of edge strength of the material, ideally formed to create an angle of 90 degrees. However, occlusal margins may be compromised to about 70 degrees where necessary (Fig. 7-6).*

3 Extend the cut into the mesial pit and buccolingually to establish the mesial wall with an obtuse mesiopulpal line angle in the same manner described for establishing the distal wall. By tilting the handpiece, place slight retentive undercuts toward the mesial portions of the buccal and lingual walls.

Mandibular first premolar. If the mandibular first premolar presents a transverse ridge, it should be preserved for strength unless cariously involved (Fig. 7-7). The pits are prepared with a No. 170 bur, extending the margins only sufficiently to facilitate condensation of the amalgam. The pulpal wall in mandibular first premolars is made parallel to a line connecting cusp tips (Fig. 7-8). If the occlusal walls are prepared so they are parallel with the long axis of the tooth, the buccopulpal line angle may come dangerously close

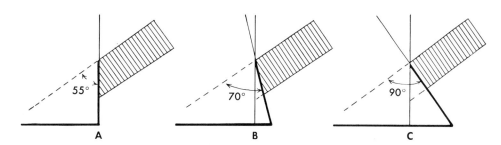

Fig. 7-6. Comparison of angles of prepared occlusal cavosurface margins on comparatively steep cusps. **A,** Completed amalgam margin will be too thin and subject to fracture. **B,** Acceptable preparation. It is desirable to have completed amalgam margins of at least 70 degrees. **C,** Although an ideal 90-degree cavosurface angle is created, such a preparation sometimes necessitates excessive tooth removal and undercutting of the cusp.

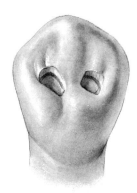

Fig. 7-7. Mandibular premolar, Class 1 amalgam preparation.

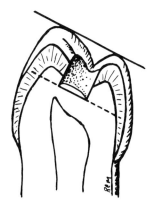

Fig. 7-8. Buccolingual cross section of mandibular first premolar amalgam cavity preparation.

to, or even expose, the pulp (Fig. 7-9). In addition, this alignment of the lingual aspect will often result in a thin, weak lingual wall that might easily fracture and shorten the life of the restoration. Retention is also established by tilting the tip of the bur bucally and lingually to slightly undercut the buccal and lingual walls.

Mandibular second premolar. Occlusal cavities in mandibular second premolars (Fig. 7-10) are prepared in a manner similar to the procedure described for mandibular molars.

Maxillary premolar. Maxillary premolars are prepared in the manner described for the mandibular molars, the cut being made from distal pit to mesial pit (Fig. 7-11) and extended buccally and

lingually to include the deep portions of the developmental grooves. Extension buccolingually should only be sufficient to properly condense the amalgam unless the extent of caries dictates greater extension.

Maxillary molar. The maxillary molar cavity is prepared following the same general procedure as that described for mandibular molars, except that the oblique ridge should not be involved (Fig. 7-12) unless undermined by caries. Occlusal Class 1 restorations in maxillary molars are normally prepared in two parts—the mesial portion including the mesial and central pits and the distal portion including the distal pit and, when indicated, the lingual groove.

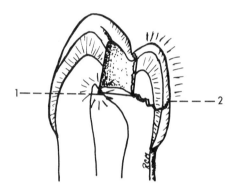

Fig. 7-9. Possible errors created by improper angulation of preparation in a mandibular first premolar. *1*, Exposed pulp; *2*, fractured lingual cusp.

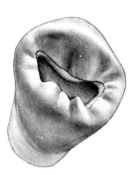

Fig. 7-10. Class 1 amalgam preparation, mandibular second premolar.

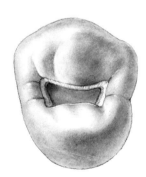

Fig. 7-11. Class 1 amalgam preparation, maxillary premolar.

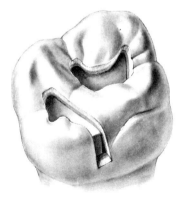

Fig. 7-12. Class 1 amalgam preparations, maxillary molar.

Pit cavities
Cavity preparation

Enter the cavity with a small fissure bur and extend its margins only far enough to establish them in sound enamel and dentin and to facilitate placement of the restorative material (Fig. 7-13). It should be deep enough to enter dentin. The outline form must be smooth and may be round, eliptical, or slightly triangular as the case requires. A No. 34 bur may be used to establish slight retentive areas occlusally and gingivally in the dentin (Fig. 7-13). Use of an inverted cone bur may not be essential since the directions of the walls may be slightly undercut with the fissure bur without weakening enamel.

Fissure cavities

Restoration of a developmental groove is usually an extension from a developmental pit and is most common in the lingual groove of upper molars and occasionally buccal grooves of lower molars.

Cavity preparation

1 Start the cut in the pit and extend it through the groove, the walls being extended only far enough to establish them in sound enamel and far enough apart to facilitate condensation of the amalgam (Fig. 7-12).

2 Additional retentive undercuts may be established with a No. 34 bur at each end of the groove,

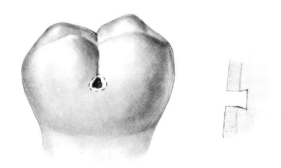

Fig. 7-13. Buccal pit cavity preparation, mandibular molar.

or the dentin of the walls of the cavity may be very slightly undercut. If the cavity is wide, a flat gingival wall should be established with retentive areas carefully placed mesially and distally in dentin with a No. 168 (169L) bur in a manner similar to the placement of proximal retention in a Class 2 cavity. These may be sharpened using gingival margin trimmers.

COMMENT: *When cavosurface angles are established, it is absolutely essential that no unsupported enamel prisms remain. The anatomy of the tooth must be considered relative to direction of enamel prisms, and retentive factors (undercuts) must be developed accordingly.*

CLASS 2 AMALGAM CAVITY PREPARATIONS
General considerations

1 It is a complex cavity form involving two or more tooth surfaces including proximal and occlusal.

2 The occlusal outline is similar to a Class 1 in that it includes all carious areas and enamel defects but should not end in a functional wear facet (include or stay away from any wear facets).

3 The proximal outline blends smoothly into the occlusal outline and roughly parallels the silhouette outline of the adjacent teeth.

4 The proximal walls extend beyond the proximal contact area, so they can be easily finished, polished, and maintained. (The amalgam-tooth junction is a potential retention area for plaque and starting point for recurrent caries.)

5 The proximal walls converge occlusally to preserve marginal ridge strength and to provide retention and conservation of tooth structure.

6 The gingival wall is perpendicular to the long axis of the root and must extend apically far enough to be below the contact area and to provide a clearance of at least 0.5 mm. from the adjacent tooth; 0.5 mm. clearance will generally result in the gingival wall extending below the free gingival margin except in cases of gingival recession.

7 The proximal box form has its own distinct resistance and retention forms.

8 The gingival wall is flat and forms a right angle or slight acute angle with the axial wall.

9 The axial wall is parallel to the long axis of the tooth and is of uniform depth into the dentin (0.5 mm.).

10 The pulpal wall parallels the cusp tips (to avoid pulp horns), is flat, and 0.5 mm. into the dentin.

11 The axiopulpal line angle is beveled or rounded to minimize stress in the amalgam.

12 All internal line angles are made definite and smooth.

13 Generally, walls of the cavity meet the cavosurface angle at 90 degrees; exceptions are occlusal walls owing to the slope of triangular ridges.

14 The proximal wall is made parallel to enamel prisms—nearly at a right angle to the cavosurface.

15 There are no bevels on cavosurface margins. The cavity margins must be definite with no loose or unsupported enamel prisms.

16 The preparation must be free from debris before the amalgam can be placed.

Reverse curve

The occlusal outline of a typical Class 2 amalgam preparation is made following *smooth flowing curves* with the absence of any sharp irregularities or deviations. The outline includes the area of caries plus any adjacent enamel defects such as pits and fissures. There are two distinct areas of the preparation:

1. Occlusal form
2. Proximal box form

The proximal outline must blend smoothly into the occlusal, forming one continuous outline. (This is done as the cavity form reaches its final stages of completion.) Often a "reverse curvature" in the buccal and/or lingual wall is formed as a necessary result of blending the buccoproximal and linguoproximal walls with the already existing occlusal form. The degree of curvature is a result of five cavity features:

1. The isthmus width adjacent to the proximal box
2. The extension of the buccoproximal and linguoproximal walls
3. Access to the buccoaxial and linguoaxial line angle
4. Occlusal and axial depth
5. The 90-degree alignment of the buccal and lingual proximal walls to the cavosurface

Keep in mind these important rules:

1. The proximal walls are very near 90 degrees to the cavosurface of the tooth to provide strength to the tooth, maximum marginal bulk of amalgam, and the greatest degree of resistance and retention for the silver amalgam.
2. The proximal walls are straight and in one plane, not warped or twisted like a ribbon.
3. The proximal walls converge occlusally to a greater degree than the occlusal walls.

In an ideal size preparation with the tooth in normal alignment and using hand instruments to refine the proximal box to the correct shape and form, we leave a nearly right-angle irregularity at the junction of the proximal and occlusal outline (Fig. 7-14). This irregularity is then smoothed, leaving a slight concavity (reverse curve) that blends in with the remaining outline (Fig. 7-15).

In a restoration with a greater occlusal isthmus width (that is, where the buccal triangular ridge has been included owing to decay), we will see a lesser degree of concavity or reverse curve (Fig. 7-16).

Generally, the lingual wall requires very little, if any, reverse curvature in an ideal preparation. Should the lingual wall be extended because of more extensive proximal decay, a more definite reverse curve may be seen (Fig. 7-17).

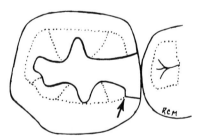

Fig. 7-14. Example of the irregularity created by the junction of the proximal box and the occlusal portions of a Class 2 amalgam cavity preparation prior to properly joining them by smoothing the buccal wall into a reverse curve.

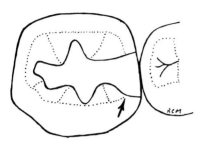

Fig. 7-15. Reverse curve form of a Class 2 amalgam cavity preparation.

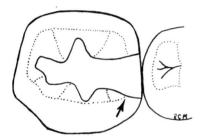

Fig. 7-16. Wider than normal Class 2 amalgam cavity preparation (compare with Fig. 7-15).

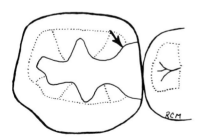

Fig. 7-17. A wider than normal proximal box resulting in reverse curves in both the buccal and lingual proximal walls.

Cavity preparation

ARMAMENTARIUM

No. 170 (57) bur
No. 168 (169L) bur
Spoon excavator
Enamel hatchets
Gingival margin trimmers

Mandibular second molar

1 Prepare the occlusal portion of the preparation as described for a Class 1 amalgam preparation (Figs. 7-1 through 7-5).

2 Extend the preparation toward the proximal surface to be restored. Make the cut toward the contact area, still using the No. 170 bur. The cut is then extended buccolingually while at the same time cutting into the marginal ridge. Care must be taken not to overextend this cut buccolingually. Do not cut entirely through the marginal ridge, but leave a thin plate of enamel to serve as a guide and to protect the adjacent tooth while making the axial cut.

3 Make the axial cut gingivally (Fig. 7-18) using the remainder of the marginal ridge as a guide. The tip of the bur is tilted alternately buccally and lingually as the cut is deepened. The depth of this cut is made to the level at which the gingival wall is to be established.

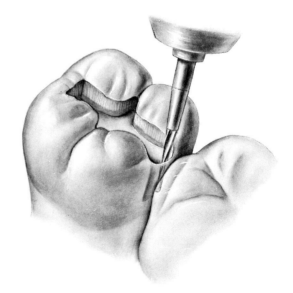

Fig. 7-18. Axial cut made gingivally and buccolingually.

4 Break out the remaining enamel using a spoon excavator or suitable hand instrument (Fig. 7-19). Frequently this enamel plate will fall away as cuts are made toward the surface of the tooth after desired extension has been established.

5 With an enamel hatchet or gingival margin trimmer, plane the gingival and proximal walls, establishing the desired outline form (Fig. 7-20).

6 Place slight retentive grooves (pyramids) in the axiolingual and axiobuccal line angles using a No. 169L or ½ round bur (Fig. 7-21). The groove may extend above the level of the pulpal floor, but the cut is made mainly with the tip of the bur by tilting it slightly toward the direction in which the cut is made. This cut must be placed entirely in dentin and not cut toward the pulp. However, contour of the tooth must be considered, since the axial wall is convex.

7 Use a gingival margin trimmer to sharpen the pyramids, and at the same time slope the dentin portion of the gingival wall slightly by sharpening the axiogingival line angle (Fig. 7-22).

COMMENT: *Some operators prefer not to sharpen the pyramids with gingival margin trimmers. However, optimal resistance form cannot be established without planing the gingival wall with a gingival margin trimmer, thereby sharpening the axiogingival line angle to create a slight inclination toward the axial wall (Fig. 7-22).*

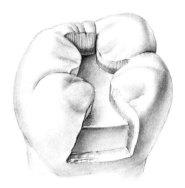

Fig. 7-20. Lingual wall and lingual one half of the gingival wall after planing with enamel hatchet.

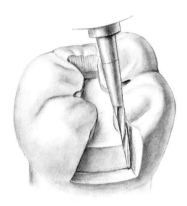

Fig. 7-21. Placement of proximal retentive grooves.

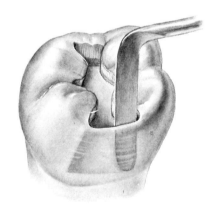

Fig. 7-19. Breaking out the proximal enamel.

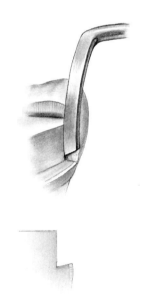

Fig. 7-22. Gingival margin trimmer used to define retention grooves and axiogingival line angle.

8 Using the opposite margin trimmer, lightly plane the gingival enamel. Care must be taken not to establish a true bevel, but this area should be planed sufficiently to remove all loose or weak enamel prisms (Fig. 7-23).

9 With the same gingival margin trimmer, plane or round the axiopulpal line angle (Fig. 7-24).

10 Wash the cavity thoroughly, dry, and apply cavity liner. If any liner should reach a cavosurface angle, it must be removed by planing with hand instruments. (Some operators prefer placing the liner before planing the proximal and gingival walls* [Fig. 7-25].)

COMMENT: *The completed cavity preparation should be extended buccolingually only sufficiently to place the proximal cavosurface margins in an area that may be readily reached by toothbrushing. When a broader area of decalcification is present, the cause of this problem should itself be dealt with.*

A common tendency is to prepare amalgam cavities too wide in the occlusal area. It must be remembered that tooth structure must support and retain the restoration, and a large, widely extended amalgam restoration is more subject to breakdown from the forces of stress than a small one adequately supported by sound tooth structure and proper cavity design. Strength of sound tooth structure is far greater than that of amalgam. Therefore, cavities should be extended to include caries and faulty tooth structure, both for prevention of recurrent caries and to facilitate condensation of amalgam.

---

*Evidence exists that covering the cavosurface margin of amalgam preparations with copal-type varnish may be beneficial.[7-9]

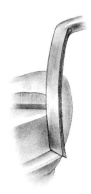

Fig. 7-23. Gingival margin trimmer used to plane gingival enamel.

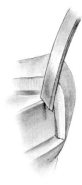

Fig. 7-24. Rounding the axiopulpal line angle.

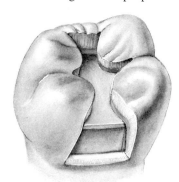

Fig. 7-25. Completed Class 2 mandibular molar amalgam cavity preparation.

Maxillary molar

Class 2 cavity preparations for amalgam in maxillary molars follow the same general procedure as that described for the mandibular molar. An MO (Figs. 7-26 and 7-28) cavity preparation includes both the mesial and central pits, and it is extended into the buccal groove to restore that part of the groove that is sharp or carious. The distal wall is placed slightly into the oblique ridge, but only enough to include the area of the buccal groove.

DO cavities in maxillary molars (Fig. 7-27) include the distal pit and are extended to include the sharp portion of the lingual groove. the mesial wall is usually placed slightly into the oblique ridge.

Binangle chisels and angle formers can sometimes be more conveniently used in maxillary molars than enamel hatchets and gingival margin trimmers.

Maxillary premolar

The same principles described previously are used for maxillary premolars. MO, DO, or MOD cavity preparations include both the mesial and distal pits and central groove (Figs. 7-29 and 7-30). Binangle chisels are generally used to plane the proximal and gingival walls. Gingival margin trimmers or angle formers may be used to place pyramids and plane line angles and gingival enamel.

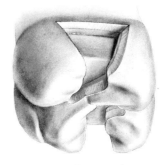

Fig. 7-27. Distal view of Fig. 7-26.

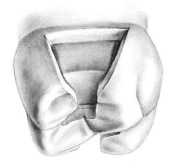

Fig. 7-28. Mesial view of Fig. 7-26.

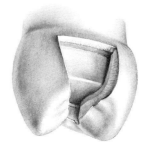

Fig. 7-29. Class 2 amalgam preparation in a maxillary premolar.

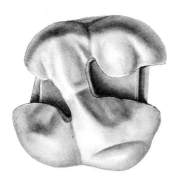

Fig. 7-26. MO and DO amalgam cavity preparations in a maxillary molar.

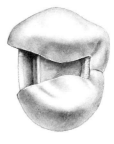

Fig. 7-30. Occlusal view of Fig. 7-29.

Mandibular first premolar

Class 2 amalgam preparations in mandibular first premolars (Figs. 7-31 and 7-32) follow the steps outlined for the mandibular molar, except that the approach for instrumentation will be more from the lingual aspect than for other posterior teeth. (See also Figs. 7-8 and 7-9.) Place the pulpal wall as described for a Class 1 preparation. If the transverse ridge is highly developed, it should be preserved. MO cavities include the mesial pit, and DO cavities include the distal pit. Only when the central groove is unusually deep or otherwise defective is it included.

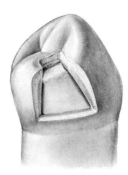

Fig. 7-31. DO amalgam cavity preparation in a lower first premolar.

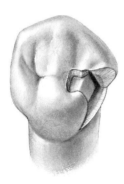

Fig. 7-32. Occlusal view of Fig. 7-31.

CLASS 3 AMALGAM CAVITY PREPARATIONS

The distal sufaces of canines should always be restored with a material that will not deteriorate in the oral environment. Resin materials are therefore seldom indicated. Loss of the distal contact area of canines allows the premolars to shift, thus affecting the integrity of the posterior occlusion. From an esthetic standpoint the restorative material is easily hidden by the normal bold contour of these teeth.

Two procedures are outlined, one for normal and one for short canines. The lingual dovetail, recommended for short canines, removes considerable lingual tooth structure but conserves the tooth structure immediately under the incisal edge, which is an advantage in some types of occlusion.

Maxillary canine, normal distolingual procedure

ARMAMENTARIUM

No. 170 bur
No. 168 (169L) bur
No. 33½ bur
Gingival margin trimmers (angle formers)
Wedelstaedt chisel

Some general similarities exist between this preparation and Class 2 preparations. However, the lingual surface must be extended for convenience form only to allow proper condensation of the amalgam.

1 On the lingual surface make an axial cut using a No. 169L bur. Establish the cut to the desired gingival level and carefully extend the gingival wall labiolingually. This cut should be made through the contact area and placed mainly in enamel.

2 The extension of the lingual outline should be conservative, only large enough to facilitate instrumentation and condensation of amalgam.

3 Break out the remaining enamel plate using a spoon excavator.

4 Plane the gingival wall and proximal walls with a binangle chisel, enamel hatchet, or Wedelstaedt chisel.

5 Place retentive pyramids using a No. 169L or ½ round bur in the labial and lingual gingival point angles (Figs. 7-33 and 7-34). The tip of the bur may be extended slightly into the gingival wall if desired.

6 Tilt the contra-angle to cut a retentive area in the incisal dentin (Fig. 7-35).

7 Plane the internal portion of the gingival wall to provide resistance form using a gingival margin trimmer.

8 Apply cavity liner.

9 Lightly plane the gingival margin with a gingival margin trimmer or angle former to remove unsupported enamel prisms.

10 With a small Wedelstaedt chisel, plane the labial and lingual enamel.

Figs. 7-36 and 7-37 illustrate a completed cavity preparation.

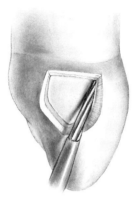

Fig. 7-33. Placing labial retention in distal Class 3 amalgam preparation, maxillary cuspid.

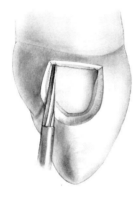

Fig. 7-34. Placing lingual retention.

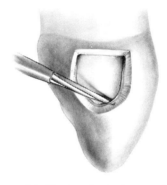

Fig. 7-35. Placing incisal retention.

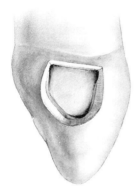

Fig. 7-36. Completed Class 3 amalgam preparation, maxillary cuspid.

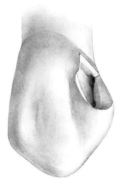

Fig. 7-37. Lingual view of Fig. 7-36.

Maxillary canine, distolingual dovetail procedure

Cavity preparation

1 Make an axial cut in the lingual surface with a No. 169L bur. Establish the gingival wall.

2 Outline the dovetail area (mesial wall). Do not extend the incisal outline more than necessary since the object is to retain as much incisal bulk as possible (Fig. 7-38). Establish a step in dentin only deep enough to allow placement of retentive areas.

3 Break out the enamel plate with a spoon excavator.

4 Plane the gingival floor with binangle chisels, enamel hatchets, or Wedelstaedt chisels.

5 Plane the labial and lingual pyramids with a No. 169L bur (Figs. 7-33 and 7-34).

6 Place retentive areas in the incisal and gingival dentin areas of the dovetail with a No. 33½ bur. Do not undercut the mesial wall.

7 Sharpen the gingivoaxial line angle with a gingival margin trimmer or angle former.

8 Apply cavity varnish.

9 Plane the gingival cavosurface margin to remove unsupported enamel prisms.

10 Plane the labial enamel and the lingual proximal enamel with a Wedelstaedt chisel.

CLASS 5 AMALGAM CAVITY PREPARATIONS

Outline forms for Class 5 amalgam restorations vary but may be generally compared with Class 5 gold foil preparations.

Fig. 7-39 shows the outline of the older or kidney-shaped cavity. Such a cavity is prepared with fissure burs and retention placed with an inverted cone bur. The newer outline with straight walls conserves tooth structure and creates a more desirable esthetic result (Fig. 7-40). When the rubber dam is placed (Fig. 3-65), the desired outline is made evident by the carious or eroded area. The normal gingival line may often be seen on the tooth when the gingiva is retracted. Outline form ideally places the mesial, distal, and gingival margins below the crest of the gingiva when the restoration is complete.

Fig. 7-41 shows a horizontal section through the middle of a prepared Class 5 cavity and demonstrates proper angulation of the mesial and distal walls and the convex axial wall.

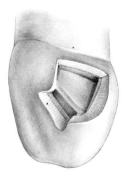

Fig 7-38. Lingual dovetail Class 3 amalgam preparation, distal of short maxillary cuspid.

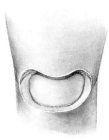

Fig. 7-39. Kidney-shaped Class 5 amalgam preparation, premolar.

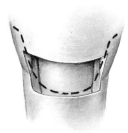

Fig. 7-40. Relationship of outline form of a Class 3 amalgam preparation to crest of gingiva.

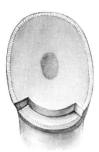

Fig. 7-41. Cross section of a Class 5 amalgam preparation showing proper angulation of the mesial and distal walls and the convexity of the axial wall.

Premolars

Cavity preparation

ARMAMENTARIUM

No. 33½ (34, 35) bur
Straight chisel
(Wedelstaedt chisel)
(Angle former)

1 With an inverted cone bur in the slow speed handpiece, establish the distal wall (Fig. 7-42).

2 Using the same bur, establish the mesial wall (Fig. 7-43).

3 Establish the occlusal (or incisal) wall using the side of the bur, taking care not to undercut the enamel (Figs. 7-44 and 7-45). The cavosurface margin must be a right angle. The occlusal outline may in some cases be curved to conserve tooth structure but will normally be straight.

COMMENT: *If the occlusal wall is located in the gingival third of the tooth, it is not necessary to undercut the dentin to establish additional retention. However, to keep the prepared enamel wall at right angles to the tooth surface when the occlusal wall is high on the tooth, it becomes necessary to place an undercut in the dentin.*

4 With the end of the bur toward the axial wall establish the gingival wall using the side of the bur (Figs. 7-46 and 7-47). Prepare the gingival wall with a slight inward slope toward the axial floor to provide retentive factor.

COMMENT: *The step is frequently described as being accomplished with the end of the bur facing the gingival wall. Although this may be possible in some cases, it will frequently be found awkward and will establish the wall with an extreme slope toward the gingival margin. Time is eventually lost by having to establish the correct internal form.*

5 Lightly smooth the axial wall with the end of the bur (Fig. 7-48). The completed axial wall should be convex, in harmony with the surface of the intact tooth.

COMMENT: *Care in executing the foregoing steps will have established the entire outline form and most of the retention form. Using a "painting" or "brushing" action with the bur, the axial wall will have been planed and the walls smoothed so as to require minimal planing with hand instruments.*

6 With a straight chisel or monangle chisel sharpen the point angles and plane the walls, paying particular attention to the cavosurface margins (Fig. 7-49).

7 If the gingival wall is established above the cementoenamel junction, plane the cavosurface

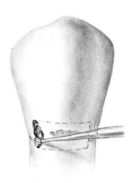

Fig. 7-42. Establishing the distal wall of a mandibular premolar Class 5 cavity preparation.

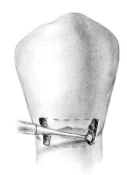

Fig. 7-43. Establishing the mesial wall.

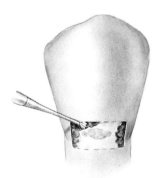

Fig. 7-44. Cutting the occlusal wall.

margin sufficiently to remove all unsupported enamel (Fig. 7-50). If it is terminated in cementum, the cavosurface margin need not be planed in the same manner as it would with enamel present; it should be planed only sufficiently to render it smooth and distinct.

COMMENT: *Only two instruments are actually essential to this preparation: the inverted cone bur and the straight chisel. Some operators prefer to sharpen line and point angles with angle formers, and Wedelstaedt chisels may be used to plane the occlusal wall, particularly if it is curved.*

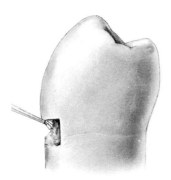

Fig. 7-45. Side view of establishing the occlusal wall.

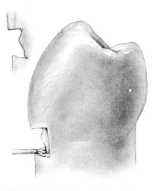

Fig. 7-46. Gingival wall.

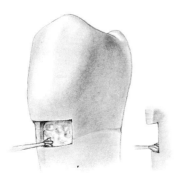

Fig. 7-47. Removal of bulk and smoothing the axial wall.

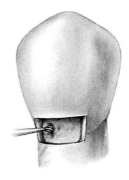

Fig. 7-48. Smoothing the axial wall.

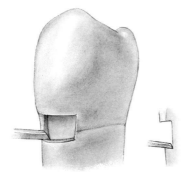

Fig. 7-49. Planing the cavity with a straight chisel.

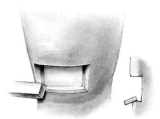

Fig. 7-50. Planing the gingival enamel.

Variations in outline form. All operative procedures must be adapted to the situation they are to serve. Figs. 7-51 through 7-56 show a few variations in outline form to illustrate this point.

If the bulk of the lesion to be restored can be treated with the typical trapezoidal outline, but a line of caries (or decalcification) extends along the gingiva (Fig. 7-51), it can often be included with an extension from the cavity preparation (Fig. 7-52). The occlusal wall of this extension may be flat in harmony with the main portion of the occlusal outline, or it may be rounded if to do so is more conservative. Creation of a sharp point in such an area is sometimes possible. However, in such cases it is usually difficult to condense the restorative material adequately.

A curved occlusal cavosurface outline (Figs. 7-53 and 7-54) is sometimes indicated.

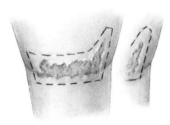

Fig. 7-51. Outline form for a Class 5 cavity with an occlusal extension.

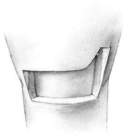

Fig. 7-52. Completed cavity preparation for Fig. 7-51.

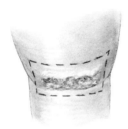

Fig. 7-53. Outline form for a Class 5 cavity preparation with a curved occlusal wall.

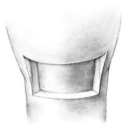

Fig. 7-54. Completed cavity preparation for Fig. 7-53.

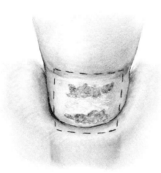

Fig. 7-55. Outline form for an extensive Class 5 cavity preparation.

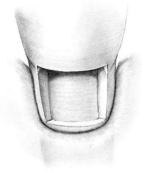

Fig. 7-56. Completed cavity preparation for Fig. 7-55.

Molar buccal restorations

Restoration of Class 5 lesions in molars frequently requires a deviation from the procedure outlined for premolars. However, the principles previously outlined should be borne in mind.

Cavity preparation

ARMAMENTARIUM

No. 34 (35) bur (for straight handpiece or contra-angle)
No. 170 (171) bur in contra-angle
Straight chisel
Wedelstaedt chisels

1 Where it is not practical to use an inverted cone bur to establish outline form, use a No. 170 bur in a contra-angle. Include only defective areas, and establish pulpal depth into dentin only deeply enough to facilitate the establishment of retentive form and condensation of the amalgam. Keep the axial wall convex in harmony with the surface of the tooth (Fig. 7-57, *A*).

2 With a No. 34 bur sharpen the occlusoaxial and gingivoaxial line angles. Be extremely careful not to involve enamel or unduly undercut the occlusal wall (Fig. 7-57, *B*).

3 Plane the enamel walls with a straight chisel or Wedelstaedt chisel.

COMMENT: *The convex form of the buccal surface of mandibular molars sometimes requires that the occlusal enamel be planed in such a manner that the occlusal and gingival walls are quite divergent. It must be planed, however, to establish a proper cavosurface angle at 90 degrees, and the internal or retention form must be established accordingly to adequately retain the amalgam. Maxillary molars present a flatter buccal surface.*

Extended Class 5 cavities

Gingival cavities may frequently be abutted to proximal restorations (Fig. 7-58); this is common in mouths in which recurrent caries is a problem. Good practice requires placement of proximal restorations, where indicated, prior to placement of such gingival restorations.

Gingival cavities in molars sometimes include the buccal pit area (Fig. 7-59) or may extend entirely through the buccal groove to the occlusal surface. Care must be taken to conserve tooth structure since the buccal cusps of molars are the working cusps, and sound dentin must be maintained to preserve them from fracture.

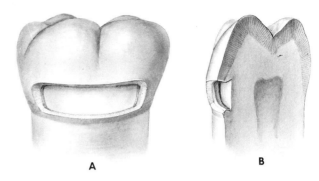

Fig. 7-57. A, Typical molar Class 5 amalgam cavity preparation. **B,** Cross section of a Class 5 molar amalgam cavity preparation.

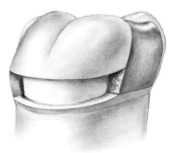

Fig. 7-58. Extension of a Class 5 amalgam cavity preparation to abut a Class 2 amalgam restoration.

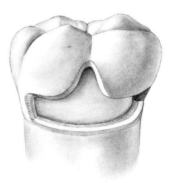

Fig. 7-59. Extended outline of a Class 5 amalgam cavity preparation to include the buccal pit area.

Lingual Class 5 molar restorations

A most trying procedure is the preparation of Class 5 cavities on lingual surfaces of mandibular molars. The procedure is generally as follows.

Cavity preparation

1 Before placing the rubber dam, rough in the outline with a No. 170 (171) bur. Retract the tongue with a mouth mirror or other large instrument. Some cases permit direct downward displacement of the tongue.

2 Rough in retention form with a No. 34 inverted cone bur.

3 Place the rubber dam, placing a clamp below the gingival margin of the cavity.

4 Use off-angle hatchets (18-10-16) to plane enamel walls (Fig. 7-60).

5 Plane retention form with gingival margin trimmers (13-80-8-14).

6 Place cavity varnish.

7 Lightly replane cavosurface margins.

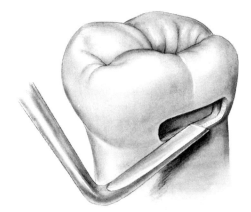

Fig. 7-60. Lingual Class 5 cavity preparation, mandibular molar. An off-angle hatchet may be used to plane the cavity walls.

RESTORATION OF EXTENSIVE LESIONS

It is not generally recommended that cusps be restored with amalgam. However, it is frequently done and with a high level of success if skillfully accomplished. When amalgam cannot be contained by four walls of sound tooth structure to provide maximum resistance form, its bulk must be increased. Missing or overlayed cusps must therefore provide sufficient bulk of amalgam ($2\frac{1}{2}$ to 3 mm. on a wall prepared perpendicular to the line of occlusal force) so that occlusal forces will not fracture it away from the tooth structure.

Lingual cusps of mandibular molars are probably the most frequently lost (Fig. 7-61).

If fracture is minimal, sufficient tooth structure may remain and adequate retention can be gained through strategic placement of undercuts (Figs. 7-61 and 7-62).

Fig. 7-63 illustrates a MOD preparation for a tooth with an extensively fractured mesiolingual cusp. If minimal tooth structure remains after preparing cavity form and inadequate mechanical retention is available through normal retentive undercuts, additional retention must be obtained by carefully placing retentive pins into solid tooth structure (Fig. 7-63). See Chapter 9 for details of pin procedures.

Restoration of cusps

ARMAMENTARIUM

Same as for Class 2

1 Prepare the Class 2 areas of the cavity as usual.

2 Extend the gingival wall to the distolingual cusp (Fig. 7-63).

3 Establish the mesial wall on the distolingual cusp, placing a retentive pyramid.

4 Plane the gingival wall and cavosurface margin.

5 Place a pin in the dentin in the area of the missing cusp.

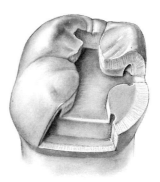

Fig. 7-61. MO amalgam cavity preparation in a mandibular molar including overlaying the mesiolingual cusp.

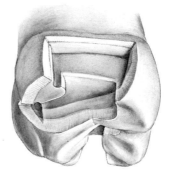

Fig. 7-62. DO amalgam cavity preparation in a maxillary molar including overlaying the distolingual cusp.

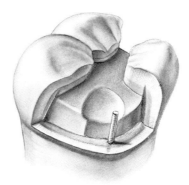

Fig. 7-63. MODL amalgam cavity preparation including restoration of the mesiolingual cusp. A pin is placed for added retention and resistance.

CEMENTOPROXIMAL CAVITIES

Sometimes carious lesions develop below the enamel in periodontal situations owing to lack of proper home care (Fig. 7-64). Restoration of these areas, if the normal Class 2 technique is utilized, demands removal of considerable amounts of tooth structure. When cast gold restorations are placed, long bevels may be utilized. However, again, a great amount of tooth structure must be removed. The type of restoration shown is most easily accomplished on the premolars. It is less often indicated in molars because of their anatomical form and lack of access.

Great care must be exercised to protect the pulp, since as the apex of the tooth is approached, the depth of tooth structure between the tooth surface and the pulp diminishes.

Cavity preparation

ARMAMENTARIUM

No. 33½ bur
Angle former (gingival margin trimmers)

1 Using a No. 33½ bur in the slow speed range, establish the lingual, occlusal, and gingival walls (Figs. 7-65 and 7-66).

COMMENT: *It is essential to remove only enough tooth structure to gain access to the carious area, remove the caries, and facilitate placement of the restorative material. Although it is not recommended that the outline form of these cavity preparations be extended for prevention, the outline form will normally be extended well lingually.*

2 Establish occlusal and gingival axial line angles using an angle former (Figs. 7-67 and 7-68). For situations in which an angle former cannot be conveniently used, use gingival margin trimmers.

3 With an angle former or gingival margin trimmer, plane the cavosurface angles. These margins may also be planed with a hoe, chisel, or enamel hatchet, whichever the situation demands.

4 Establish the buccoaxiocclusal and the buccoaxiogingival point angles with the angle former (Fig. 7-68). The buccal and axial walls may be planed with a 6½-2½-9 hoe.

Fig. 7-69 illustrates a completed cavity preparation.

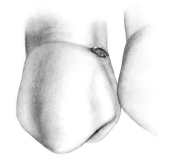

Fig. 7-64. Cementoproximal caries.

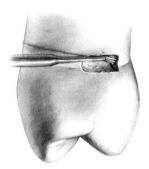

Fig. 7-65. Outlining the cavity using an inverted cone bur.

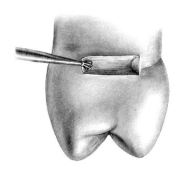

Fig. 7-66. Establishing the facial wall.

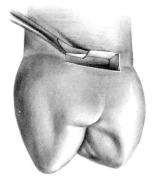

Fig. 7-67. Planing the gingival wall using an angle former.

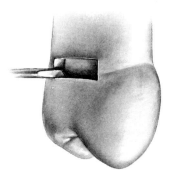

Fig. 7-68. Sharpening the line and point angles.

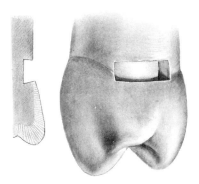

Fig. 7-69. The completed cavity preparation.

REFERENCES

1. Research Commission: Excessive expansion of amalgam, J. Am. Dent. Assoc. **29:**292, 1942.
2. Healy, J. H., and Phillips, R. W.: A clinical study of amalgam failures, J. Dent. Res. **28:**439, 1949.
3. Nadel, R.: Amalgam restorations, cavity preparations, condensing, and finishing, J. Am. Dent. Assoc. **65:**66, 1962.
4. Black, G. V.: Operative dentistry, ed. 4, Chicago, 1920, Medico-Dental Publishing Co.
5. Markley, M. R.: Personal lectures.
6. Sturdevant, C. M., et al.: The art and science of operative dentistry, New York, 1968, The Blakiston Division, McGraw-Hill Book Co.
7. Phillips, R. W.: New concepts in materials used for restorative dentistry, J. Am. Dent. Assoc. **70:**652, 1965.
8. Dolven, R. C.: Micromeasurement of cavity lining, using ultraviolet and reflected light, and the effect of the liner on marginal penetration evaluated with Ca45, J. Dent. Res. **45:**12, 1966.
9. Phillips, R. W., Swartz, M. L., and Norman, R. D.: Materials for the practicing dentist, St. Louis, 1969, The C. V. Mosby Co.

CHAPTER 8

AMALGAM INSERTION AND FINISHING

After trituration amalgam is in a plastic condition, which can be forced under pressure into the details of a tooth preparation designed for it. Filling Class 1, 5, and 6 preparations is a fairly simple matter of placing small increments into the cavity and packing (condensing—Figs. 8-1 to 8-3) it against the cavity walls and into line angles and point angles.

The proximal portion of Class 2 and Class 3 amalgam preparations presents special problems when condensing amalgam. The amalgam will be forced into the interproximal area where there is no tooth remaining to confine the amalgam to the preparation (Fig. 8-4). With no wall present to confine the amalgam during condensation, porosity or voids will result at margins where good adaptation of amalgam is necessary for sealing the tooth against bacterial invasion and sensitivity caused by leakage. To provide a "wall" to contain the amalgam in such cases a matrix is used.

A matrix is a thin metal band that is placed in the interproximal area to help confine the amalgam to the preparation during condensation. It helps to shape the amalgam to the original contour of the tooth, and it serves as a wall against which amalgam can be properly condensed. There are many types of amalgam matrices. Three basic types will be discussed in the text to follow.

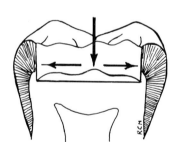

Fig. 8-1. Forces used to condense amalgam into a Class 1 cavity.

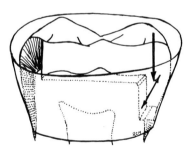

Fig. 8-2. Forces used to condense amalgam into a Class 2 cavity.

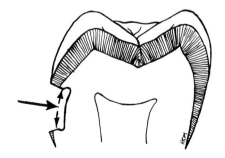

Fig. 8-3. Forces used to condense amalgam into a Class 5 cavity.

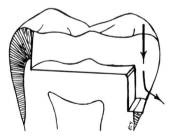

Fig. 8-4. Illustrates the necessity of a strong matrix against which to condense amalgam in the proximal portion of a Class 2 cavity.

Matrix types

TOFFLEMIRE MATRIX*

ARMAMENTARIUM

Tofflemire retainer
Universal Tofflemire band No. 1
Wedges
Explorer
Contouring pliers or burnisher

The Tofflemire matrix is probably the most popular matrix used for Class 2 restorations. It is easily and quickly applied and when properly placed, provides satisfactory proximal contour as well as adaptation to the prepared tooth.

The retainer (Fig. 8-5) has an adjustment knob that moves a sliding car to adjust the size of the band and tighten it to the tooth, a locking knob to hold the matrix band in the retainer, and a slotted guide. The universal matrix band (Fig. 8-6) is a boomerang-shaped strip of stainless steel (0.002 or 0.0015 inches thick). When approximated, the two ends produce a tear-shaped loop with one flared and one constricted opening (Fig. 8-7). The con-

---

*Getz Teledyne.

stricted opening will form the most gingival portion of the band, while the flared portion forms the occlusal portion of the matrix.

Procedure

1 The two ends of the matrix band are brought together (Fig. 8-7) and placed in the single slot of the sliding member.

2 The middle portion of the band is placed into one of the three slots (Fig. 8-8). Select one of the three slots at the end of the retainer to accommodate the direction the band should extend to surround the tooth. It is usually more convenient to put the band through a side slot so the matrix retainer, when applied and tightened, will be parallel to the dental arch with the adjusting knobs pointing anteriorly. This will also keep the retainer out of the way and help prevent dislodgment.

3 The small outer knob is tightened to lock the band into the retainer (Fig. 8-9).

4 Adjust the band to the approximate size of the tooth by turning the larger inner knob (Fig. 8-10).

5 The loop is expanded and rounded, with the handle of the beavertail burnisher or other instrument, tried on the tooth, and tightened to the approximate size noting the location of the proximal contact areas (Fig. 8-11).

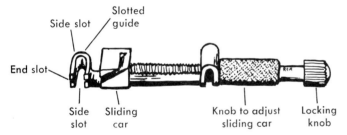

Fig. 8-5. Tofflemire matrix retainer.

Side slot
Slotted guide
End slot
Side slot
Sliding car
Knob to adjust sliding car
Locking knob

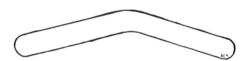

Fig. 8-6. Matrix band.

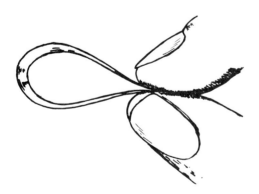

Fig. 8-7. Matrix band ends held together prior to insertion into the matrix retainer.

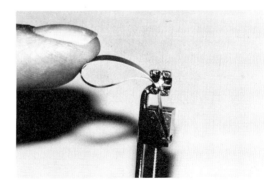

Fig. 8-8. Loop of matrix is placed through one of the slotted guides at the end of the retainer.

6 The proximal contact areas are marked so proximal contour can be shaped. The band and retainer are removed, and with the burnisher over two or three layers of squeeze cloth the proximal area is expanded out, forming a slight convexity at the proximal contact (Fig. 8-12).

7 The band is placed back on the tooth and tightened. Make sure the band extends beyond the gingival margin and that it makes contact with the adjacent tooth. If the band is too tight:

   a. Gingival enamel may fracture.
   b. Proximal contact may be open.
   c. Contact area may be high.
   d. Proximal contour may be flat.
   e. Tooth may be deformed.

A burnisher or an amalgam condenser may be used to enhance the proximal contact by forcing it against the adjacent tooth.

8 A wedge may be necessary to adapt the matrix band at the gingival margin (Fig. 8-13) and also to separate the teeth slightly to compensate for matrix band thickness. The wedge is inserted from either the buccal or lingual embrasure, depending on which area requires the greatest closure. Inserting the wedge into the largest embrasure (usually the lingual) often provides optimum adaptation of the band.

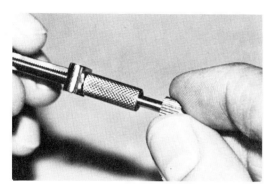

Fig. 8-9. Small outer knob is tightened to lock the matrix band into sliding car of retainer.

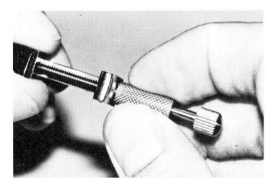

Fig. 8-10. Large inner knob is used to adjust size of the matrix loop.

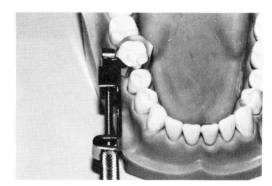

Fig. 8-11. Matrix band and retainer are fitted around prepared tooth.

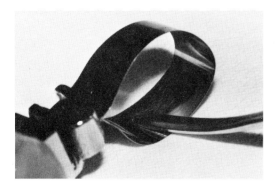

Fig. 8-12. Contouring band in the proximal contact area using a burnisher.

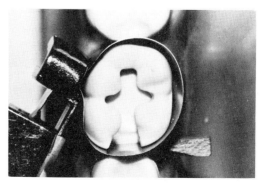

Fig. 8-13. Wedge can be used to adapt the matrix band at the gingival margin.

9 Cotton pliers or serrated pliers may be used for handling the wedge, and an amalgam condenser can be used for seating the wedge.

Make sure the wedge is apical to the gingival margin of the preparation. If it is placed coronal to the gingival margin, the proximal contour of the restoration will be severely indented, and excess amalgam may be forced out at the gingival margin.

Check the preparation to make sure the gingival margin is sealed and the matrix band is stable. If loose enamel rods are present at the cavosurface margin, remove them with a G-3 explorer or scrape with a gingival margin trimmer or other suitable instrument.

Buccal and lingual proximal margins do not need to be sealed as tight as the gingival margins since these areas can be easily carved.

Clean the preparation with an air syringe and an explorer. The preparation is now ready for amalgam insertion.

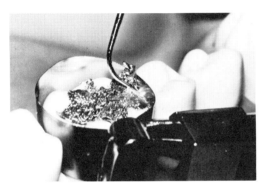

Fig. 8-14. Explorer being used to relieve flashing of amalgam at marginal ridge.

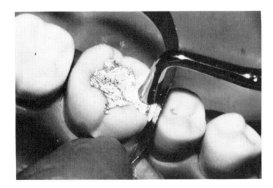

Fig. 8-15. Large condenser is used to support the amalgam in the proximal contact area when removing matrix band.

10 After the amalgam is condensed, relieve the flashing of amalgam at the marginal ridge(s) to minimize the possibility of proximal amalgam fracturing when removing the matrix band (Fig. 8-14).

11 Loosen the gnurled knobs and remove the matrix holder from the band.

12 Remove the wedge and while supporting the amalgam occlusal to the contact area with a large condenser, grasp and remove the band with a hemostat or serrated pliers (Fig. 8-15).

Precautions

1 Make sure the open end of the slot of the retainer faces the gingival tissue. This is necessary for easier application and removal of the retainer and band.

2 If the wedge is above the gingival cavosurface margin, it may indent the band causing faulty proximal contour.

If the wedge cannot be placed below the margin, then leave the wedge out and tighten the band. Make sure to check and carve the gingival margin to remove overhanging amalgam.

3 Use fresh bands to aid in placement and removal and to create smooth contours.

CUSTOM AMALGAM MATRIX

ARMAMENTARIUM

Explorer
Scissors
Stainless steel matrix material
Greenstick compound
F-2 burnisher
Serrated amalgam condenser
Wood wedges
Ivory No. 1 matrix retainer (Fig. 8-16)
Bunsen burner or alcohol flame

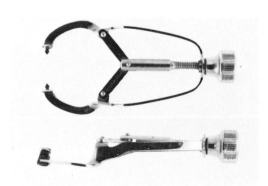

Fig. 8-16. Ivory No. 1 matrix retainer.

The custom amalgam matrix is superior for condensing amalgam in teeth where it is difficult to adapt a Tofflemire matrix (that is, barrel-shaped teeth, cusp reduction). In two-surface Class 2 amalgam restorations the custom matrix has the advantage of not requiring compensation for two thicknesses of matrix material in the proximal contact areas, whereas additional care must be taken to assure tight proximal contacts when a circumferential matrix (Tofflemire or T-Band) is used. It provides excellent adaptation to the tooth contours. The retention is not dependent on the tension on the band, but instead the band is held in place by greenstick compound and stabilized with the Ivory No. 1 matrix retainer. Since there is no tension on the stainless steel band, there is less tendency to flatten the contoured proximal area of the band.

Procedure

1 About ¹/₂ inch length of 0.0015-inch stainless steel matrix material is cut from the spool and trimmed into a "kidney" shape with a crown and bridge scissors (Fig. 8-17). The narrowest dimension is adjusted to approximately the occlusal height of the tooth. The band must not extend more than 1 to 2 mm. above the marginal ridge; otherwise, the amalgam condenser tip may be prevented from reaching the gingival floor. If it is too short, it will be difficult to properly condense the amalgam to the height of the marginal ridge because there will be no support for the soft amalgam (Fig. 8-18).

2 The longest dimension of the band must extend 2 to 3 mm. beyond the buccal and lingual walls of the proximal box. This provides enough material to seal the margins but not so much material as to prevent or hinder the greenstick compound from being applied.

3 The band is now shaped to restore the proximal contour using the F-2 beavertail burnisher (Fig. 8-19). The kidney-shaped matrix material is placed on a couple thicknesses of squeeze cloth or paper towel and burnished in the area where the proximal surface of the tooth is to be restored. This action expands the band in the contact area and also causes the band to curl.

4 The band is returned to the tooth to check for proximal contour and contact (Fig. 8-20).

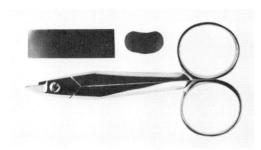

Fig. 8-17. Matrix material and crown shears used to form a kidney-shaped matrix.

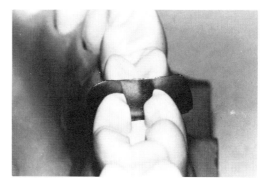

Fig. 8-18. Proper occlusal height for the matrix.

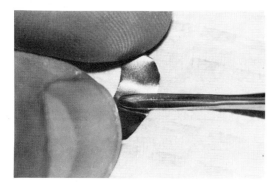

Fig. 8-19. Contouring the matrix.

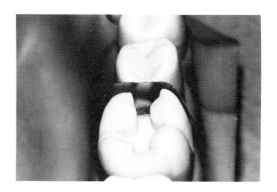

Fig. 8-20. Check the matrix adaptation.

5 The wood wedge is selected and inserted into the largest proximal embrasure using the cotton pliers and amalgam condenser. The position of the wedge is checked from both proximal and occlusal directions to make sure it is located below the gingival margin and that the middle two thirds of the margin is tightly sealed and adapted (Fig. 8-21). Do not wedge the matrix if the gingival margin of the preparation is too extended to allow the wedge to rest apical to the gingival floor. Instead, look at the degree of matrix adaptation and remember to carefully carve away any excess amalgam.

6 Next the matrix band is reinforced with greenstick compound. Small cones of compound can be prepared beforehand (Fig. 8-22). Two of these are warmed on the flat side until shiny; one is stuck to the thumb and the other to the index finger so they may be applied to the tooth simultaneously. The pointed end is then warmed lightly to soften the compound (it should be heated only enough to soften the outer layer of the cone), leav-

ing a harder inner core to act as a plunger (Fig. 8-23). The compound is now applied to the buccal and lingual embrasure areas, adapting the matrix band to the tooth and sealing the proximal margins (Fig. 8-24).

7 The compound is allowed to cool and harden slightly before stabilizing it with the Ivory matrix retainer.

8 Open the jaws of the retainer wide enough to fit over the compound. The jaws are lightly warmed in a Bunsen burner so that when they (Fig. 8-25) are closed the jaws will slightly penetrate into the compound. The body of the retainer is allowed to rest on the anterior teeth. Once the compound has cooled and hardened, tighten the retainer a few more turns to make sure the matrix is well adapted and stable (Fig. 8-26).

9 A sharp instrument may be used to remove excess compound, particularly material occlusal to the band.

10 A warm instrument may be used to readapt or contour the internal portion of the matrix band.

11 Check and remove any loose enamel prisms on the cavosurface margins. Clean and dry the preparation before inserting the amalgam.

12 After condensation the matrix is removed. First carve the amalgam at the marginal ridge (Fig. 8-27). Loosen the knob on the Ivory matrix retainer, which will open the jaws, and remove the retainer from the mouth. The compound is removed carefully with an instrument, chisel, or hoe. The wedge is removed with cotton pliers or serrated pliers (Fig. 8-28). The matrix band is carefully removed to the buccal or lingual side (Fig. 8-29) while holding the amalgam with a condenser so as not to fracture the marginal ridge.

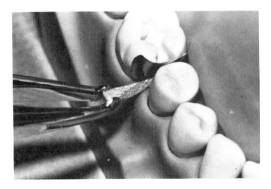

Fig. 8-21. Placement of the wood wedge.

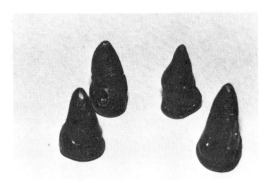

Fig. 8-22. Green compound cones.

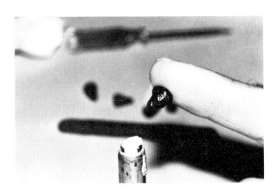

Fig. 8-23. Top of the compound cone heated.

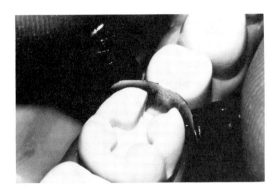

Fig. 8-24. Compound forced in place.

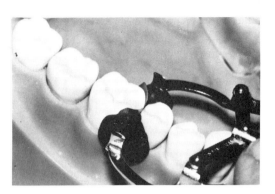

Fig. 8-25. Retainer in place.

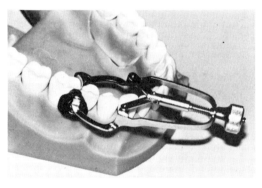

Fig. 8-26. Retainer in place and resting on anterior teeth.

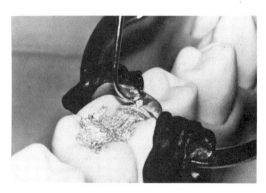

Fig. 8-27. Carve away excess amalgam over the enamel ridge.

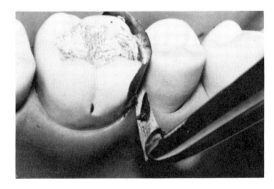

Fig. 8-28. Remove the wood wedge.

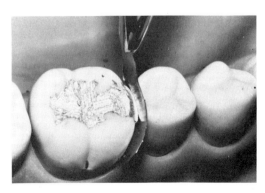

Fig. 8-29. Slide the matrix bucally or lingually.

T-BAND MATRIX

A T-Band is a curved brass strip approximately 2 inches long and ¹/₄ inch wide (Fig. 8-30). At one end there are two wings that give this matrix its characteristic T shape. The T-Band matrix has the advantage of surrounding a prepared cavity without having an interfering seam (such as the Tofflemire matrix does at the point of attachment to the retainer) that may make condensation difficult.

The T-Band does not gain support by tension in the band. Therefore it can be contoured more closely to the desired tooth shape. This allows better condensation because of less bulk of amalgam, and the preparation also takes less amalgam to fill. If the preparation involves all the cusps and extends far below tissue, it is easier to place and support the T-Band matrix than a Tofflemire matrix.

Application procedure

1 The T-Band fits like a belt around the tooth. The buckle being the T portion of the band.

2 The band is curved to allow for the gingival convergence of the tooth when the T-Band is made into a loop. The constricted opening fits closest to the gingiva.

3 Form the band into a loop with the T portion inside. Fold the wings over the other end of the band securely so the band will hold its circular shape and form a sliding joint. A loop is thus formed, which may be varied in diameter by pulling the free end.

4 Try the band on the tooth and adjust the size to closely fit the cervical portion of the tooth (Fig. 8-31).

5 Fold the free end back on itself at the sliding joint (Fig. 8-32) and trim off the excess, leaving

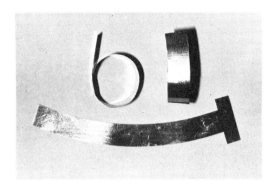

Fig. 8-30. T-Band matrix.

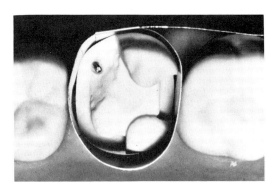

Fig. 8-31. Try the loop over the tooth.

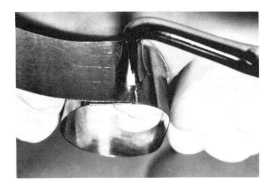

Fig. 8-32. Fold the free end at the sliding joint.

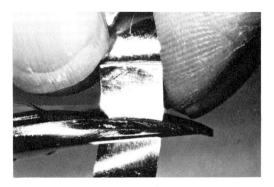

Fig. 8-33. Cut off the excess material leaving approximately ¹/₄ inch of band material.

approximately $1/4$ inch (Fig. 8-33). This will maintain the band diameter and prevent it from expanding.

6 Remove the band from the tooth and if necessary trim the gingival portion to follow the contour of the gingiva. Contour the contact areas with a burnisher on a compressible surface (several thicknesses of squeeze cloth [Fig. 8-34]).

7 Replace the band on the tooth; check gingival contour and adaptation, and check that contact is present in the proximal portions.

8 If necessary, a crimp or tuck may be made to more closely contour the band in the occlusal areas.

9 Wedge the interproximal areas when possible to compensate for matrix band thickness and to help prevent amalgam from being forced out at the gingival margins (Fig. 8-35).

10 The T-Band may be reinforced by compound bars across the buccal and lingual surfaces. The compound enhances the stability of the matrix and allows better condensation of amalgam.

11 After the compound bars are placed, attach the Ivory No. 1 matrix retainer to stabilize the compound and matrix (Fig. 8-36).

12 Check the gingival areas for adaptation and remove any debris from the preparation with an explorer and air before filling.

13 When condensation is completed, remove the retainer and compound and loosen the band. Grasp each end of the band, and while supporting the amalgam with the condenser at the marginal ridge, gently pull it through the proximal contacts (Fig. 8-37).

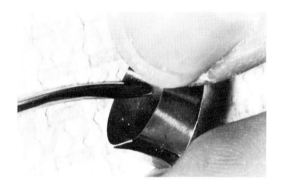

Fig. 8-34. Burnish the matrix to contour.

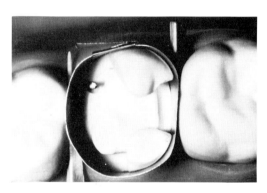

Fig. 8-35. Matrix in place supported by wedges.

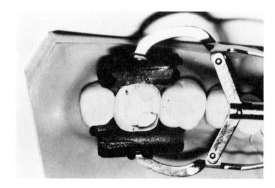

Fig. 8-36. Ivory No. 1 matrix retainer in place to stabilize the compound and matrix.

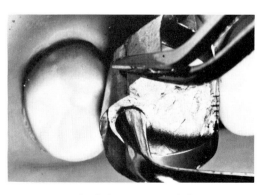

Fig. 8-37. Removal of the matrix while supporting the amalgam.

Insertion of amalgam
CLASS 2 AMALGAM RESTORATIONS
Insertion

ARMAMENTARIUM

Matrix retainer and band
Condensers
Wedges
Contouring pliers (or egg burnisher)

1 Select a matrix band of proper width and place it in the retainer.

2 It is often desirable to slightly contour the band using contouring pliers (Fig. 8-38) or by burnishing with an egg burnisher (Fig. 8-39) or contouring pliers. Care must be taken to establish contour in harmony with the tooth being restored, with particular care being paid to the contact area.

3 Place the matrix on the tooth (Fig. 8-40). Be certain the edge of the band is placed gingival to the gingival cavosurface angle. Care in preparation and placement of the matrix is far more important than having it tight. Screwing a band tightly around the tooth does not mean an overhang will be prevented or desired contour will be created.

4 Place a wood wedge between the teeth (Figs. 8-40 and 8-41). Be certain the wedge is supported by both teeth and *not* occlusal to the gingival cavosurface margin.

5 Compound may be used to support the matrix and wedge.

COMMENT: *Placement of compound is particularly desirable for "barrel-shaped" or highly contoured teeth. The most common cause of overhanging restorations is lack of care in wedging and fixation of the matrix. Particular care must be taken to observe the adaptation of the matrix to the gingival cavosurface margin. If any space exists between the band and the tooth in a proximal concavity at the gingival cavosurface margin, particular care must be taken to remove the excess amalgam immediately after the matrix is removed.*

6 Mix the amalgam using the method of choice. Avoid moisture contamination such as mulling in the palm of the hand.

7 Using an amalgam carrier, inject a load of the mix into the proximal portion of the cavity and condense to the gingival floor (Fig. 8-42).

8 Using a diamond or triangle end condenser, condense the amalgam to the gingival wall. The mix must be condensed laterally into the retentive undercuts (Fig. 8-43) and against the proximal cavosurface margins, rotating the condenser appropriately to fit into these angles or corners.

9 Use a larger condenser as the occlusal surface is approached (Fig. 8-44).

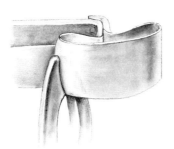

Fig. 8-38. Contouring matrix using contouring pliers.

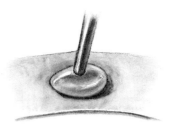

Fig. 8-39. Contouring matrix by burnishing.

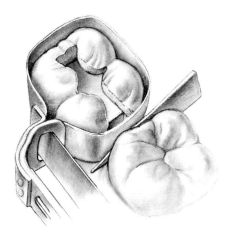

Fig. 8-40. Matrix in place supported by wedge.

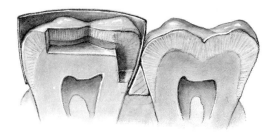

Fig. 8-41. Cross section of matrix supported by wedge.

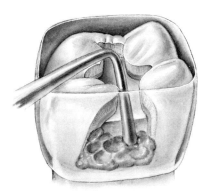

Fig. 8-42. Initial condensation.

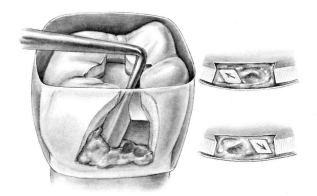

Fig. 8-43. Condensation into angles.

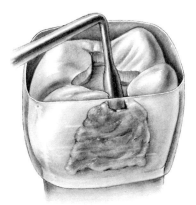

Fig. 8-44. Larger condenser point for occlusal area.

10 Place successive masses of amalgam in the cavity and condense as appropriate. When the proximal portion of the cavity is filled, a small round condenser is used to condense into the prepared grooves (Figs. 8-45 and 8-46) and angles on the occlusal surface. Lateral as well as apical force must be used to assure maximum condensation. Final condensation is made with a large condenser.

11 For final condensation use a large condenser (Fig. 8-47).

COMMENT: *Considerable force must be used to condense amalgam even when mechanical condensers are used. As the buildup is accomplished, excess mercury should be expelled from the amalgam. This mercury-rich material should be scraped free and eliminated as the cavity is filled. The condenser must be stepped, each particle of amalgam being condensed forcibly in place. If the restoration is fairly large, it is advisable to use more than one mix since proper mixing, manipulation, and condensation time should not exceed three minutes.*

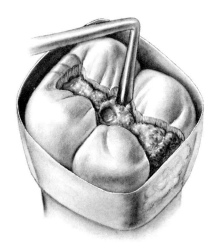

Fig. 8-45. Smaller condenser point to reach groove ends.

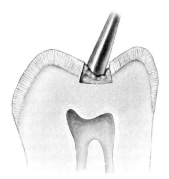

Fig. 8-46. Cross section, large condenser point.

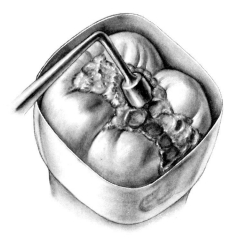

Fig. 8-47. Large condenser for final condensation.

Carving

ARMAMENTARIUM

Sharpened double-end explorer (sickle and contra-angle)
Double-end carver (cleoid and discoid)
Cotton pliers
Cotton

Amalgam should be carved when it has begun its initial set.

1 Before removing the matrix band use a sharpened sickle explorer to remove the excess amalgam over the marginal ridge area (Fig. 8-48).

2 With the discoid and cleoid roughly carve the occlusal anatomy (Figs. 8-49 to 8-51). Quickly remove the excess with a large discoid, starting at the distal margin and allowing it to reach both buccal and lingual margins (Fig. 8-50).

3 Loosen the matrix retainer. Support the amalgam above the proximal contact with a large condenser and remove the matrix laterally toward the lingual (or buccal) margin. Avoid removing it occlusally because it may fracture the amalgam.

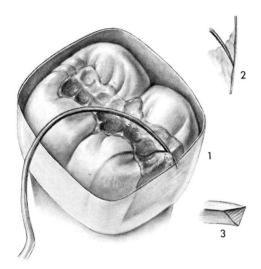

Fig. 8-48. Sharpened explorer used as carver to remove excess over marginal ridge.

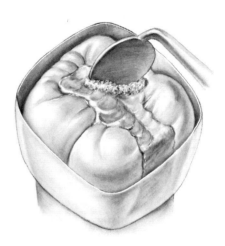

Fig. 8-49. Large discoid carver to remove surface excess.

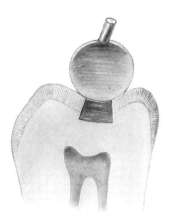

Fig. 8-50. Cross section, large discoid carver reaches buccal and lingual margins.

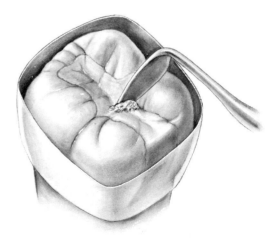

Fig. 8-51. Cleoid carver used to carve anatomy.

4 Immediately remove excess amalgam from the gingival margin, using a sharpened explorer (Fig. 8-52). The finished amalgam must be precisely flush with the tooth surface. The sickle explorer illustrated has been sharpened on three sides so that it will cut rather than burnish.*

5 Carve the proximal areas to contour with a sharpened sickle explorer (Fig. 8-53).

6 Finish carving the occlusal surface.

COMMENT: *While carving amalgam, it is helpful to allow the carving instrument to rest partially on tooth structure and carve from the margins toward the amalgam. Grooves established on the occlusal surface should restore proper anatomy to provide proper occlusion but must not be exaggerated. They should be quite definite but smooth enough to clean easily. All carving instruments must be kept sharp so that they will cut cleanly.*

7 Remove the rubber dam and check the occlusion by assisting the patient to very carefully close. Occlusion is checked with typewriter ribbon (or carbon paper if preferred) and corrected by further carving.

8 Carefully rub the occlusal surface occasionally with cotton to smooth it during final carving. A little time spent at this point will greatly reduce the amount of time required to finish and polish the restoration.

---

*Evidence of the possible desirability of burnishing amalgam should be considered. Before it is accepted a great deal of information regarding this concept is needed, such as technique, percentage of residual mercury in the burnished area, and clinical results.[1,2]

CLASS 3 AMALGAM RESTORATIONS
Insertion and carving

Insertion of the amalgam in prepared Class 3 cavities is very similar to that of Class 2 procedures using a narrow bicuspid band. Insertion may be facilitated if the incisal third of the band is trimmed away with a crown shears. The majority of the carving is done before the band is slipped out labially.

CLASS 5 AMALGAM RESTORATIONS
Insertion and carving

ARMAMENTARIUM

Amalgam carrier
Condensers
Sharpened sickle explorer

1 Inject a mass of amalgam into the cavity.

2 Condense with appropriate condensers. First condense toward the distal margin, then the mesial margin, next the gingival margin, and finally toward the occlusal margin, being sure all angles are condensed. Step the condenser point along each margin and eliminate excess mercury-rich amalgam.

3 Build the amalgam up until it is slightly overcontoured and is condensed over all margins.

4 With a sharpened sickle explorer establish the desired contour. Always rest a part of the carving instrument on tooth structure to prevent overcarving along margins.

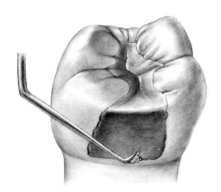

Fig. 8-52. Explorer used to remove gingival excess.

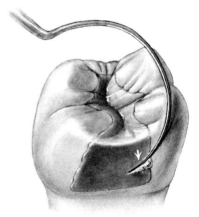

Fig. 8-53. Explorer used to remove excess from proximal margin.

Polishing amalgam restorations

Just as all surfaces of the teeth should be highly polished, so should all restorations. A highly finished amalgam restoration with properly polished margins will resist tarnish and corrosion, will be easier for the patient to clean, and does not contribute to recurrence of caries.

CLASS 1 AND CLASS 2 AMALGAM RESTORATIONS

ARMAMENTARIUM

High-speed handpiece	Bristle brush
Contra-angle	Rubber cup
Inverted cone stone	Flour of pumice
Finger stone	Tin oxide
Rubber abrasive points	High-speed finishing burs
Abrasive disks	

Amalgam must be allowed to set for at least twenty-four hours before the following steps are undertaken. It cannot be overemphasized that the most important factor in easily producing beautiful, highly finished amalgam restorations is proper and adequate carving and smoothing at the time the amalgam is placed.

1 Use the cleoid and discoid carver to smooth all carved anatomy.

2 Using a finishing bur of appropriate shape, lightly smooth the entire occlusal surface amalgam (Fig. 8-54).

COMMENT: *In the use of any polishing instrument and materials it is recommended that the polishing instrument be kept in motion to avoid establishing low spots, pits, undesirable grooves, or flat spots. Finishing burs should be run at a stall-out speed and kept moving in a brushlike motion while they are applied to the surface of the amalgam. The same principle applies to abrasive disks and rubber cups.*

Stones should be avoided on the surface of a tooth. It is sometimes easy, especially with a rough or unbalanced stone, to "pound" the enamel, thereby loosening some prisms and spoiling a margin.

3 Use a $^3/_8$-inch abrasive disk to smooth the proximal areas, taking care not to "ditch" the amalgam (Fig. 8-55).

4 Check the gingival margin for possible roughness. (Files and knives may be used to plane this area, but if properly placed and carved in the beginning, it is usually better not to risk roughening this area with instruments.)

5 A shaped rubber abrasive point may be used to polish occlusal anatomy (Fig. 8-56). Air and water cooling is in order to prevent overheating.

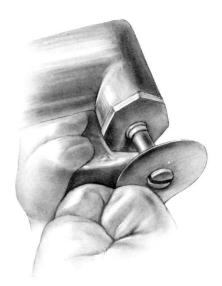

Fig. 8-55. Disking proximal area.

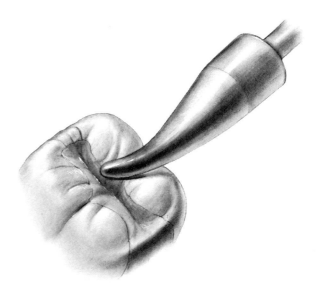

Fig. 8-56. Rubber point used to smooth surface.

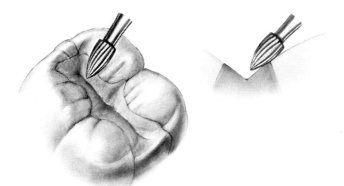

Fig. 8-54. Large twelve-blade finishing bur used to smooth surface.

6 With a brush, polish the entire surface with a wet mix of flour of pumice (Fig. 8-57).

7 Polish the entire surface with a rubber cup using flour of pumice (Fig. 8-58).

COMMENT: *This step can be accomplished most ideally with a comparatively soft small flexible rubber cup. Hard rubber cups are more likely to generate heat and do not adapt easily to the contour of the tooth. Again, slow speeds are essential to avoid generating heat.*

8 To establish the highest polish (Fig. 8-59) dry the restoration and with a rubber cup apply dry tin oxide (many commercial products are available), using slow speed and light pressure.

ADJUNCTS TO FINISHING

Some operators prefer to use various rubber finishing burs different grades, sizes, and shapes. Extreme caution must be exercised with these rubber items to prevent heat generation, which is not only painful but may permanently damage the pulp and also damage the strength of the amalgam.

CLASS 5 AMALGAM RESTORATIONS

It is not essential to place a rubber dam for this procedure, but without it care must be exercised not to injure the gingiva, and difficulty may be encountered in reaching the gingival margin.

1 Smooth the surface with a ³/₈-inch extra fine garnet disk. When using disks, keep them in constant motion and use light pressure and slow speed.

2 Smooth with an extra fine sand disk.

3 Polish with a rubber cup using flour of pumice.

4 Polish is completed with tin oxide.

COMMENT: *When finishing any Class 5 restoration, extreme care must be exercised not to ditch the tooth gingival to the restored area. Utmost care must also be used to establish and preserve proper contour.*

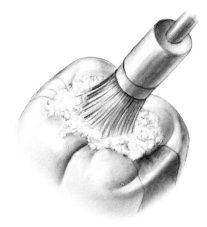

Fig. 8-57. Pumice and brush used to polish grooves.

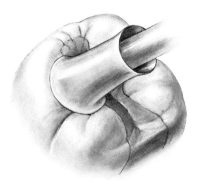

Fig. 8-58. A rubber cup is used for final pumice finish and high shine.

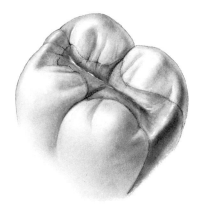

Fig. 8-59. Completed restoration.

Guidelines for carving large amalgam restorations

In practice dentists are often confronted with the necessity of restoring function to extensively broken down posterior teeth. When cusps are missing and surrounding tooth structure is scarce, the ideal restorative material is usually a gold casting. However, when the patient is unable to afford the higher cost of a crown or an inlay, only one other choice for treatment is left—amalgam. Composite resins could be used to restore grossly involved teeth, but the response of the soft tissue around these restorations has not been favorable. Composite resins readily leak after a short period of use, and they do not maintain adequate occlusion because of occlusal wear. If the cavity preparation for such teeth is properly designed and sufficient, retention is provided; amalgam, even though a brittle material, will serve the patient for many years.

Carving a large amalgam restoration to proper form and function is not easy but can be facilitated by careful observation of certain details before beginning, during, and after cavity preparation. Before discussing these details, the objectives of carving amalgam will be reviewed.

1. *Restore normal arch form and occlusion.* Carving amalgam to normal occlusion must often be done by estimating the original position and length of cusps, fossa location, and depth of grooves. The opposing dentition is often obscured by the presence of a rubber dam and cannot be brought into close approximation to the tooth being restored until the rubber dam is removed. The rubber dam is not removed at this time, however, since good access and visibility are needed to properly carve the restoration (particularly the interproximal areas). In spite of this, it is important to carve the restoration so that it is neither too long nor too short. If too long, the restoration will not allow the opposing teeth to occlude properly; if too short, there may be supereruption of the opposing dentition causing interfering contacts and loss of arch integrity. Clinically, the tooth is carved as nearly as possible to the estimated height and shape, the rubber dam is then removed, and any minor adjustments for occlusion are done.

2. *Restore normal proximal contact and embrasure form.* To minimize chances of food impaction and drifting, every effort should be made to provide a solid proximal contact area. The dimensions and precise location of the proximal contact varies somewhat throughout the mouth depending on tooth size, shape, and position. In general, the contact area is oval in shape, approximately 1.5 mm. long buccolingually and 1 mm. high occlusogingivally, and located between the middle and buccal thirds of the crown buccolingually (Figs. 8-60 and 8-61).

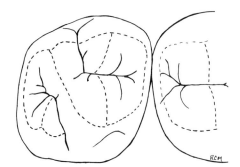

Fig. 8-60. Occlusal view of maxillary molars showing proper embrasure form and location of proximal contact area.

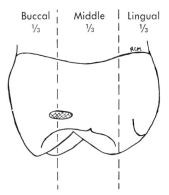

Fig. 8-61. Proper location of proximal contact area.

Care must be used to provide adequate room for the interproximal papilla by carving the gingival embrasure so it blends into the root form. The gingival embrasure may actually have a slight concavity (Fig. 8-62) or negative contour apical to the contact area owing to the presence of flutings or furcations on the root surface.

The buccal and lingual embrasures emante from the proximal contact; the lingual embrasure is usually the largest. Too small an embrasure form leaves a rather broad contact with a stagnant area adjacent to the gingiva that tends to collect plaque and food debris. The occlusal embrasure forms one side of the marginal ridge; the other wall emanates from the adjacent occlusal pit. The occlusal embrasure is rounded in such a way as to eliminate a potentially weak ridge of amalgam above the contact (Fig. 8-63). It is often difficult to thread floss through a contact such as this (Fig. 8-63). It usually shreds the floss beyond usefulness.

3. *Restore proper axial contours.* Axial contours should be smooth without excess bulges. In general, the height of contour of the buccal cusps is near tissue level. The lingual height of contour is near the middle third of the tooth. Axial contours should smoothly blend into the remaining tooth structure and approximate normal tooth shape. Care must be taken to avoid bulky axial contours. Overcontoured axial areas will trap plaque, and gingival inflamation will result.

4. *Reestablish basic occlusal anatomy.* It is important to simulate normal tooth anatomy on the occlusal surface. If cusps and grooves are left flat, increased occlusal forces will be required to adequately break up food. The patient may also have problems because definitive centric contact is lacking. Restore occlusal anatomy to follow remaining triangular ridges, cusp ridges, supplemental grooves, and so forth. Avoid making too many supplemental ridges and grooves (chicken scratches). These weaken the surface amalgam, are difficult to polish, and consequently trap plaque. Proper occlusal anatomy should be neither deep nor shallow. If deep, thin amalgam margins may result; if shallow, occlusion may be high. Heavy occlusal forces may result in tooth sensitivity or fracture of the restoration. It is relatively easy to finish a restoration that has smooth flowing anatomy. Allow one strong triangular ridge per cusp delineated by one supplemental groove on each side, one central groove, one buccolingual groove, a central pit (if a molar), mesial and distal

pits, and full rounded marginal ridge with one spillway into the largest embrasure. Marginal ridges should be carved to the same height as those of the adjacent teeth to maintain proper dental arch form. Likewise, cusp height should follow the normal curve of the arch and be positioned to avoid excursive interferences with opposing dentition. Avoid carving mesial or distal pits too deep. This will present a potential fracture site near the axiopulpal line angle (Fig. 8-64). If mesial and distal pits are carved too close to the marginal ridge, the marginal ridge will be weakened and may fracture.

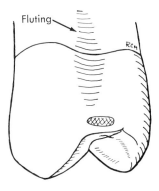

Fig. 8-62. Concavity or fluting gingival to the contact area of a maxillary premolar.

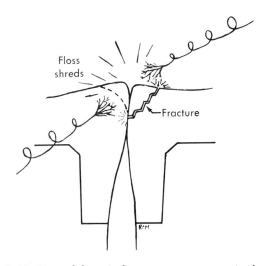

Fig. 8-63. Dotted line indicates proper marginal ridge contour. Excessive contact area and sharp marginal ridges may fracture easily and/or make introduction of floss difficult.

5. *Remove all excess amalgam (flashings) from beyond the cavosurface margins.* The amalgam should blend smoothly into remaining tooth structure. A rough or irregular finish of amalgam margins leaves areas for plaque accumulation that may lead to secondary decay and restoration failure. Excess amalgam in areas adjacent to soft tissue (overhangs) will cause tissue irritation and resultant bone loss.

6. *Extend amalgam up to the margins without voids or deficiencies.* These deficiencies or submarginal areas will accumulate plaque causing secondary decay and failure. Shallow submarginal areas can be eliminated by enamoplasty during polishing, provided that the defect does not extend to more than one third of the thickness of the enamel in that area. Deeper defects necessitate complete removal of the amalgam and reinsertion of a new mix. (Once amalgam has reached its initial set, it is not possible to add to it, even with a fresh mix. Layering or a weak bond often results between the two layers, which will eventually fracture off.) If an attempt is made to plasty the enamel around a deep deficiency, chances of tooth sensitivity, exposing dentin, producing an easy inroad for future decay, and disrupting the patient's occlusion may be increased.

There are certain observations that can be made prior to cavity preparation to aid in reestablishing the proper occlusion and tooth form when restoring a tooth with a large amalgam restoration.

1. *Make a set of study models.* These serve as a very helpful guide; however, they must be made before treatment. Stone casts of the patient's dentition will show the original shape of the teeth, the opposing teeth, and the centric occlusion of the patient's dentition. These features can be related back to carving the restoration.

2. *Examine the patient's occlusion before preparation.* Note any supereruption of the opposing dentition into the area to be restored. This should be corrected by reducing the opposing cusps and reshaping them according to the guidelines for occlusal adjustment. Note the height and position of the opposing teeth so that the occlusion can be carved to avoid interferences in lateral excursions.

3. *Look at the same tooth on the opposite side of the arch.* This tooth may give some valuable clues as to tooth shape.

4. *Note the relationship of cusps and axial contours to the adjacent teeth.* A mental note of the relative cusp height and groove depths will serve as a useful guide to reestablishing the proper occlusion while the rubber dam is still in place. Actually measuring the relative cusp heights by placing the handle of an instrument across the cusp tips mesiodistally and noting the relative heights will also be helpful.

The following is a list of aids that can be used after the preparation is cut:

1. Knowledge of normal tooth morphology, dental arch form, and function
2. Remaining cusp tips (Knowing the position of one or two cusps greatly facilitates location of those that are missing by visualizing normal tooth morphology superimposed on it.)
3. Remaining axial contours (If these are followed using relatively straight carving instruments, such as the D-3 Hollenback, and the amalgam is made to blend into the existing axial contours, the boundaries of the occlusal table can be established.)
4. Location of all preparation margins by removing gross excess as soon as matrix is removed (This would also include eliminating gingival excess and carving embrasures. By removing the gross excess amalgam, the boundaries of the preparation can be seen.)
5. Lightly scribing the position of the grooves on the surface of the amalgam before beginning any definitive carving (This gives a good idea of the layout and proportions of the occlusal anatomy and prevents carving pits or grooves midway between opposing walls of the preparation to minimize thin amalgam margins.)

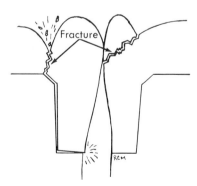

Fig. 8-64. Anatomy carved too deep resulting in potential fracture.

6. Carving parallel to the margins of the preparation to minimize chances of producing submarginal areas

7. Establishing the general planes of cusps where no tooth structure remains to serve as a guide (Triangular ridges should be most prominent and lead from the central groove to the cusp tip. Avoid making triangular ridges too steep; otherwise the occlusal surface will have deep anatomy and cusps and margins will be weak.)

8. Location of the marginal ridge height at the same level as the adjacent teeth, except where the adjacent tooth is grossly out of alignment and/or is to be restored in the near future

9. Establishment of developmental grooves and pits last (These are carved to follow cusp form. Avoid making pits too close to the marginal ridge since this will weaken this area and may result in later fracture.)

10. At least 2 mm. of amalgam overlaying cusps that are to be covered (If cusps have been reduced because of undermined enamel, be sure to reduce them sufficiently to allow a minimum of 2 mm. of amalgam to cover them. If insufficient reduction was made, this cusp will be too high when adequate thickness of amalgam is added. The resultant occlusion will be high, or if this amalgam is reduced, insufficient bulk will remain to have a strong restoration.)

11. Making all preparation margins definite and as close to a 90 degree angle at the cavosurface as possible (This will allow easier location of the margins as well as minimizing thin weak amalgam or enamel margins.)

12. Cavity instrumentation
    a. Carve embrasure form and eliminate proximal overhangs with amalgam knife working toward the contact area from the buccal, gingival, lingual, and occlusal surfaces (Figs. 8-65 and 8-66), or use sharpened shepherd crook explorer to carve these areas (Figs. 8-67 and 8-68).
    b. Use a carving instrument that closely approximates the shape of the surface to be carved. If the surface is fairly flat, that is, axial contours and some occlusal areas, use a Hollenback carver or the back of an amalgam knife (Fig. 8-69).
    c. The discoid-cleoid can be used to carve curved areas of the occlusal surface such as grooves and pits. A Hollenback carver can sometimes be used if it is aligned parallel to the ridges and grooves (Fig. 8-70).
    d. Always use sharp carving instruments. A dull instrument will require excess pressure to carve amalgam adequately. Oftentimes this excess pressure is all that is necessary to fracture the freshly inserted amalgam.

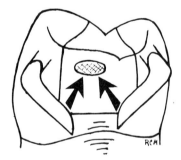

Fig. 8-65. Amalgam knife used to carve embrasure area.

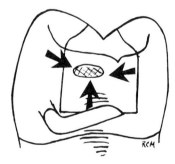

Fig. 8-66. Amalgam knife used to carve embrasure area to conform to tooth surface.

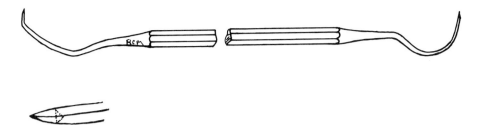

Fig. 8-67. Sharpened explorer (formed like a scaler) to carve proximal margins.

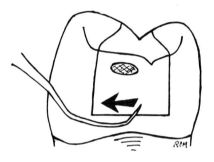

Fig. 8-68. Sharpened explorer to carve gingival margin.

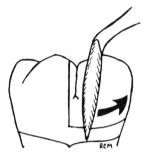

Fig. 8-69. Hollenback carver.

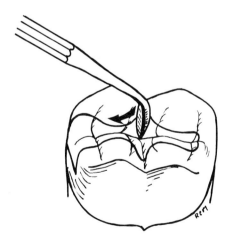

Fig. 8-70. Cleoid carver.

REFERENCES

1. Kanai, S.: Structure studies of amalgam. II. Effect of burnishing on the margins of occlusal amalgam fillings, Acta Odont. Scand. **24:**47, 1966.
2. Kato, S., Okuse, K., and Fusagama, T.: The effect of burnishing on the marginal seal of amalgam restorations, J. Prosthet Dent. **19:**393, 1968.

CHAPTER 9

PINS

Uses of pins in restorative dentistry

Many techniques are currently available that enable dentists to restore extensively destroyed teeth, even to the extreme of the entirely missing clinical crown. It has been customary to resort to endodontic therapy and the use of posts or dowels to stabilize a crown to the remaining root. Other procedures now seem desirable for many cases or can be used in conjunction with an endopost.

It is difficult to generalize about the uses of pins since so many variables are encountered, not only from one patient to another but from one tooth to another in the same mouth. Intermaxillary stress, age of the patient, length of the crown, tooth morphology, and pulp size are only a few of the factors that must be considered. Also, a great deal of research is indicated on the uses of pins. Current concepts of their uses are based largely on clinical or empirical experience, clinical judgment being the final factor in determining how and where they should be placed.

A *pin*, as used in restorative dentistry, is an extension of a restoration into a prepared hole, or a metal rod secured in a hole drilled in the dentin for the purpose of retaining a restoration in or on the tooth.

Types of pins

Many types and sizes of pins are currently available for restorative procedures. They can be classified into the following general outline:
1. Nonparallel pin techniques
   a. Cemented pins
   b. Friction-retained pins
   c. Self-threading pins (not cemented)
   d. Threaded pins used in conjunction with castings to provide retention
2. Parallel pin techniques—procedures for producing castings with pins to enhance retention
   a. Simple indirect procedures
   b. Plastic pin techniques
      (1) Direct
      (2) Indirect
   c. Preformed metal pins
      (1) Direct
      (2) Indirect
   d. Root canal posts (dowels)

Indications

One or more pins may be indicated to supplement inadequate retention for a restoration. If a vital tooth is broken down by caries or trauma to the gingival level, pins must be placed to create a foundation of some type to retain a restoration. If half a clinical crown, either buccal or lingual, is missing and the remaining tooth structure may be of doubtful strength, pins may be indicated. If an angle of an anterior tooth is missing, pins may be helpful in establishing retention for the restorative material.

Pins should be placed if, in the judgment of the operator, the restoration might fail if they are not used. They should not be used indiscriminately.

An additional principle is the use of pins to conserve tooth structure. If a choice exists between a possible necessity of utilizing a full crown to restore a posterior tooth and retaining an amalgam or cast gold restoration using pins, for example, the pins should be used if tooth structure will be conserved by their use. A rather common restorative problem is the restoration of a lingual cusp of a maxillary premolar with the buccal cusp intact. Rather than sacrifice the buccal surface to place a full crown, a much more conservative procedure is the placement of pins to retain a three-quarter crown restoration. (See Figs. 9-11 and 9-12.)

Friction-retained or self-threading pins should not be placed in devital teeth or teeth of older people. Elasticity of dentin decreases with age, and use of these types of pins frequently induces crazing and fractures. Cemented pins are preferable in such teeth.

There are several biological factors that must be considered when contemplating the use of pins including the following:
1. Tooth vitality (elasticity of dentin).
2. Location of the pulp
3. Morphology of the tooth (crown and root)
4. Bulk (thickness) of available dentin
5. Size of the tooth
6. Intermaxillary strength (occlusion)

In addition to the biological factors the following should be considered in pin selection:
1. Type
2. Size
3. Length
4. Depth of holes (channels)
5. Location of holes
6. Distribution
7. Number to be used
8. Restorative materials used

Tooth vitality (elasticity of dentin)

Dentin of nonvital teeth is brittle compared to the relative elasticity of normal dentin. Pins that must rely on inducement of stress on dentin or the elasticity of dentin to enhance retention may cause crazing. Crazing is the formation of small cracks in the tooth structure induced by internal stress.

It is, therefore, generally recommended that cemented pins be used in devital or teeth of older people suspected of having brittle dentin. Friction-retained and self-threading pins[1] may induce crazing in such teeth. In such cases cemented pins may be used to increase retention and better distribute the load since they do not induce stress.

Placement of pins

Proper placement of pins is very important from the standpoint of pulpal and periodontal health. A pin placed into the pulp chamber threatens pulp vitality. A pin that perforates into the periodontium may cause serious periodontal complications.

Some of the factors that must be considered in the placement of pins, regardless of what type is used, are (1) depth of placement, (2) diameter, (3) the number used, (4) desirable locations in which they may be placed, (5) direction of the drilled hole, and (6) length of the pin extended into the restorative material.

PIN DEPTH

It is desirable to use a type of pin that will achieve its maximum retentive factor with as short an extension into dentin as possible. Self-threading pins (Whaledent) achieve their maximum practical retention at 2 mm. in dentin. Cemented pins placed the same depth have less than half the retentive factor as the self-threading pins; thus for comparable effectiveness they must be placed deeper and/or more pins should be placed. In so doing they grasp more of the remaining tooth structure, which is most desirable.

PIN SIZE (DIAMETER)

Pins larger in diameter have greater retentive strength than those of smaller diameters of the same length. For example, cemented pins that are 0.025 inch in diameter and 3 mm. in dentin require about 18 pounds of tensile load to remove them from the dentin.[1] Cemented pins that are 0.018 inch in diameter of the same depth require only approximately 12 pounds of tensile load to remove them.

Self-threading pins that are 0.031 inch in diameter and 2 mm. in depth require about 59 pounds of tensile strength to fracture them from dentin,[1] whereas pins 0.023 inch in diameter fracture at approximately 34 pounds of tensile strength.

NUMBER OF PINS

The number of pins desirable in each given circumstance must be a matter of clinical judgment. Such judgment, however, can be based on the relative retentive power of each pin placed as noted under *Pin depth* earlier. A large molar in a mouth exhibiting a strong bite should obviously receive more pins than a small tooth in a situation subjected to relatively inactive occlusal function.

A suggested rule of thumb is at least *one pin for each missing cusp*. This, however, must depend on the type of pin used and strength requirements. Self-threading pins exhibit the greatest retentive power; thus fewer should be required than for cemented pins. Anterior teeth should receive at least two and up to four pins if most of the crown is missing.

LOCATION (DISTRIBUTION)

Placement of the pins will depend largely on the morphology of the tooth. Thus areas of furcations should be avoided unless they are clearly an adequate distance from the starting point. The starting point should usually be midway between the pulp and the tooth surface.

Friction-retained and self-threading pins should not be placed closer to enamel than 0.5 mm. if crazing is to be avoided.

All pins must be placed to avoid injury to the dental pulp or perforation of the periodontal membrane.

When two or more pins are placed, they should be distributed in a manner to enhance stability, not grouped together.

DIRECTION

As the hole is drilled, it must be directed midway between the pulp and root surface. It is not desirable to have the holes parallel for pin-retained amalgam or resin. Holes drilled for pins to be cast as part of the gold restoration must be parallel, of course. More complex procedures exist for utilization of pins in cast restorations. Devices for paralleling two or more pins are in relatively common use but find their greatest value in crown and bridge procedures; therefore, these are not included here, except as noted.

Three general types of pins used for restorative purposes are (1) cemented pins, (2) friction-retained pins, and (3) those cast as part of the restoration.

Cemented and friction-retained pins are used primarily for retaining amalgam (or resin) foundations, over which a cast restoration may be placed. The advantages and disadvantages of the placement of pins for amalgam restorations are obvious. However, cases that are so extensive as to require their use may justify placement of cast restorations.

It is generally considered safest to locate pin holes at the line angles of the tooth. Usually there is adequate thickness of dentin between the den-

tinoenamel junction and the pulp chamber to
safely place pins. In addition, there are seldom
any flutings or furcations in the line angles of a
tooth that might possibly complicate placement.

Relatively safer areas for pin placement in a
molar are toward line angles or corners of the
crown as indicated in Fig. 9-1. Avoid furcation
areas (Fig. 9-2), flutings (Fig. 9-3), and areas of
pulp proximity (Fig. 9-4). Also avoid placement of
pins too close to enamel (Fig. 9-5) because crazing
of the enamel may be induced.

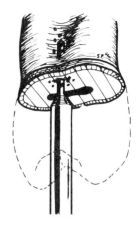

Fig. 9-3. Fluted areas on tooth roots should be avoided.

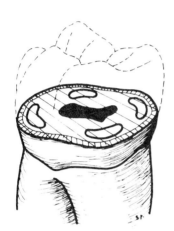

Fig. 9-1. Indicated areas near tooth line angles for
placement of pins.

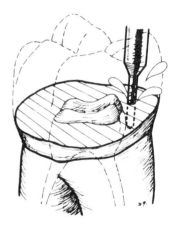

Fig. 9-4. Proximity to the dental pulp must be avoided.

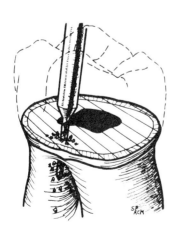

Fig. 9-2. Furcation areas should be avoided for placement of pins.

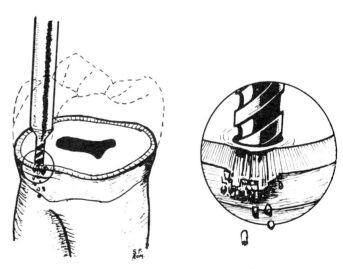

Fig. 9-5. Proximity to dentinoenamel junction must be
avoided.

PIN LENGTH

Pins do not reinforce amalgam or increase its compressive strength. Fracture tests show that fracture lines emanate from the pins. This is in part due to incomplete condensation around pins, thereby introducing weak spots in the amalgam. The optimal pin length in amalgam has been found to be approximately 2.0 mm.[1] Increased length weakens the amalgam and does not contribute to retention.

TECHNIQUE OF DRILLING PINHOLES

1 Consider the following points (while establishing the basic cavity preparation):
    a. Inspect radiographs for the anatomical features of the tooth.
    b. Probe the root surface adjacent to the pin site for shape of the root.
    c. Recall the normal morphology of root shape and size and shape of the pulp cavity.
    d. Estimate the amount of available dentin from the dentinoenamel junction to the pulp chamber.

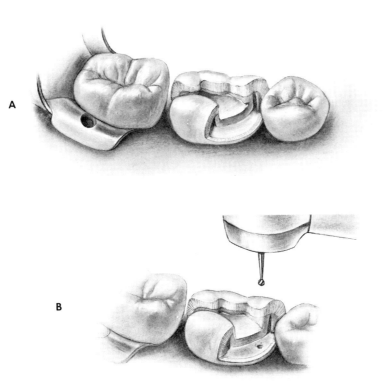

Fig. 9-6. Preliminary steps prior to drilling holes for pins. **A,** Basic preparation completed. **B,** Starting point placed using a No. ¼ (½) bur.

2 Using a ¹/₂ round bur in a high-speed hand-piece, make a small depression in the appropriate location at the line angle of the tooth. This will prevent skidding of the twist drill.

3 Inspect the location of the depression. Relocate, if necessary, before using the twist drill.

4 Select the proper size twist drill and place it in the low-handpiece (a reducing gear contra-angle is preferred).

5 Align the twist drill to avoid the pulp or perforation of the root. (Bisect the distance between the pulp and root surface.)

6 In stages, with air coolant, drill the pin hole 2 to 3 mm. deep into dentin. When the twist drill is removed from the hole, the air will remove the dentin chips and cool the point before reinsertion and deeper drilling.

7 Avoid stopping the handpiece while the twist drill is in the hole since it may become stuck and fracture off in the hole.

8 When two or more pins are placed, they should be distributed in a manner to enhance stability, with as much separation between them as possible.

Cemented pins

Markley[2] cautions against the use of friction-retained pins because of the possibility of creating undue internal stress in the dentin that may cause subsequent fracture. He therefore recommends the following general procedure for placing threaded steel pins.

ARMAMENTARIUM

No. ¹/₂ (¹/₄) bur
0.027-inch drill (0.021-inch for anterior teeth or other small teeth)
0.025-inch steel wire (0.020-inch when the 0.021 drill is used)
Crown and bridge cement
Spiral
Amalgam and appropriate instruments

1 Place a rubber dam.

2 Reduce the marginal enamel to sound dentin and desired outline form as indicated for the particular situation.

3 Remove all caries and treat the pulp region as appropriate (Fig. 9-6, *A*).

4 With a No. ¹/₂ (¹/₄) bur establish steps or starting points midway between the pulp and the tooth surface (Fig. 9-6, *B*). Without these the drill may tend to "run" or move as the hole is started.

5 Drill holes with a 0.027-inch drill at very slow speed (Fig. 9-7, *A*). Depth of holes should be minimum of 2 mm. and as deep as 4 mm. Direction of the holes should generally be paralled with the surface of the tooth, but the holes are more retentive if not placed parallel with each other. Placing the drill on the surface of the tooth to determine its contour aids evaluation of the proper direction to drill.

6 Cut and bend lengths of 0.025-inch threaded steel wire as appropriate, and arrange them on the bracket table to facilitate rapid placement after the cement is introduced into the holes.

7 Paint the prepared tooth with cavity varnish only if deemed essential to protect the pulp. Moffa, Rozzano, and Doyle[1] demonstrated that varnishing the pinholes induces retention by approximately 46%. Pinholes can be varnished using wisps of cotton formed on the tips of root canal broaches (Fig. 9-7, *B*).

8 Mix zinc phosphate cement to a consistency desirable for inlay cementation. Pick up a quantity of cement with a spiral (Fig. 9-7, *C*). Most spirals are easier to manage if shortened. Place the spiral into a pinhole and run it slowly to force the cement inward (Fig. 9-7, *D*). Revolve the spiral slowly while withdrawing it.

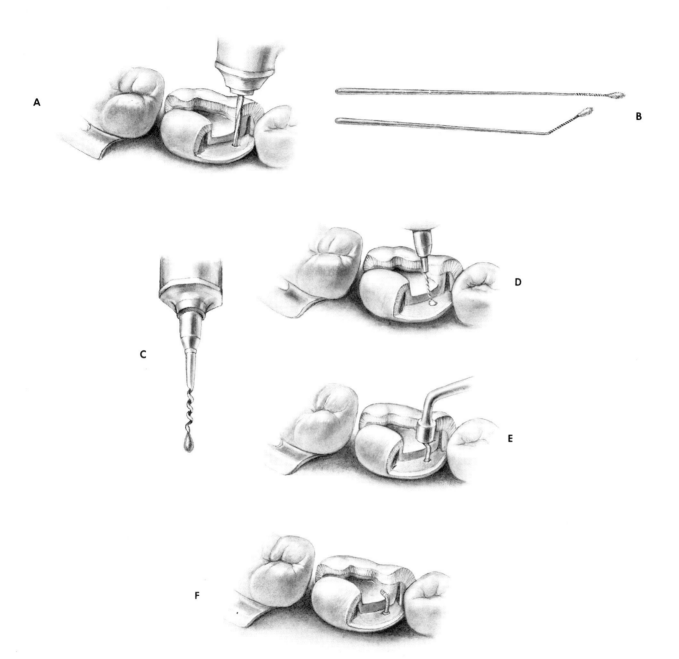

Fig. 9-7. Cemented (Markley) pins being placed. **A,** Holes being drilled. **B,** Cotton swab on barbed broach for varnishing the pinholes. Varnish is not recommended unless deemed essential for pulp protection. **C,** Spiral with droplet of cement to be placed into the pinhole. **D,** Placement of the cement. **E,** Treaded steel pin being pressed in place using an amalgam condenser. **F,** Pin in place.

9 Place the pins one at a time as the cement is placed in each hole, forcing them firmly to the bottom of each hole with a serrated amalgam condenser (Fig. 9-7, *E*). The slab should be cooled to retard the set of the cement remaining on it, thus allowing the operator to place a pin in each hole as it is filled with cement.

10 While the cement is setting, place a matrix band.

11 Pin in place (Fig. 9-7, *F*).

12 Condense the amalgam.

13 Remove the matrix band and carve the amalgam to the desired contour.

COMMENT: *It is recommended that the amalgam be allowed to set at least one day before proceeding with the final preparation for a cast restoration. The newer alloys, however, if properly managed may allow preparation at the same appointment.*

14 Prepare the tooth as indicated for the cast restoration. Prepared margins should normally be established in sound tooth structure.

COMMENT: *Cemented pins have been proved, beyond question, to be of great value clinically. One of the writers, during his senior year in dental school, restored one of his father's upper first premolars, which was fractured off cleanly level with the gingiva. Two iridioplatinum staples, as taught by the late Dr. John Kuratli, were cemented and the body of the crown built up with amalgam fillings incorporated in cement, over which a full cast gold crown was placed. The restoration served twenty-nine years, surviving in a mouth exhibiting unusually heavy stress.*

Friction-retained pins (Unitek*)

ARMAMENTARIUM

As provided by the manufacturer

1 Place a rubber dam.

2 Remove all old restorative material and caries. Place a base if indicated (Fig. 9-8).

3 Place starting points with a ½ (¼) bur (Fig. 9-8).

4 Drill holes, observing precautions noted in step 5 in the cemented pin technique (Fig. 9-8, *A*).

5 Press or mallet the pins in place (Fig. 9-8, *B*).

6 Cut off the excess length with a high-speed bur. Always cut the pin using a tiny (no. ¼ or 33¼) bur in a manner that will not allow the bur to vibrate or "grab" the pin, thereby dislodging it. The rotational direction of the bur should be toward the base of the pin. A recommended alternative is cutting the pin to its proper length before it is placed.

7 Proceed as outlined in the preceding technique.

COMMENT: *The holes for this procedure must be drilled with extreme care. An eccentric or oversized drill will not create a hole with adequate retentive factor. Rapid drilling may also create an oversized hole. After a pin is placed it should be firmly tested to be certain of its stability.*

---

*Unitek Corp., Monrovia, Calif.

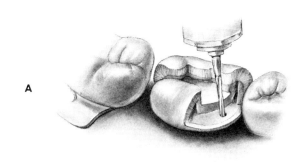

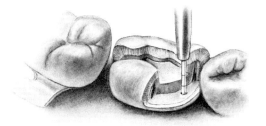

Fig. 9-8. Placement of Unitek pin. **A,** Hole being drilled. **B,** Pin driven in place.

TMS (Whaledent*) pins

ARMAMENTARIUM

As provided by the manufacturer

1 Perform the appropriate steps to prepare the tooth for pin placement.

2 Place starting points with a No. $^1/_2$ ($^1/_4$) bur.

3 Place the holes with the drill (Fig. 9-9, *A*). Whaledent markets a 1:10 ratio, slow-speed contra-angle for this purpose.

4 Screw the pins in place with the wrench provided (Fig. 9-9, *B*) The pins may also be placed with the contra-angle, using the attachment provided.

5 Bend the pins to accommodate placement of the amalgam (Fig. 9-9, *C*) and cut off any excess length if necessary (Fig. 9-9, *D*). A length of 2 mm. is adequate.

6 Place the amalgam as outlined in the preceding techniques.

A wide variety of armamentaria are available for self-threaded pin procedures. Pins are now available in several diameters, and self-limiting drills (2 mm.) are recommended; 2-in-1 pins, each section 4 mm. in length, are convenient.

*Whaledent, Inc., Brooklyn, N.Y.

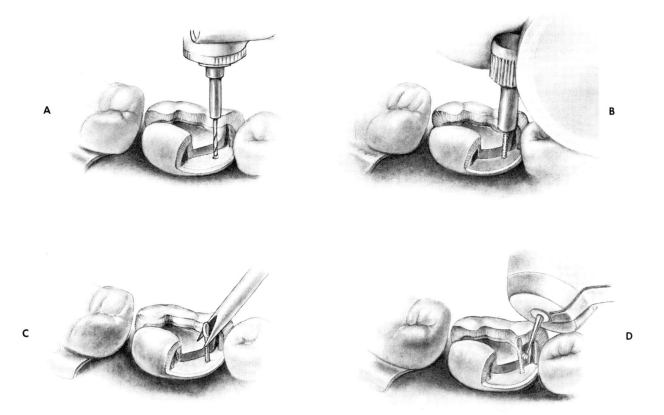

Fig. 9-9. Placement of TMS (Whaledent) pins. **A,** Drilling the hole with a 1:10 ratio contra-angle. **B,** Screwing the pin in place. **C,** Bending the pin to desired position with the instrument provided in the kit. **D,** Cutting off excess length using a No. $^1/_4$ bur.

Pin castings (parallel pins)

Methods of casting retentive pins as part of the casting include (1) reproduction of the pinhole prepared with a No. 169L or larger bur by means of impression material for an indirect procedure, and (2) drilling the holes and placing slightly smaller plastic pins in them for the purpose of reproducing them either in a direct pattern or an impression for an indirect procedure.

IMPRESSIONS OF PINHOLES

Pinholes as small as No. 169L burs can easily be reproduced using conventional impression materials. Hydrocolloid can be introduced into such holes using a syringe with a small needle (approximately 23 gauge). Rubber base or silicone impression materials can be easily introduced into small holes. Spirals are recommended since they accomplish the desired results most efficiently. (See Fig. 9-7, *C.*) A pattern lubricant introduced into the holes and then well blown out of them with air will facilitate removal of the impression pins.

PLASTIC PIN TECHNIQUES

Twist drills are available in several sizes for which nylon bristle stock is available.

1 Drill holes of the desired size (Fig. 9-10, *A*).

2 Place slightly smaller nylon bristles into the hole (Fig. 9-10, *C*). These should have been previously prepared by cutting to the desired length and creating a head on one end with a hot instrument (or by heating the pin and pressing it to a cold metal surface). These pins must extend far enough out of the holes to ensure that they will be stable in the impression as it is removed and poured, and the portion of the pin in the hole must be clean to be certain it will not bind when the impression is removed from the tooth. Sometimes, however, in upper teeth the pins may tend to fall out. In such cases wipe the pin with a small amount of a soft wax so it will stay in place while the impression is taken.

3 Take an impression using the desired material.

4 Pinholes for this procedure should be slightly countersunk, using a round bur prior to cementing the inlay. This is to accommodate discrepancies that frequently occur in the casting adjacent to the pin.

5 Pour the impression in an acceptable manner to enable individual dies to be created and trimmed.

6 Using slotted pliers, carefully draw each nylon pin out of the die in the direction of its long axis.

7 Lubricate the die, place a smaller sized nylon pin in each hole, and wax the pattern.

8 Complete the remaining steps as for routine castings.

Obviously, the foregoing concept can be applied to a direct technique, in which case heads do not have to be created on the nylon pins.

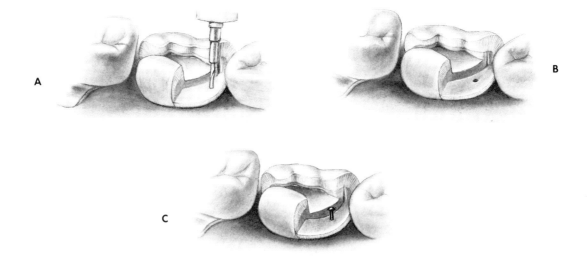

Fig. 9-10. Nylon pin technique to produce pins on a gold casting. **A,** Hole is drilled. **B,** Completed hole and preparation. **C,** Nylon pin is placed in the hole prior to taking the impression.

Amalgam foundation for cast three-quarter crown

The proved value of using pins to retain extensive restorations makes possible the restoration of extensively missing crowns without resorting to endodontic therapy in teeth with vital, healthy pulps.

A pin-retained amalgam core usually simplifies the preparation of such cases to receive cast restorations, and the impression procedure is greatly simplified. Placement of an amalgam foundation for such cases is therefore strongly recommended.

PLACEMENT OF PINS AND AMALGAM

The restoration procedure for a maxillary premolar with a fractured lingual cusp (Fig. 9-11, *A*) follows.

ARMAMENTARIUM

No. 170 (171) bur
No. ½ (¼) bur
Drill and pins of choice
Amalgam
Amalgam matrix band and holder
Amalgam condensers
Carving instruments

1 Place a rubber dam. It is essential that as much of the tooth as possible be exposed to view.

2 Remove all of the old restorative material and caries with a No. 170 bur, being careful not to undercut the buccal cusp unnecessarily (Fig. 9-11, *B*).

3 With a No. ½ (¼) bur place starting points as indicated (Fig. 9-11, *C*).

4 Drill the type of holes desired (Fig. 9-11, *D*).

5 Place the pins and bend as indicated. Fewer pins than shown in Fig. 9-11, *E*, may be indicated in the majority of cases of this type.

6 Reduce the length of pins if necessary.

7 Place the amalgam matrix and carefully condense the amalgam, using small condensers around the pins.

8 Remove the matrix and carve to contour to eliminate occlusal interference (Fig. 9-11, *F*).

Allow the amalgam to set at least one day before proceeding with the final preparation.

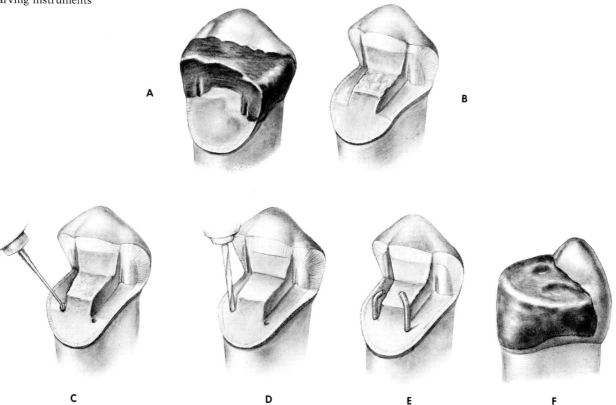

Fig. 9-11. Building an amalgam foundation for a cast restoration. **A,** Fractured lingual cusp and MOD amalgam in a maxillary premolar. **B,** Restorative materials and caries eliminated. **C,** Starting points for pinholes placed with a No. ½ (¼) bur. **D,** Holes being drilled. **E,** Pins in place. **F,** Amalgam in place.

FINAL PREPARATION

ARMAMENTARIUM

No. 170 (171) and 699L burs
Torpedo-shaped diamond point
Torpedo-shaped white finishing stone
Finishing disks

1 With a No. 170 (171) bur reduce the mesial, lingual, and distal surfaces. This reduction should extend gingivally only sufficiently to allow a chamfer to be placed gingival to it in tooth structure (Fig. 9-12, *A*).

2 Reduce the occlusal amalgam to sound enamel along the remaining cusp (Fig. 9-12, *B*).

3 Place retentive grooves on the mesial and distal surfaces (Fig. 9-12, *B*). If possible, they should be placed in sound tooth structure. However, they should not be placed buccally to the extent that the final preparation is overextended to gain their placement in sound tooth structure.

4 Place a gingival chamfer slightly below the crest of the gingiva, terminated in sound tooth structure (Fig. 9-12, *C*). Extend this cut buccally to join and/or prepare the proximal walls. The junction of the chamfer and the proximal walls should be rounded and smooth.

5 Reduce the lingual incline of the buccal cusp with the torpedo-shaped diamond point or fissure bur (Fig. 9-12, *D*).

6 Place a bevel on the buccal margin of the lingual reduction (Fig. 9-12, *E*).

7 Polish the chamfer (Fig. 9-12, *C*), the lingual plane of the buccal cusp (Fig. 9-12, *D*), and the buccal bevel (Fig. 9-12, *E*) with a white finishing stone.

8 Polish the proximal walls with ⅜-inch finishing disks (Fig. 9-12, *F*).

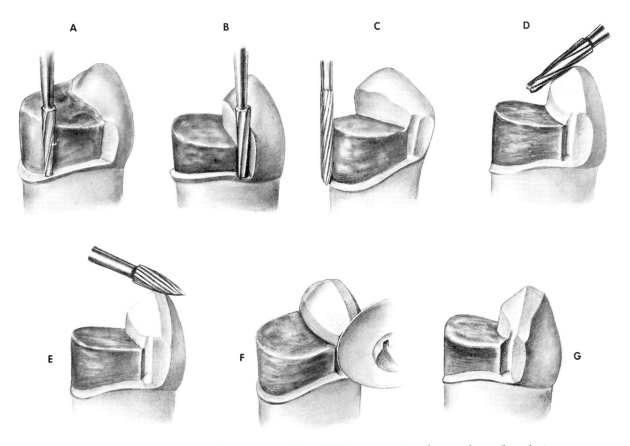

Fig. 9-12. Preparation of a three-quarter (four-fifth) crown using the amalgam foundation placed in Fig. 9-11. **A,** Reduction of the mesial, distal, and lingual surfaces. **B,** Occlusal amalgam reduced and the proximal grooves being placed. **C,** Gingival chamfer being established. **D,** Reduction of the lingual incline of the buccal cusp. **E,** Placement of the buccal bevel. **F,** Polishing the proximal walls with ³/₈-inch finishing disks. **G,** Completed preparation.

REFERENCES

1. Moffa, J. P., Rozzano, M. R., and Doyle, M. G.: Pins—a comparison of their retentive properties, J. Am. Dent. Assoc. **78:**529, 1969.
2. Markley, M. R.: Pin retained and reinforced restorations and foundations, Dent. Clin. North Am., p. 229, March, 1967.

CHAPTER 10

CAST GOLD

Cast gold restorative procedures enable the operative dentist to rebuild teeth extensively destroyed, improve function, and provide preventive services relative to periodontal therapy.

Indications

Indications for cast gold restorations include the following: (1) extensively destroyed teeth, (2) occlusal reconstruction, (3) cracked teeth, (4) endodontically treated teeth, and (5) splinting. Additional indications may include use of cast gold to maintain color harmony and to avoid possible electrolysis where amalgam restorations may not be compatible with gold previously placed.

EXTENSIVELY DESTROYED TEETH

Cast gold is generally resistant to deformation by stress and must be considered as the material of choice if cusps are missing, weak, or extensively worn.

Amalgam relies largely on the remaining tooth structure to contain and support it and, even when retained by pins, does little toward strengthening or protecting remaining tooth structure from stress. Extensive restorations using cast gold can, on the other hand, protect the remaining tooth structure. It must be remembered, however, that the design of the preparation determines the retention of the restoration, as with all restorative materials. The design must incorporate retentive factors such as parallel walls, grooves, and/or pins to create resistance and retention form. Other restorative materials rely on opposing undercuts to retain them in their prepared cavities.

OCCLUSAL RECONSTRUCTION

In general, when cusps must be covered, a gold casting is superior to amalgam. If a patient is suf-

fering from occlusal disharmony, where adjustment by selective grinding alone is not adequate to achieve a stable occlusion, then cast restorations should be placed.

A gold casting allows one to accurately control tooth contours and occlusion when teeth are rotated, supererupted, intruded, or extensively broken down.

All phases of a cast gold restoration must be well planned and meticulously executed. No procedure in restorative dentistry demands more careful attention to detail than that of placing cast gold.

The many steps involved before the casting is taken to the mouth require consideration when preparing the cavity. The procedure involves (1) preparing the tooth, (2) taking the impression, (3) pouring the impression, (4) finishing the die, (5) waxing the pattern, (6) drawing and investing the pattern, (7) casting the gold, (8) finishing the casting prior to cementation, and (9) cementation. The cavity must be designed with all these steps and the physical factors involved well in mind.

CRACKED TEETH

Frequently patients are seen who complain of pain caused by cracks. Such cracks are often obscure, even when existing restorative materials have been removed. Typically, the patient with a cracked tooth will complain that it often hurts to bite on it. Such teeth, if vital, usually become hypersensitive to thermal change. Occasionally the cusp or part of the tooth affected by the crack can be located by percussion. Great care should be taken to ensure that teeth suspected of being cracked are not in hyperocclusion.

Cracked teeth should be restored by overlaying cusps to prevent further development of the crack. (See Figs. 10-20 and 10-24.)

ENDODONTICALLY TREATED TEETH

A major indication for restoration of and/or protection of pulpless teeth is cast gold. Endodontically treated teeth are normally subject to fracture if the root canal opening is large or if the tooth has been restored in such a way as to contribute to fracture of cusps.

It is strongly recommended that pulpless posterior teeth be protected by castings overlaying cusps (See Fig. 10-20.) as protection against fracture by means of a cast restoration that will tie the cusps together.

In addition to pin-retained foundations (Fig. 9-11) teeth with missing cusps may be restored as shown in Fig 10-24.

Retention of the casting can also be enhanced by use of a dowel-type preparation. Dowels (or posts) should be considered for short teeth or teeth with one or more missing cusps. Maximum retention may be created by placing pins in conjunction with dowels.

SPLINTING

In selected cases teeth with weakened periodontal support can be splinted for stabilization by placing cast restorations and soldering adjacent castings together.

COMPARISON OF INLAY AND AMALGAM PREPARATIONS

When engineering a particular preparation, careful consideration must be given to the type of restorative material that will be used. What are its physical properties, its strengths and weaknesses? How is it to be manipulated and inserted? How will it be retained? To what type of forces will it be subjected? Equally important is knowledge of tooth histology, morphology, and occlusion as well as mechanical strengths and weaknesses of the tooth structure.

In comparing one restoration type with another, a logical way of thinking is helpful. One of the easiest ways of comparing or contrasting two different preparations is to follow the order in which the tooth is prepared—namely, the seven steps of cavity preparation as described by Black. The following is a comparison of typical Class 2 inlay and amalgam cavity preparations.

INLAY PREPARATION

General considerations
1. May support the tooth structure; for example, the cusps are covered.
2. Preparation is tapered such that there is draw. Retention is achieved by nearly parallel opposing walls, close adaptation of the casting, and a cementing medium.
3. There is good resistance to occlusal forces and function when there is adequate thickness of gold in the areas of occlusal contact.

Outline form
1. The occlusal outline includes pits, fissures, and other enamel defects such as decay.
2. There is a smooth, flowing outline with no sharp irregularities.
3. Isthmus width may be narrower than amalgam, since gold is not as brittle as amalgam.
4. Reverse curve is not normally found since bulk of gold is not necessary. In fact, all margins are beveled to allow ease of finishing. There is also sufficient access into the proximal area owing to the divergent walls.
5. The proximal outline is slightly more extensive than an amalgam preparation (between 0.5 mm and 1.0 mm) to provide:
   a. Access for disking the preparation
   b. Access for finishing the gold
   c. Extension for ease of home care and maintenance
6. The gingival cavosurface point angles are rounded for ease of finishing gold.

AMALGAM PREPARATION

1. Preparation is supported by the tooth.
2. Preparation is designed to create retention from parallel walls and undercuts.
3. There is poor resistance to forces of occlusion.

1. This feature also holds true for amalgam preparations.
2. There is a smooth, flowing outline with no sharp irregularities.
3. Amalgam is a brittle material and requires right angle margins to withstand the forces of occlusion.*
4. Reverse curve is often found because amalgam requires bulk at the margins for strength and for convenience form into the proximal surface.
5. The proximal outline provides approximately 0.5 mm. clearance from the adjacent tooth at the level of contact for ease in finishing and home care.
6. Gingival cavosurface point angles form a definite angle for ease of condensing amalgam.

Continued.

*Markley teaches that an occlusal step is not necessary for amalgam that can rely on proximal locks or pins for retention.

INLAY PREPARATION
Outline form—cont'd

7. The proximal outline provides for a uniform display of gold, is harmonious with adjacent tooth contours, and diverges occlusally.
8. The proximal outline blends into the occlusal outline at the marginal ridge.

Internal form

1. The preparation must draw. There are no undercuts. Buccal and lingual walls diverge occlusally.

2. All internal line and point angles are formed to provide a definite line of draw, better resistance, and retention form.
3. The axial wall converges toward the occlusal side.
4. The axial and pulpal walls are straight in an occlusogingival direction and into dentin 0.5 mm.
5. Axial walls follow axial contours of the tooth when viewed from the occlusal side.
6. The pulpal floor is parallel to the occlusal table of the tooth.
7. The gingival wall is straight buccolingually and in two planes, providing a definite axiogingival line angle as a seat for the casting.
8. Groove extensions are obtuse to the pulpal wall to prevent undermining the enamel wall, to conservatively include the enamel defect, and to provide draw.
9. The axiopulpal line angle is beveled to prevent voids in the working die and nodules in the casting that would provide difficulty in seating the casting.

AMALGAM PREPARATION

7. The proximal outline provides uniform extension beyond the adjacent tooth and converges occlusally.

8. The proximal outline blends into the occlusal outline at the marginal ridge.

1. The preparation must *not* draw. There are retentive undercuts in the proximal, parallel buccal, and lingual walls or slightly convergent occlusally.
2. All internal line and point angles are made definite to provide the best resistance and retention and allow ease of condensation.
3. The axial wall is parallel to the long axis of the tooth.
4. The axial and pulpal walls are straight in an occlusogingival direction and into dentin 0.5 mm.
5. Axial walls follow the contour of the tooth when viewed from the occlusal side.
6. The pulpal floor is parallel to the occlusal table of the tooth.
7. The gingival wall is flat and makes a right angle or slightly acute angle with the axial wall. It provides a definite seat when condensing amalgam.
8. Groove extensions are generally obtuse to the pulpal wall to prevent undermining the enamel wall and to conservatively include the enamel defect.
9. The axiopulpal line angle is beveled to reduce stress on the amalgam.

INLAY PREPARATION
Internal form—cont'd

10. All margins are beveled:
    a. For ease of finish—30 to 45 degrees in gold
    b. To protect the remaining enamel prisms
    c. To provide a lap-sliding fit of the casting to the tooth (especially at the gingival surface)
    d. To include deep grooves and yet conserve tooth structure
    e. To develop circumferential retention

Class 1 gold inlays

Class 1 lesions are not normally restored with cast gold. Other materials usually lend themselves more ideally to restoration of these lesions with conservation of tooth structure. Also, from an economic standpoint the possible development of proximal caries, especially in younger people, must be borne in mind.

AMALGAM PREPARATION

10. There are no cavosurface bevels. All margins should be as close to 90 degrees as possible to provide a butt joint for bulk of amalgam.

Class 2 gold inlays

Most inlays are placed to restore proximal surfaces. All of the considerations such as extension for prevention, conservation of tooth structure, and so forth must be observed. The main advantages to restoring proximal surfaces with gold castings are their ability to effectively maintain or improve occlusion and to maintain or improve proximal contours.

BASIC PREPARATION, MANDIBULAR RIGHT SECOND MOLAR

The following procedure is a fairly standard technique for preparing a routine, simple Class 2 cavity and will apply to most posterior teeth, the only variations being use of binangle chisels on upper premolars and molars when accessible.

ARMAMENTARIUM

No. 170 bur
No. 169L bur
Spoon excavator
Enamel hatchet (binangle chisel)
Gingival margin trimmers
Finishing disks

1 Place the rubber dam.
2 Prepare the occlusal portion of the cavity with a No. 170 bur, extending the preparation into the grooves adequately to include those that are defective or deep (or polish out groove defects). Place the distal margin only slightly onto the marginal ridge, keeping the distopulpal line angle obtuse. The buccopulpal and linguopulpal line angles are also slightly obtuse, thereby avoiding the creation of undercuts to create a "line of draw."

3 Extend the occlusal cut toward the contact area, into the marginal ridge, and then buccolingually, but do not rock the handpiece to create undercuts.
4 Extend this cut gingivally with a No. 169L bur as for amalgam (Fig. 7-18), but without undercuts.
5 Break out the proximal enamel with a spoon excavator (Figs. 10-1 and 10-2).
6 Begin refining the proximal walls and gingival wall with the No. 169L (170) bur (Fig. 10-3). The proximal walls for inlays should be decidedly flared buccolingually, creating obtuse proximal-cavosurface angles that permit conservation of tooth structure internally. However, the proximal walls should not be cut out completely with burs unless the case demands or access allows it since this may result in overextension or damage to the adjacent tooth.

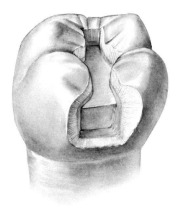

Fig. 10-2. Outline form of Class 2 cavity preparation.

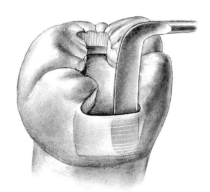

Fig. 10-1. Breaking out the proximal enamel using a large spoon.

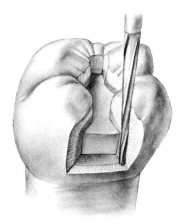

Fig. 10-3. Planing the walls with a tapered fissure bur.

7 Plane the proximal and gingival walls with an enamel hatchet (Fig. 10-4).

8 Place a gingival bevel with a gingival margin trimmer (Fig. 10-5). The bevel should usually terminate just below the crest of the normal gingiva.

9 With ³/₈-inch extra fine garnet or sandpaper disks in a contra-angle, smooth the proximal walls (Fig. 10-6). This should highly finish the cavosurface margins (Fig. 10-7).

COMMENT: *Should the operator wish a definite cavosurface bevel placed on the occlusal margins, it should be relatively slight and may be placed as the cavity is prepared with the No. 170 bur. When the proximal margins are disked, the disk should be moved into the occlusal portion of the cavity, which should place an adequate and well-finished bevel in these areas.*

VARIATIONS FOR EXTENSIVE CASES

Many inlays are placed to restore teeth extensively damaged by caries or in which overextended amalgams have failed. Following are a few principles that may be applied in such cases:

1 Remove all amalgam and caries. Place a base if indicated.

2 Extend the preparation to its indicated outline; that is, all walls should be established in sound dentin and enamel.

3 Place retentive proximal grooves with a No. 169L bur (Fig. 10-8).

4 Place a retentive slot at the distal wall (Fig. 10-9). This distal retention is normally about 1.5 or 2 mm. deep and must not be placed near the pulp (Fig. 10-13).

5 Bevel the gingival cavosurface angle with gingival margin trimmers (Fig. 10-5) or, if access permits, with a finishing bur (Fig. 10-10).

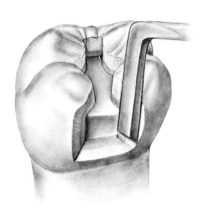

Fig. 10-4. Planing the proximal walls using an enamel hatchet.

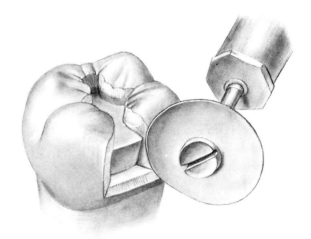

Fig. 10-6. Disking the proximal walls.

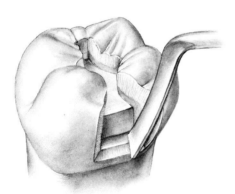

Fig. 10-5. Planing the gingival bevel using a gingival margin trimmer.

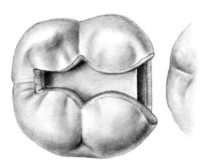

Fig. 10-7. Completed Class 2 gold inlay preparation.

6 Place a short bevel on the occlusal margin with a No. 170, 171, or finishing bur (Fig. 10-11).

COMMENT: *The steps involved in producing a cast gold restoration utilizing indirect techniques require consideration of several factors. Sharp margins on the proximal walls are desirable, but they should not be formed in a manner that will cause them to cut the underlying impression material as it is removed from the tooth. Also, sharp gingivobuccal and gingivolingual line angles should be avoided since the gingival bevel should meet each proximal wall on a curve to avoid a sharp point angle on the tooth surface. Reproduction of the tooth with impression materials is difficult if the proximal wall extend outward sharply, as is possible on a bell-shaped tooth, thus cutting the impression as it is withdrawn from the mouth.*

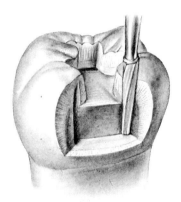

Fig. 10-8. Placing slight proximal grooves, extensive Class 2 inlay preparation.

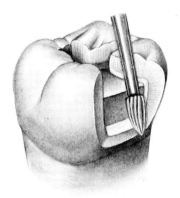

Fig. 10-10. Placing the gingival bevel.

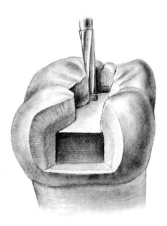

Fig. 10-9. Placing a distal slot or pin.

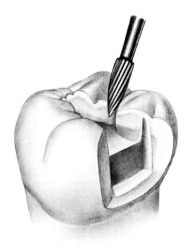

Fig. 10-11. Placing the occlusal cavosurface bevel.

7 Polish the proximal walls and cavosurface angles with finishing disks (Fig. 10-12). The gingival bevel should meet the proximal walls in a curve, and the occlusal bevel should also be continuous onto the proximal wall, disappearing as the margin of the proximal wall turns in a gingival direction.

8 The finished preparation is shown in Fig. 10-13 and 10-14.

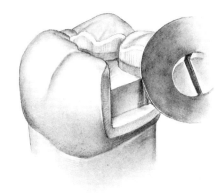

Fig. 10-12. Disking the proximal walls.

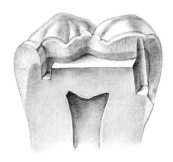

Fig. 10-13. Cross section of Class 2 gold inlay cavity preparation showing proximal groove and distal slot.

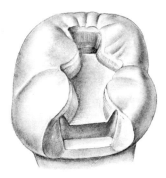

Fig. 10-14. Completed preparation.

OCCLUSAL OVERLAY

The terms *overlay* and *onlay* are generally used to denote the extension of a restoration to include the occlusal portion of a cusp or cusps. The term *overlay* is included in *Current Clinical Dental Terminology* as "a cast intracoronal restoration that includes the restoration of one or more cusps. May also designate the extension of another material to include one or more cusps."*

Onlay refers to a part of a removable prosthesis. Common usage, however, has made the two terms synonymous when used in operative dentistry.

Overlaying (or onlaying) cusps is desirable when (1) a fracture of the cusps is possible because of extensive loss of tooth structure supporting them, (2) when occlusal function may be improved, (3) when a crack is suspected, and (4) for pulpless teeth.

Some practitioners may question the justification for overlaying cusps in the case illustrated. It must be emphasized that the operator's clinical judgment must include a careful evaluation of the reasons for including the cusps. The case shown is basically diagrammatic to demonstrate a procedure that may be routinely applied to a wide range of requirements.

Cavity preparation

ARMAMENTARIUM

Nos. 170 and 169L burs
Gingival margin trimmers
Flame-shaped finishing bur
11A wheel diamond
Pear-shaped finishing bur
Finishing disks

1 Remove all caries and old restorative materials.

COMMENT: *Operators possessing experienced clinical judgement may, in selected cases, leave a small amount of carious dentin or old restorative material in an undercut area. It must be removed prior to placement of the final restoration, preferably while the anesthesia is still effective immediately after taking impressions.*

2 Extend the buccal and lingual occlusal walls into sound dentin with a No. 170 (171) bur.

3 Straighten up the proximal walls, placing them in sound tooth structure and extending to self-cleansing areas.

*From Boucher, C. O., editor: Current clinical dental terminology, ed. 2, St. Louis, 1974, The C. V. Mosby Co.

4 With a No. 169L bur place retentive grooves in the proximal walls (Fig. 10-15).

5 Place the gingival bevel using a gingival margin trimmer (Fig. 10-16) a small flame-shaped diamond point, or finishing bur (Fig. 10-17) where access permits. Cases of this type frequently are extensive to a degree that use of a small diamond point is possible. However, it is obvious that great care must be taken to avoid damage to the adjacent tooth, unless it is being restored also.

6 Reduce the internal inclines on the cusps using a small wheel-shaped diamond point (Fig. 10-18) or a flame-shaped diamond point. The wheel is usually indicated only when extensive cutting is required. It reduces enamel rapidly and should be followed by the finishing bur to smooth the cut. The depth of these cuts should create about 1 to 1.5 mm. of occlusal clearance over the lingual cusp and 0.5 mm. on the buccal cusp.

7 Place the occlusal bevels with a No. 170 bur using a low speed or finishing bur (Fig. 10-19). Keep the buccal extension to a minimum to avoid displaying gold.

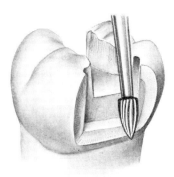

Fig. 10-17. Alternate method of placing gingival bevel, twelve-blade bur.

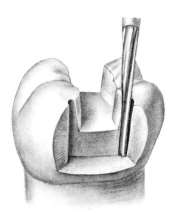

Fig. 10-15. Placement of proximal grooves using a 169L bur.

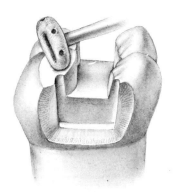

Fig. 10-18. Occlusal reduction.

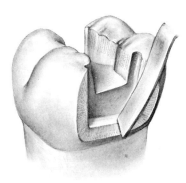

Fig. 10-16. Plane gingival bevel using a margin trimmer.

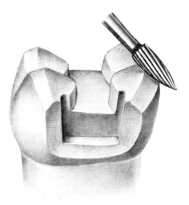

Fig. 10-19. Occlusal bevels placed using twelve-blade bur.

8 Finish all margins, including the gingival bevel where accessible, with a small finishing bur.

9 Polish the proximal walls with finishing disks (Fig. 10-20).

The completed preparation (Fig. 10-21) should provide adequate space between the tooth being restored and its antagonists in the opposing arch to create adequate thickness in the casting to allow for placement of proper anatomy. All margins should be smooth and definite, with proximal and gingival margins meeting in a smooth curve.

For an unusually short crown it is sometimes extremely desirable to conserve the buccal and lingual tooth structure rather than resort to full coverage of the clinical crown. A preparation such as shown (Fig. 10-22) is recommended. Placement of pinholes bucally and lingually adds greatly to retentive factor and stability. They can be placed with a No. 169L bur and should be 2 or 3 mm. deep. A nylon pin technique may also be used of course. (See Chapter 6.)

VARIATIONS FOR EXTENSIVE CASES

Patients with completely destroyed or broken cusps require variations in the designs of the prepared cavities to comply with the requirements of resistance and retention form. Use of pins and grooves usually facilitates this.

Fig. 10-23 shows a lost distolingual cusp of a maxillary molar and amalgam restorations that will be presumed faulty for the purpose of demonstration. Fig. 10-24, shows the old restorations removed, and Fig. 10-25 shows the completed preparation for the overlay restoration.

A pinhole has been placed using a No. 169L bur to a depth of 2 to 3 mm.

COMMENT: *It must be noted that nearly parallel walls are desirable for retentive factor for cast restorations. However, when short teeth or cases in which the prepared walls are necessarily short are encountered, pins and/or grooves are highly desirable, if not essential, to gain adequate retentive factor for the restoration.*

Fig. 10-26 shows a mandibular molar extensively damaged. The preparation (Fig. 10-27) results in what common usage terms a *three-quarter crown*, a misnomer in the case of posterior teeth since four of the five surfaces are included in the restoration.

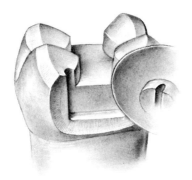

Fig. 10-20. Disking proximal walls.

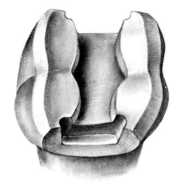

Fig. 10-21. Completed preparation.

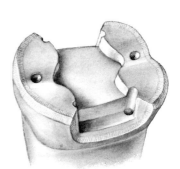

Fig. 10-22. Short MOD overlay preparation utilizing pins for stability.

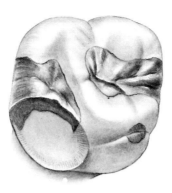

Fig. 10-23. Extensive restoration needed.

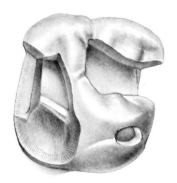

Fig. 10-24. Amalgam removed.

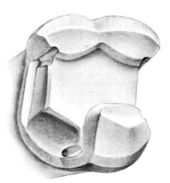

Fig. 10-25. Completed preparation.

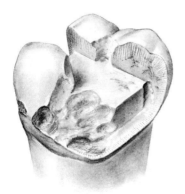

Fig. 10-26. Extensively broken down molar.

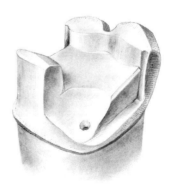

Fig. 10-27. Completed preparation (³/₄ crown).

Class 3 gold inlays

Cast gold procedures for restoration of single proximal surfaces of anterior teeth seem to be used relatively infrequently by the average operator. Indications are for large restorations when they may be placed without an undue display of gold. Insertion should normally be from the lingual aspect.

SIMPLE CLASS 3 INLAY

Cavity preparation for a simple Class 3 inlay is similar to that for a porcelain Class 3 inlay except that the margins are beveled. They should not be placed where the incisal angle is weak or may be endangered.

ARMAMENTARIUM

No. 170 (171) bur
Jeffery hatchets

1 Open the cavity with a No. 170 (171) bur.
2 Establish the indicated outline. Extend the cavity labially only enough to allow adequate extension to be established by planing to place a bevel.
3 Place opposing incisal and gingival retentive grooves in dentin (Fig. 10-28).
4 Bevel accessible margins with the bur (white finishing stone).
5 Bevel the remaining margins and walls with Jeffery hatchets.

The impression procedure, if the wax pattern is not carved directly, may be the same as that described for a Class 3 porcelain inlay. (See Figs. 16-13 to 16-17.)

LINGUAL DOVETAIL INLAY

Replacement of large lingually extended silicate restorations can often be accomplished with a lingual dovetail inlay. The procedure usually allows retention of tooth structure that supports the incisal angle.

ARMAMENTARIUM

No. 170 (171) bur
Jeffery hatchets
Wedelstacdt chisel

1 Open the cavity with a No. 170 (171) bur, removing all caries and/or silicate material.
2 Establish desired outline form of the proximal preparation to create a line of draw. Do not undercut the incisal angle.
3 Cut the dovetail. The dovetail should not be created at great expense of tooth structure but should be cut only large enough to facilitate retention of the restoration (Fig. 10-29).
4 Bevel the lingual margins.
5 Plane the gingival and labial walls with Jeffery hatchets and place appropriate bevels.
6 Plane the incisal margins with a Wedelstaedt chisel.

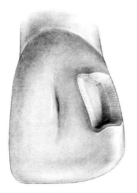

Fig. 10-28. Class 3 inlay preparation.

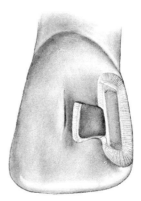

Fig. 10-29. Class 3 lingual dovetail inlay preparation.

Class 4 gold inlays

The proximal surfaces of anterior teeth with weak or broken incisal angles may be restored with gold inlays. It is preferred that such restorations not be extended labially, creating a display of gold.

CLASS 4 PIN INLAY

The conventional Class 4 pin inlay involves the incisal edge to gain adequate retention. It is indicated only in teeth that are thick labiolingually.

ARMAMENTARIUM

Torpedo-shaped diamond point
No. 35 inverted cone bur
No. 170 (171) bur
No. 169L bur
Binangle chisel (15-8-8)
Angle former (70-80-2½-9)
Finishing disks

1 Using a torpedo-shaped diamond point of diamond wheel, reduce the incisal edge (Fig. 10-30), involving approximately three fourths of the tooth width.

2 Cut an incisal stop using a No. 35 bur (Fig. 10-31). Do not remove the dentin from the labial enamel. If the tooth is abraded through the incisal enamel, the labial extension of this cut should stop short of the enamel and a bevel should be placed into the enamel.

3 Cut the proximal box with a No. 170 (171) bur, creating the desired line of draw, usually perpendicular to the labial surface of the tooth (Fig. 10-32).

4 Plane the labial proximal enamel (Fig. 10-33), preparing it as a bevel using a binangle chisel (15-8-8).

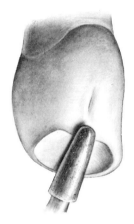

Fig. 10-30. Incisal reduction.

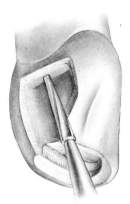

Fig. 10-32. Proximal box prepared.

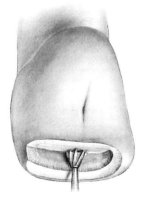

Fig. 10-31. Incisal step.

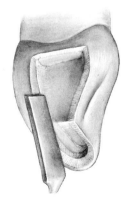

Fig. 10-33. Plane proximal walls.

5 Bevel the lingual margins with a bur (Fig. 10-34).

6 Place a bevel on the gingival wall (Fig. 10-35) with an angle former (7-80-2½-9).

7 Using a No. 169L bur (at slow speed), place pinholes in each end of the gingival wall, approximately 1 to 2 mm. deep (Fig. 10-36).

8 Place a pinhole in the incisal wall near the opposite end from the proximal box.

COMMENT: *In placing two or more pinholes by eye it is helpful to drill the first hole to part of its depth. Start the second hole, drilling only part of its desired depth. Then return to the first hole, realign the bur to it, then step to the third hole, and establish part of depth. Return again to the first hole, establish its depth, then step alternately to the second and third holes, deepening them a little at a time, checking with the others for parallel alignment as they are deepened.*

9 Disk the labial wall with finishing disks.

10 The completed preparation shown in (Fig. 10-37). The pattern may be carved, placing plastic pins directly into the pinholes, or the indirect procedures employed as desired.

PARTIAL ANTERIOR VENEER

A variation from the preceding restoration that has the advantage of preserving the incisal edge may be performed as follows. It is especially indicated on many canines to restore distal incisal angles.

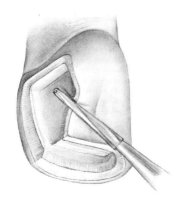

Fig. 10-34. Bevel lingual cavosurface angles.

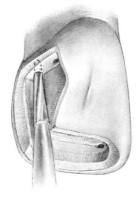

Fig. 10-36. Pinholes in gingival wall.

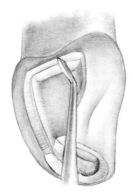

Fig. 10-35. Bevel gingival cavosurface angle.

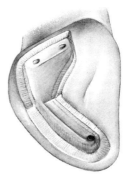

Fig. 10-37. Completed Class 4 preparation.

ARMAMENTARIUM
Torpedo-shaped diamond point
No. 170 bur
No. 169L bur
Torpedo-shaped white finishing stone
Finishing disks

1 Prepare the proximal groove (or box) as indicated with a No. 169L bur, usually parallel with the labial surface (Fig. 10-38, *C*). In canines this groove may be extended well labially on the distal aspect of the tooth without unduly displaying gold.

2 Place the mesioincisal pinhole with a No. 169L bur (Fig. 10-38, *A* and *B*).

3 Place the mesiolingual groove (Fig. 10-38, *A*) with the No. 169L bur. This groove should normally be placed on the lingual border of the mesial surface.

4 With a small torpedo-shaped diamond point, place a chamfer from the mesiolingual groove to the distolabial proximal wall. This reduction usually needs to be slight on mandibular canines (and mandibular incisors). The chamfer should include the gingival ends of the grooves.

5 Using a No. 170 bur (or an inverted cone bur, if preferred) place an incisal groove or finish line extending from the mesioincisal pinhole, below the incisal edge, to the distal proximal groove. Also place a groove or finish line from the mesioincisal pinhole to the mesiolingual groove.

COMMENT: *Placement of the groove or finish line from mesial to distal can usually conserve considerable incisal tooth structure. Also, it is seldom necessary to reduce the lingual surface of a mandibular anterior tooth more than illustrated (Fig. 10-38), the enamel being left intact except for margin reductions.*

The same general preparation can be applied to maxillary anterior teeth with the variation that the lingual surface must be reduced to allow for an adequate thickness of gold when required by occlusion.

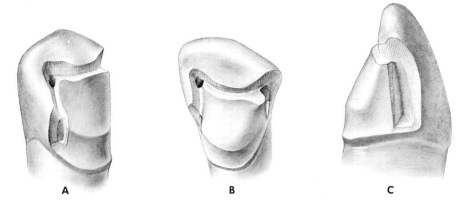

Fig. 10-38. Partial veneer crown preparation, lower right canine.

Class 5 gold inlays

Placement of gingival gold inlays is generally indicated when the size of the lesion does not make placement of cohesive gold or amalgam practicable.

Cavity preparation

ARMAMENTARIUM

No. 170 (171) bur
Wedelstaedt chisel

1 Establish the outline indicated, keeping the occlusal and ginigval walls slightly divergent to permit a line of draw (Fig. 10-39).
2 Plane the peripheral walls with a Wedelstaedt chisel, placing slight bevels. Finishing disks, where accessible, may be helpful in creating a sharp, well-finished margin.
3 Smooth the axial wall with a Wedelstaedt chisel.

Impression and finishing

Most Class 5 gold inlays lend themselves easily to direct waxing. Indirect procedures, where de-sired, are the same as for a Class 5 porcelain inlay as far as the impression is concerned.

Finishing is the same as that for any cast gold restoration. It is suggested that part of the sprue be left on the casting for trying the inlay in place. The sprue pin should facilitate removal of the inlay from the cavity, after which it may be removed prior to cementation.

CLASS 5 INLAY WITH PINS

Should the lesion be extensive, it may be desirable to add pins for increased retention.

Pin holes may be placed using a No. 169L bur (Figs. 10-40 through 10-42) or drilled for a nylon pin procedure. Placement obviously must avoid the pulp. Alignment may be accomplished by using a Chayes Loma Linda parallelometer, which can quickly be attached to a No. 212 or No. 16 clamp with compound (Figs. 10-43 and 10-44). The holes are then quickly drilled and the parallelometer removed (Fig. 10-45). The pattern may be waxed directly using nylon pins, or an indirect procedure may be elected.

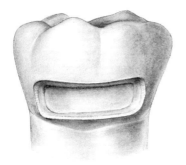

Fig. 10-39. Class 5 gold inlay preparation.

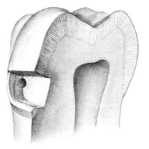

Fig. 10-41. Buccolingual cross section of Fig. 10-40.

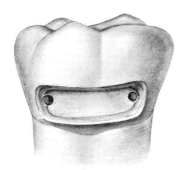

Fig. 10-40. Class 5 gold inlay preparation with pins.

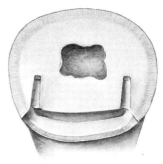

Fig. 10-42. Transverse cross section of Fig. 10-40.

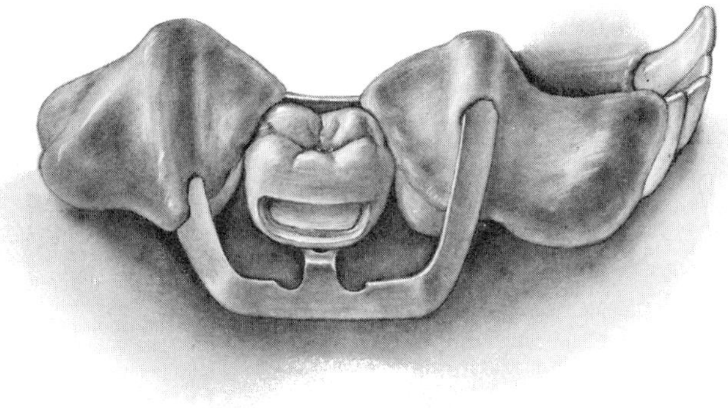

Direct wax pattern procedure

Since the introduction of elastic impression materials of various types, less emphasis is being placed on carving wax patterns directly in the mouth. For relatively simple cases, however, the procedure has merit, especially for single-surface restorations. Access for such cases generally allows the creation of the wax pattern in less time than that required to perform the steps necessary in an indirect procedure.

CLASS 2 DIRECT PATTERN

Obtaining a direct pattern for a Class 2 inlay is similar in some respects to an amalgam procedure in that it may utilize the same type of matrix bands and holders and carving instruments. In general, instruments for carving amalgam should be sharp, but they should not be so sharp for carving wax.

ARMAMENTARIUM

Matrix bands and holder
Contouring pliers or egg burnisher
Inlay wax
Explorer

1 Adapt a matrix band to the tooth, leaving it loose enough to slip easily onto the tooth. A copper band may also be used if preferred.
2 Contour the band in the area of the proximal restoration if indicated, using the contour pliers.
3 Lubricate the band lightly with a light oil.
4 Soften a stick of inlay wax slowly in a flame and fill the band. Place a thumb or finger on one open end of the matrix to contain the wax.
5 Lubricate the prepared tooth lightly with saliva.
6 Slowly heat the wax-filled matrix band. The wax must be heated slowly to allow the heat to penetrate it throughout. If the wax acquires a gloss, let it cool until the gloss disappears and the surface appears frosty.
7 Press the band and wax in place on the tooth and tighten the matrix slightly while firmly holding the wax and band in place with a finger.
8 Chill the wax with cold air.
9 Carve the occlusal surface. Use a large discoid carver to eliminate the bulk of the excess wax and use a sickle explorer or small Ward or Hollenback type of carver to remove the excess between the band and the marginal ridge, similar to carving amalgam. Refine the carving to the degree possible with the band in place using preferred instruments.

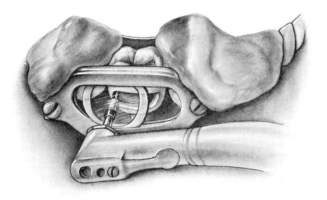

Fig. 10-43. No. 212 clamp in place and Class 5 inlay preparation.

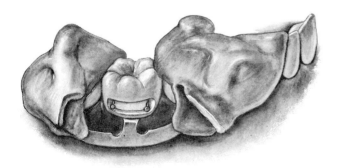

Fig. 10-44. Loma Linda parallelometer in place.

Fig. 10-45. Nylon pins in pinholes.

10 Loosen and remove the matrix band. Slip it out buccally or lingually while firmly holding the occlusal portion of the pattern with a finger.

11 Using a sickle explorer or a small Hollenback or Ward type of carver, remove the excess wax from the proximal margins.

12 The wax may be refined still further by carving. Polish it lightly with wet cotton. Always work and carve the wax toward the margins. The height of the marginal ridge should usually correspond to that of the adjacent tooth.

13 Use the explorer to remove the excess gingival wax. Use a regular sickle rather than a sharpened one as for amalgam. The rounded instrument will burnish the wax as well as carve it. Always hold the wax in place while carving, and always rest the carving instrument partly on tooth structure while carving along margins.

14 Pass a very fine thread between the wax pattern and adjacent tooth.

15 Warm a small gold staple (made from small-gauge gold wire), holding it with cotton pliers, and sink it into the occlusal surface of the wax. Allow it to cool.

16 Pass a ligature through the staple and gently remove the pattern. Inspect it for detail.

17 It is usually desirable to add a quantity of soft wax to the contact area. This is done carefully to avoid disturbing the pattern or involving the margins.

18 Sprue the pattern appropriately and carry out proper casting procedures.

Indirect inlay procedures

The advent and continued improvement in elastic materials that allow the accurate fabrication of dies have made it possible to perform much dentistry on the laboratory bench that was previously more difficult, if not impossible. These techniques are of great value, especially for crown and bridge procedures and extensive oral reconstruction.

It is because of extensive use of these procedures in crown and bridge techniques that, as applied to the operative field, they are relatively briefly outlined here. Excellent brochures on cast gold procedures are available from commercial companies, and much may be gained from studying them.

SOFT TISSUE RETRACTION

Reduction or retraction of the gingival tissue is essential when the margin of the preparation has been established below it. Techniques for accomplishing this include (1) rubber dam, (2) cotton pledgets and yarn in conjunction with chemicals, (3) surgery, and (4) electrosurgery.

Rubber dam

The ideal method of retracting soft tissue from the prepared margins is with a rubber dam. For operative purposes this is frequently possible. It is not always practicable, however, when, for example, full arch impressions are required or multiple teeth have been prepared.

Cotton pledgets and yarn

Probably the most popular procedures for tissue retraction use cotton material of some type impregnated with epinephrine. Commercially prepared pellets and yarns are available and are effective and efficient. Epinephrine (1% solution is recommended) may be used with four-strand cotton yarn, which can be obtained in department or variety stores.

For the Class 2 case the following routine is generally followed.

1 Remove the saliva from the gingival crevice with compressed air.

2 Moisten an elongated small cotton pledget with a 1% solution of epinephrine (commercial pellets may be used).

3 Gently press the cotton in place along the prepared margin, extending it beyond the proximal walls. Use a blunt-end blade of a large plastic instrument to place the cotton.

COMMENT: *Two paramount precautions must be observed during management of the soft tissue for impressions: (1) Do not use excessive pressure to gain tissue retraction. Various degrees of firmness are, of course, necessary in different cases, and it is essential that the margin be cleanly exposed to view to obtain a clear impression of it. However, excessive retraction is not desirable since permanent damage to the gingiva may result. Moreover, hemorrhage may be avoided if time is taken to gently induce the required retraction. Time is as important an ingredient as the materials used. (2) Excessive use of epinephrine may overexcite some patients. A very small amount may bring forth an untoward reaction in some individuals. Caution is suggested with people who are inclined to be overtense or who have organic problems that may contraindicate the use of epinephrine, which is rapidly absorbed through the mucosa and gingival tissues.*

If inflamed tissue is present, it may be helpful to precede the placement of the epinephrine pledget with a quick application of 1% zinc chloride as a styptic. Leave it only a few seconds, and thoroughly wash it off the tissues.

4 Leave the cotton in place for several minutes while the impression material is being readied.

5 Dry the area to be recorded with compressed air, and gently tease the cotton out.

6 Quickly inject the impression material, and proceed with the chosen impression procedure.

More difficult cases or preparations with extended prepared margins (three-quarter crowns) will usually require use of cord of some type. Following is a typical procedure.

1 Place an elongated wisp or pledget of cotton, moistened with epinephrine, along the prepared margin.

2 Over the cotton place two or three strands of cotton cord moistened with epinephrine. Loop the cord around the tooth, tie the first half of a knot to allow the cord to be retained when tightened slightly, and then gently, using plenty of time, press the cord in place around the margin. Tighten the cord and cut off the two ends close to the half knot on the buccal side of the tooth.

COMMENT: *Placement of the first cotton should aid in providing deeper retraction where indicated. If more bulk is desired, use three or all four strands of the cord. Sometimes a second, bulkier cord loop may be placed over the first.*

Electrosurgery

Electrosurgery and other similar techniques are advocated by some operators, but definite hazards accompany their use. They are likely to destroy more tissue than is desired, such loss occurring even after the restoration is completed.

Use of electrosurgery instruments seems contrary to the concept that all periodontal involvement should be under control prior to initiating restorative procedures.

Surgery

Again, periodontal problems should be corrected prior to restorative procedures. However, occasionally a difficult situation may be encountered in which the restorative dentist must operate well below the crest of the soft tissue. In such cases surgery can be decidedly helpful. Hemorrhage can be controlled by use of epinephrine and cotton procedures. When tissue is removed surgically, periodontal principles must be observed and the area of surgery protected during healing with an adequate dressing.

COMMENT: *Use care not to extend a preparation beneath the crest of the gingiva when the gingiva has recently received periodontal surgery and virtually no gingival sulcus remains. To attempt to do so may induce gingival recession.*

HYDROCOLLOID IMPRESSIONS

One of the most widely used materials for impressions by those operators engaging in extensive use of cast restorative procedures is hydrocolloid. Hydrocolloid is an extremely accurate material, economical to use, and easily controlled for use to reproduce extensive, multiple, or intricate restorations. Compared with other popular impression materials it also has the advantage of being functionally compatible with moist tissues where a rubber dam cannot be placed.

Following is the procedure commonly used for hydrocolloid.

ARMAMENTARIUM

Hydrocolloid conditioning unit with three adjustable tanks
Hydrocolloid
Selection of trays (solid rather than perforated trays are preferred)
Rubber tubing for chilling
Modeling compound (or wax)
Syringes, one with small point
Timer

The hydrocolloid is liquefied according to manufacturer's directions, usually by boiling for ten minutes. It is then stored in a tank at 160° F. The syringes are also loaded with sticks of hydrocolloid and boiled. They may be more critical and must be checked to assure adequate conditioning. They are also stored at 160° F.

1 When the tooth or teeth have been properly prepared and the tissue retraction procedure executed, prepare a suitable tray by placing hard wax or compound stops on each end. The wax- or compound-prepared tray is tried on the teeth and seated to the position desired. The stops provide stability while the hydrocolloid is chilled. Provide adequate space on all sides of the teeth to assure accuracy.

2 Load the tray with hydrocolloid and place it in the tempering tank (105° F.).

3 When the tray has been tempered for from three to five minutes, remove and wipe the surface water from the hydrocolloid.

4 As the assistant is removing the tray from the tempering bath, the operator teases out the retracting cotton, cleans the teeth with the air-water spray *leaving a film of water on the teeth,* and uses one of the syringes to inject hydrocolloid into the prepared cavity. Begin at the gingival point angles, cover the gingival wall, inject along the gingival crevice, then up into the occlusal portion of the cavity; at all times avoid trapped air.

5 Quickly place the loaded tray over the injected area and seat it onto the stops.

6 Chill the tray with cool (room temperature) water for a full five minutes, holding it absolutely stable. Temperatures below 55° F. may cause warpage.

7 Remove the tray sharply in a direction of the line of draw of the prepared teeth.

8 Inspect the impression for detail. A clear excess area around all gingival margins should be evident.

9 The operator must determine the extent of the models needed for laboratory procedures. If an extended area of occlusion is involved, full arch models are desirable, taken after sectional impressions have been obtained.

10 Paint the prepared tooth surfaces with a solution of para-monochloraphenol and corticosteroid and place appropriate interim protection on them.

MOUNTING CASTS

Face bow recordings and bite registrations are taken according to the needs of the case and ability of the operator.

If only a limited area (a tooth or two) is being restored, an excellent method of registering the bite is with the use of Duralay.* Mix a small amount of Duralay. As it becomes doughy, place a wad of it over some posterior teeth and have the patient close until set.

RUBBER IMPRESSIONS

Rubber impression materials are extensively used in cast gold procedures and have the distinct advantage of accepting silver plating. Silver plated dies are unexcelled in production of accurate casting.

Rubber impression materials must be used following the manufacturer's directions. Custom-made trays must closely conform to teeth to be reproduced. The material may be introduced into prepared cavities by means of instruments, syringes, or artists' brushes. Prepared channels (pinholes) may be easily reproduced by using Lentulo spirals to fill them with rubber.

POURING AND PREPARING THE WORKING DIE FROM HYDROCOLLOID IMPRESSIONS
ARMAMENTARIUM

Two colors of hardest setting die stones
Rubber bowl and spatula
Vacuum equipment
Brass dowel pins
Straight pins
Separating medium

As soon as the impression is completed, it should be rinsed free of saliva and placed in a 2% solution of potassium sulfate for ten minutes. It must be emphasized that no impression is ever as accurate as when it is first taken. It is therefore always advisable to pour impressions immediately.

1 Dust dry plaster into the impression and rinse it. The plaster should help in the removal of bits of saliva and blood.

2 Place straight pins from the buccal to the lingual aspect in the hydrocolloid over each prepared tooth and those adjacent.

3 Pour a layer of vacuumed stone into the impression of the teeth to a level 4 to 5 mm. above the gingival margin.

4 Place brass dowel pins adjacent to the straight pins in the direction of the long axis of the prepared teeth.

5 After the stone is set, blow the moisture off its surface and paint it with silica gel or die lubricant to ensure the separation of the dies from the next stone pour.

*Reliance Dental Mfg. Co., Shelby, N.C.

6 Pour a second layer of stone of a different color as a base to the model to a depth of the length of the brass dowel pins.

7 When the stone has reached its initial set, place it back in the potassium sulfate solution to set.

8 Separate the stone model from the hydrocolloid and allow it to dry thoroughly for at least a day or two.

9 Before trimming the model, use a thin-bladed jeweler's saw to separate the prepared die. Cut down to the level of the second stone pour.

10 Press the ends of the brass dowel pins to remove the dies.

11 Wet the remaining model and trim it as desired.

COMMENT: *Every effort must be made to avoid rinsing the dies in water. Stone is water soluble, and although difficult to observe, the fine sharp margins may be affected if washed in water. Therefore, the dies should be removed before trimming the model base, and the base should be redried before they are replaced in it. Any wetting of a stone die is undesirable.*

12 Use a large acrylic bur to remove stone below the gingival margin of the die.

13 Mount the model and its opposite member on a crown and bridge articulator.

SILVER-PLATED DIES

Although a detailed outline or production and use of silver dies is not presented here, their use is strongly recommended. A well-outlined procedure should be followed.[3]

WAXING THE PATTERN

Techniques of waxing occlusion and wax patterns are many and varied, and some are quite involved. Methods of waxing occlusion properly can use highly sophisticated procedures, which may be necessary to the needs of some cases. The procedure included here is a simple one in keeping with basic objectives of this atlas.

ARMAMENTARIUM

Inlay wax, regular or soft
Wax spatula
Die lubricant (Slickdie*)
Bunsen flame
Wax carvers

1 Lubricate the die.

2 Remove excess lubricant from the die with compressed air.

*Slaychris Products, Portland, Ore.

3 Flow wax onto the die with a wax spatula. A wax pen is highly recommended for waxing procedures of all types. Cotton pliers can also be used to carry wax to the die. Build up the bulk as indicated to the desired contour.

4 Carefully carve the proximal and gingival margins. Always use burnishing action to work the wax toward the margins. Avoid use of sharp carvers on stone die margins. The fingers can be used to condense and work the wax to the margins.

5 Lift the wax off the die to be certain it is not luted to it; reseat it.

6 Carefully establish the contact areas. Add wax or soften the wax in the contact areas and gently place the die in the model. Adjust the contacts approximately although not accurately at this time.

7 Wax the occlusal surface. "Wax-added" techniques are recommended. Occlusion can be checked with powdered zinc stearate to be certain of a balanced occlusal surface. Brush the powder onto the surface using a large soft brush. (Zinc stearate burns out cleanly with the wax during the burnout process.) Close the models together and open to observe occlusal contact through the zinc stearate dust.

8 Accurately finish the contact areas.

9 Sprue the pattern; short spruing is recommended.

10 Mount the sprue in a sprue former.

11 Line a casting ring with asbestos or other nonasbestos liner. Moisten the asbestos without compressing it.

12 Wash the wax pattern thoroughly with a detergent solution to clean it, and carefully rinse off the detergent to avoid the possibility of forming bubbles during the investing procedure.

13 Mix the casting investment, vacuumed thoroughly. Follow the manufacturer's directions precisely.

14 Pour the investment, being absolutely certain not to trap air.

15 Place the ring in a water bath at 100° F. for at least thirty minutes.

16 Remove the ring and warm the base to facilitate removal of the sprue if a metal sprue is used.

CASTING AND POLISHING

Two general concepts of casting are popular, so-called low-heat burnout and high-heat burnout. Also, differences of opinion exist as to whether the ring should be placed in the furnace with the temperature partially elevated. A great deal depends on the type of investment used and other variations in the procedure and technique up to this point.

The low-heat procedure is recommended since investments begin to break down at 1350° F.

1 Place the ring in a cold furnace.

2 Elevate the temperature to 900° F. for two hours.

3 Casting is best accomplished with use of a properly adjusted and managed gas-air flame. Use of fluxes should be minimal.

4 After casting remove the ring from the casting machine and allow it to bench cool at least until all the red color is gone.

5 Quench in water and remove the casting from the investment. Scrub the casting with a stiff toothbrush to remove all investment.

6 Boil the casting in a pickling solution, such as Prevox* or hydrochloric acid.

7 Place the casting in hydrofluoric acid for several hours to eliminate all traces of silica materials. This treatment may be reduced to several minutes with use of an ultrasonic tank.

8 Boil the casting in a soda solution.

9 Remove the sprue with a separating disk.

10 Contour the casting properly in the area of sprue removal.

11 Check all surfaces of the casting thoroughly using a magnifying glass to be absolutely certain no nodules or casting discrepancies exist. Use a found bur to remove nodules if found.

12 If stripping is desired (full or three-quarter crowns), do it at this time. Stripping is an electrolytic process of reducing the surfaces of a gold casting that abut the prepared cavity in the tooth. The margins and outer surfaces are protected by painting them with fingernail polish. The casting is then clipped to the anode of the stripping unit and dipped for several seconds into the solution contained in a tank, to which is attached the cathode.

The interior of the casting can also be reduced using aqua regia, but this process is less convenient. Stripping is recommended for full and three-quarter crowns. Fresh aqua regia will reduce a casting 25 microns, which is desirable to create space for cement. Markley feels it is more accurate and does not produce cyanide fumes. It

takes three minutes to remove 25 microns by stripping. An intimate overall fit is desirable to provide optimum cement thickness (25 microns). Excess cement thickness may reduce the life expectancy of the casting.

13 Carefully try the casting on the die. It should seat accurately.

14 Carefully seat the die in place on the model. Adjust the contact areas by polishing with rubber abrasive wheels until the desired degree of contact is established.

15 Adjust the occlusion.

16 Polish the casting using the following steps as appropriate: (a) light stoning, (b) abrasive rubber disks and points (c) tripoli-impregnated felt wheels, and (d) gold rouge–impregnated felt wheels.

17 Thoroughly clean the casting using a detergent. An ultrasonic cleaner is highly recommended.

18 Before trying the casting on the tooth or reducing (stripping) for cement it is recommended that its interior, occlusal surface, and contact areas be dulled or "frosted" using an air blast containing an abrasive powder. This may be accomplished using a device such as a Jelenko Handysander or an artist's air eraser, using powdered stone as the abrasive. (The abrasive sold with the eraser works fine, but stone is less expensive.) The frosty surface will enable the operator to easily see any high spots and make appropriate corrections. Highly polished gold is very difficult to mark while checking occlusion and contacts.

It is recommended that the areas ground to correct occlusion be repolished and the casting refrosted and left with this finish in the patient's mouth. This will enable the operator to evaluate occlusal function at subsequent visits. Over a period of time the luster returns to the casting. There seems to be no valid reason why a high glare on a finished gold casting is desirable anyway.

REFERENCES

1. Markley, M. R.: Pin retained and reinforced restorations and foundations, Dent. Clin. North Am., p. 229, March, 1967.
2. Bassett, R. W., Ingraham, R., and Koser, J. R.: An atlas of cast gold procedures, Buena Park, Calif., 1964, Uni-Tro College Press, p. 48.
3. Krug, R. S., and Markley, M. R.: Cast restorations with gold-foil–like margins, J. Prosthet. Dent. **22:**54, 1969.

---

*Williams Gold & Refining Co., Inc., Buffalo, N.Y.

FITTING THE CASTING IN THE TOOTH PREPARATION

ARMAMENTARIUM

G-2 and G-3 explorers
Dental floss (waxed)
Binangle inlay seater
Leather- or plastic-faced mallet
Articulating ribbon
B-46 gold file
Mouth mirror

1 The cavity preparation must be clean. Any debris in the preparation will prevent complete seating. It is helpful to clean the casting using an ultrasonic unit and appropriate solution.

2 Adjust proximal contacts.

a. If the contacts are too tight, relieve them carefully. If too light, the gap will need to be closed by adding solder.

(1) For slight reduction, use a $^7/_8$-inch fine garnet disk.

(2) For gross reduction, use a separating disk.

b. Continue relieving contacts until the casting can be seated properly.

c. Contact with approximating tooth must be positive but must not wedge the teeth apart. Test the location, size, and degree of contact using fine waxed floss and a mouth mirror. The floss should snap through contact with moderate apical pressure without shredding. If the floss does not meet any resistance when passing through the contact area, the contact must be built up with solder.

d. Adjustment of the proximal contacts should allow the inlay to seat completely. If there is a marginal discrepancy because of incomplete seating, one of the following may be the cause:

(1) Undercuts in preparation

(2) Distortion of the impression

(3) Nodule inside the casting

(4) Debris on the internal surface of the preparation

(5) Too much gold in the contact area

(6) Distortion of the wax pattern

e. If the marginal discrepancy of the casting on the tooth is greater than 0.1 mm., difficulty will be encountered in sealing the gold margins and an inferior clinical restoration will result.

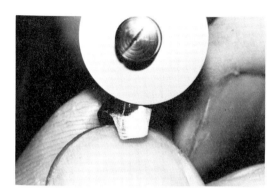

Fig. 11-8. Smoothing proximal surface.

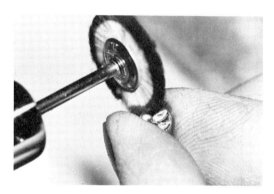

Fig. 11-9. Brush and tripoli are used to polish the occlusal anatomy.

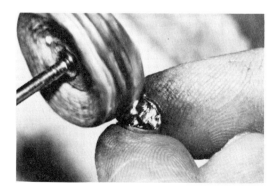

Fig. 11-10. Felt wheel and rouge used for final polish.

3 Adjust occlusion.

a. Seat the inlay completely with a mallet and a binangle inlay seater or use a wood stick.

b. Using articulating ribbon, mark areas of hyperocclusion (Fig. 11-11).

c. Remove high spots with a high-speed green stone or finishing bur. Relieve only within the anatomical form of the casting.

d. Removal of the inlay is most readily accomplished with the B-46 file by placing the serrations of the file against the casting in the interproximal embrasures and pulling in a coronal direction. A large excavating spoon may be better. It can be inserted with the flat surface of one blade on the surface of the inlay under a contact area. Tilt the blade slightly to engage the gold and life the casting.

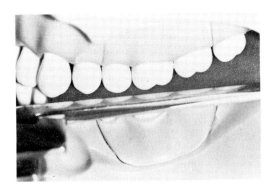

Fig. 11-11. Checking occlusion.

ADAPTATION (SPINNING) OF GOLD MARGINS

ARMAMENTARIUM

Spruole mandrel
³/₈-inch fine and medium garnet disks
F-2 burnisher
Rubber dam
Orange solvent
³/₈-inch fine cuttle disks
Instruments used to fit casting (previous section)

Adaptation of gold margins are done *on the tooth*—not on the die. (Krug and Markley, however, strongly recommend the use of silver dies, which allow finishing to be completed on the die.*) This procedure is most readily completed when the teeth are isolated under a rubber dam. Make sure the casting stays completely seated during the adaptation procedures. Any debris within the casting or preparation will cause incomplete seating and difficulty spinning margins closed. A cotton pellet with orange solvent will remove traces of rouge or tripoli from the inside of the casting (Fig. 11-12).

---

*Krug, R. S., and Markley, M. R.: Cast restorations with gold foil–like margins, J. Pros. Dent. **22**:54-67, 1969.

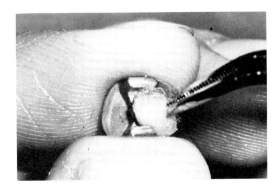

Fig. 11-12. Cotton pellet and solvent used to remove polishing media.

1. *Occlusal* (intracoronal castings, that is, MOD, MO, DO)
   a. Small, mounted stones work well to adapt gold to the anatomical form of the occlusal surface. The stone must rotate from gold to tooth (Fig. 11-13).
   b. The F-2 burnisher may be used to help smooth scratches formed by the stones.
2. *Proximal, buccal, and lingual*
   a. Use a fine 4/0 garnet disk, ³/₈-inch, mounted in a Spruole mandrel rotating from inlay to tooth (Figs. 11-14 to 11-16).
   b. If margins are accessible, use the mandrel in a straight handpiece. If not, use slow-speed contra-angle.
   NOTE: *Avoid using stones on bucco- and linguo-occlusal margins where cusps are covered, and avoid using stones interproximally. Enamel margins may be shattered and leave an inadequate gold seal.*
3. *Gingival*
   a. Marked excess can be reduced with a ⁷/₈-inch fine garnet disk in the Moore mandrel, holding the casting in the fingers.
   b. Proximogingival angles on tooth can be smoothed with a ³/₈-inch fine garnet disk rotating from gold to tooth.
   c. A gold file may be used to remove excess and to help burnish the gingival margin close to the tooth. (Fore the most part, gingival margins are finished by careful observation of fit with an explorer and by making the appropriate modifications with a cuttle disk and the casting in hand.
4. Do not place casting back on the die after reaching this point; the now friable margins may be destroyed.

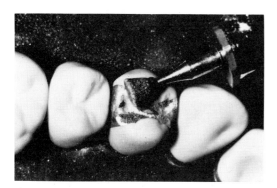

Fig. 11-13. A small stone is used to adapt gold to the occlusal margin.

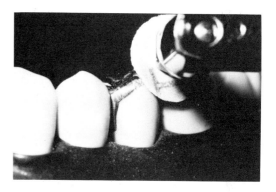

Fig. 11-15. Disking the buccal margins.

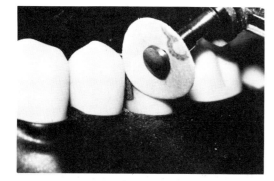

Fig. 11-14. A fine ³/₄-inch garnet disk is used to adapt proximal margins.

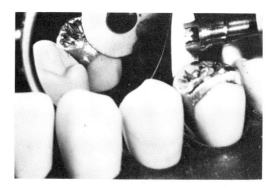

Fig. 11-16. Disking the lingual margin.

PREPARATION OF CASTING FOR CEMENTATION

1 Using a cotton pellet and chloroform, orange solvent, or ultrasonic cleaner, clean the inlay thoroughly, removing rouge and tripoli.

2 Carefully wash with soap and water and dry with air (avoid touching fragile gold margins).

3 Examine the casting for debris and curled margins.

4 The casting is now ready for cementation.

Cementation

ARMAMENTARIUM

Mallet
Inlay seater
Crown and bridge cement
Chilled glass or teflon pad
Cement spatula
E-1 or E-2 plastic instrument
Extra fine, extra narrow linen strip
F-2 burnisher
G-3 explorer
Slow-speed handpiece
Contra-angle (R.A.)
Soft rubber cup (R.A.)
Dappen dishes (3)
Polishing powders (such as, 303, 309 tin oxide)

1 Thoroughly clean the preparation. Meticulous attention must be paid to proper preparation of the tooth for cementation. All of the temporary material must be removed and the cavity scrubbed alternately with chloroform and hydrogen peroxide to remove all oil and pellicle. Then dilute acid may be used to remove pellicle, and the cavity is washed and dried. Saliva must not be allowed to cover the preparation again prior to cementation.

2 Mix cement in the prescribed manner.

3 Apply cement to all internal surfaces of casting and coat the cavity preparation (Fig. 11-17).

4 Seat casting.

a. Use heavy hand pressure.

b. Follow with light taps with a mallet and inlay seater (Fig. 11-18) until cement no longer exudes from margins. (Additional pressure may be gained by placing a cotton roll, rubber wheel, or stick on the occlusal surface of the inlay and having the patient bite.) A Medart pressure applicator is recommended.

c. With the F-2 burnisher, clear cement from the margins and burnish them down lightly to readapt the margins *before* the cement sets.

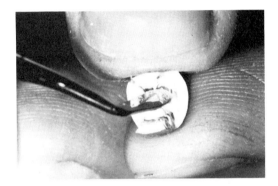

Fig. 11-17. Coating the internal surface with cement.

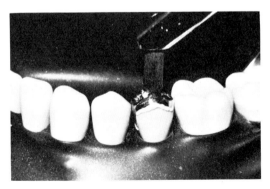

Fig. 11-18. Light mallet taps used with pressure to seat the casting.

FINAL POLISHING

1 Using an explorer, remove excess cement (Fig. 11-19). (If cement has not set, be sure to support the casting with an instrument.)

2 Clean contacts and embrasures using dental floss.

3 Final polishing

a. Smooth the proximal margins lightly using ³/₈-inch fine cuttle disks.

b. Gingival

   (1) Lightly strip the proximal margins using an extra narrow fine linen strip.

   (2) Finish with extra narrow, extra fine linen strip (Fig. 11-20).

c. Occlusal

   (1) Clean the anatomy with a cleoid carver.

   (2) Follow lightly with a burlew point.

d. Remove small scratches with wet 303 powder in a rubber cup. Cover the occlusal and proximal surfaces.

e. Complete the polish using 309 paste in rubber cup.

f. A high luster can be obtained by a final polish with dry 309 or tin oxide powder (Fig. 11-21).

g. Remove debris with explorer, air, and water (Fig. 11-22).

h. Remove the rubber dam and recheck the occlusion.

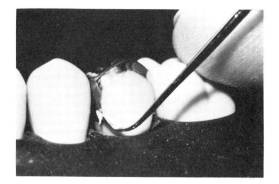

Fig. 11-19. Removing excess cement.

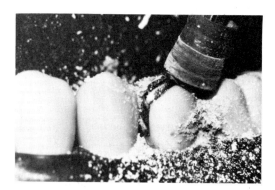

Fig. 11-21. Final polish.

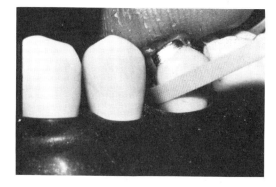

Fig. 11-20. Finishing strip on proximal surface.

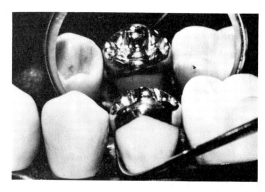

Fig. 11-22. Removal of polishing debris.

CHAPTER 12

TEMPORARY RESTORATIONS

A temporary restoration, as the name implies, is a restoration needed only for a short duration. It provides protection and function for the tooth until such time as the permanent filling material can be inserted and finished. A temporary restoration may also be used to stabilize an existing disease condition (such as rampant caries) until such time as definitive restorative procedures may be completed. Depending on the type of temporary material, its length of service may vary from a few days to several months. It should be inexpensive and easily and quickly placed and removed.

Functions

Functions of temporary restorations include:
1. Protection of dentin and pulp from thermal, chemical, and mechanical irritants that can cause hypersensitivity
2. Maintenance of occlusal relationships (prevent supraeruption)
3. Prevention of drifting (loss of mesiodistal dimension)
4. Protection and support of the gingiva (temporary restoration must have good gingival margins and axial contours)
5. Maintenance esthetics (anterior restorations)
6. Protection of margins of prepared teeth

The criteria for an *excellent temporary restoration* include:
1. Proper size and form for
   a. Patient comfort
   b. Esthetics
2. Proper axial contours
   a. Allow natural tissue stimulation by food
   b. Permit self-cleansing and patient maintenance
   c. Support gingival tissue in its natural position
3. Harmonious color (when visible—as in anterior teeth)

4. If a preparation is extended below the crest of the gingiva, the temporary restoration should terminate between the crest of the gingiva and the preparation margin to provide
   a. Support of soft tissue and to prevent food impaction (Food impaction can result in tissue recession.)
   b. Support of soft tissue to facilitate trial of final restoration
   If the margins of the temporary restoration are overextended, the gingival attachment may be damaged. If they are underextended, the tooth may become hypersensitive because of exposed dentin tubules.
5. Centric contact must be present to prevent supraeruption of prepared or opposing teeth (loss of vertical dimension)
6. Basic occlusal anatomical form should be present to allow mastication of food
7. A temporary restoration must be free from excursive interferences
   a. For patient comfort (to avoid occlusal trauma)
   b. To prevent dislodgment
8. Proximal contact is necessary
   a. To prevent drifting (loss of mesiodistal dimension)
   b. To prevent food impaction and tissue damage
9. A smooth polished surface is important
   a. For patient comfort
   b. To minimize plaque retention
   c. To minimize tissue irritation
   d. To facilitate patient and self-cleansing
10. A temporary restoration should have sufficient thickness and strength
    a. To withstand normal masticatory forces without deformation or fracture
    b. To minimize thermal sensitivity
11. A temporary restoration should be hermetically sealed (cemented) to the tooth
    a. To prevent pulpal irritation caused by tissue fluids, debris, and bacteria
    b. For patient comfort, that is, to eliminate pain caused by pulpal irritation
12. Exposed margins of the cavity preparation are covered
    a. For patient comfort (A rough surface may be irritating to tongue or adjacent soft tissue.)
    b. To prevent damage to the preparation

General categories of temporary restorations

An *interim restoration* is used when a tooth has been prepared and a second appointment is necessary to place the final restoration.

A *provisional restoration* is used as a diagnostic aid when the type or extent of the final restoration is to be determined by the patient's response to the temporary restoration that closely simulates the form or design of the intended final restoration. It is usually constructed of a less expensive material, such as acrylic, and should be easily modifiable.

An *"intermediate" restoration* is used when time to treat the patient is minimal and patient comfort and tooth protection are important. Zinc oxide and eugenol, crown and bridge cement, or any other material that is quickly placed is inserted into the tooth and definitive treatment is done at a later date.

Selection of the type of temporary restoration depends on:
1. Time (expected length of use)
2. Esthetic demands
3. Need for adjacent tooth stabilization
4. Extent of tooth involvement
   a. Amount of tooth structure remaining
   b. Whether or not missing teeth are to be replaced

Interim restorations

There are many varieties and combinations of interim restorations. These are used where the final cavity preparation is complete; therefore, the temporary restoration must:
1. Be easily inserted and removed without damage to margins or internal features of the preparation
2. Protect the cavity preparation from damage during the interim period

To comply with the requirement of ease of removal:
1. Various types of acrylic temporary restorations can be used only on preparations that draw (inlays, crowns, onlays).
2. Softer materials must be used for preparations that do not draw (that is, amalgam and foil preparations).
   a. Gutta-percha
   b. Zinc oxide and eugenol (ZnOE) preparations (Temp-Bond, Cavit)
   c. Aluminum shell (only if cusps are reduced or there is no opposing tooth)

ACRYLIC TEMPORARY RESTORATIONS

All acrylic temporary restorations must be cemented using a quick-setting zinc oxide–eugenol type of material.

Alginate impression technique (tooth generally intact or the dentist has a model for the alginate impression). This technique is useful in fabricating an acrylic temporary restoration for:

1. Full crown, onlay, and inlay preparations
2. Anterior or posterior teeth (especially where esthetics is important)
3. Single or multiple restorations
4. Short- or long-term protection

Celluloid crown form technique (for broken down teeth that have poor shape and require short- or long-term protection). The crown form is not the temporary restoration; it serves only as a matrix for the cold cure acrylic. This technique may be used when:

1. Individual anterior or bicuspid crown preparations require temporary protection.
2. There is extensive breakdown or fracture contraindicating use of the alginate impression technique.

Polycarbonate crown technique

1. Indications are the same as celluloid crown form, but the crown becomes the outer shell of this acrylic temporary restoration.
2. The polycarbonate shell is festooned to fit the tooth, filled with cold cure acrylic, and placed on the tooth to set. After it is set, it is removed from the tooth, the excess flashing is removed, and the temporary restoration is polished and cemented on the tooth preparation for short- or long-term protection.

Vacuum-form technique (used especially where there is more than one preparation). The vacuum-form technique:

1. Requires a plaster model to form the plastic matrix
2. Is useful for either short- or long-term protection

The plastic template is trimmed to cover teeth requiring temporary protection and, when possible, at least one tooth mesial and distal to area requiring the temporary restoration. The adjacent teeth serve as an index for the plastic template.

Cold cure acrylic is poured into the vacuum-formed plastic. It is inserted over the patient's prepared teeth. Similar to celluloid form, vacuum plastic serves only as a matrix and is not part of the temporary restoration. The set acrylic is festooned to fit teeth and cemented on with calcium hydroxide or zinc oxide and eugenol.

GUTTA-PERCHA (a gum rubber)

1. Gutta-percha may be used in any small Class 1, 2, 3, or 5 preparation that is not in heavy occlusion.
2. A disadvantage is that gutta-percha tends to separate adjacent teeth in Class 2 restorations.
3. Another disadvantage is that gutta-percha does not seal well, often resulting in tooth sensitivity; it must be used with eucalyptol solvent to obtain a better seal to the tooth.
4. Gutta-percha is used for short-term protection.

ZINC OXIDE AND EUGENOL (Temp-Bond, Cavit)

1. Zinc oxide and eugenol may be used in any small Class 1, 2, 3, or 5 preparations.
2. Zinc oxide and eugenol is for short term use.
3. Zinc oxide and eugenol may be reinforced with cotton fibers.
4. Zinc oxide and eugenol has the advantages of being generally sedative to the tooth and a good seal.
5. A disadvantage of zinc oxide and eugenol is that it does not stand up well under heavy occlusion.

ALUMINUM SHELL (anatomical preformed crown, anodized)

1. Aluminum shells are used primarily on posterior teeth since they are not tooth colored.
2. Aluminum shells may be used where the preparation is a three-quarters crown, full crown, onlay preparation, or amalgam preparations when cusps are to be restored or the tooth is not in occlusion.
3. An aluminum shell may be used for one or two weeks (longer depending on how well it stands up under use).
4. An aluminum shell must be shaped to protect preparation margins and provide proper occlusion.
5. Seal and retention is provided by temporary cement, either zinc oxide and eugenol or calcium hydroxide.
6. The primary disadvantage of this type of temporary restoration is the metallic taste (except for anodized varieties) or galvanic action caused by dissimilar metals in the mouth.

GOLD CROWN OR INLAY

1. A gold crown or inlay may be used if time does not permit finishing and cementation of a casting.
2. A casting may be used if it is necessary to redo the restoration.
3. Cast gold temporary restorations are cemented on with either zinc oxide and eugenol or calcium hydroxide and may be used for several months.

Provisional restorations

1. Provisional restorations usually are custom acrylic and often involve multiple restorations.
2. Provisional restorations are used as diagnostic aids usually when altering:
   a. Occlusion (decreasing or increasing vertical dimension) to determine patient acceptance
   b. Size and shape of teeth
3. Provisional restorations are used as diagnostic aids to evaluate soft tissue or tooth response when:
   a. Periodontal surgery is either contemplated or has been completed
   b. Teeth have a questionable prognosis:
      (1) Minimal tooth remaining
      (2) Deep pockets
      (3) Excessive mobility

ADVANTAGES

1. There is minimal financial investment needed to test the response before expensive castings are made.
2. The temporary restoration may be readily altered if modifications or corrections are necessary.
3. The temporary restoration simulates the form of the final restoration.
4. It may be used for anterior or posterior restorations.
5. It has a medium long–term usefulness (one to three years before remake).
6. Teeth are prepared to desired cavity form.

FABRICATION

1. Diagnostic models (study casts) are mounted on an articulator.
2. Teeth are prepared on the diagnostic model.
3. A diagnostic waxup is completed.
4. An alginate impression of the diagnostic waxup is made to make a diagnostic stone cast of the waxup.

5. The alginate impression may be used directly to fabricate the temporary restoration or a vacuum-form plastic shell can be made of the diagnostic stone cast. (Do not use diagnostic waxup directly on vacuum-form machine since the wax will melt.)
6. The temporary restoration is then made from the vacuum-form with cold cure acrylic.

Intermediate restorations

Intermediate restorations are used when the tooth is broken down because of caries or trauma.

1. Intermediate restorations may be used for moderate periods of time.
2. No definitive tooth preparation is necessary.
   a. Decay is removed and a medication is placed.
   b. Retentive undercuts or pins are placed. (Acid etch may be used if composite resin is used.)

INDICATIONS

The indications for intermediate restorations are:

1. Where there is rampant caries or poor gingival health (disease control)
2. Where pulpal or periodontal prognosis is questionable (wait until outcome is clear)
3. As a maintenance program:
   a. When patient cannot afford treatment (cost)
   b. When patient attitude is a problem (does not care about tooth, expects "to have dentures anyway")
4. For patient comfort (until a more permanent restoration can be made)—when time is a factor or when patient was seen on an emergency basis
5. When esthetics is critical (that is, fracture of an anterior tooth where composite resin is used as a temporary restoration and a crown will eventually be necessary)
6. As a buildup of extensively broken down or involved teeth that will receive a crown later
   a. Pin amalgam
   b. Pin composite

TYPES OF INTERMEDIATE RESTORATIVE MATERIALS

The following is a list of types of intermediate restorative materials:

1. Strong cements
   a. Crown and bridge cement (zinc phosphate)
   b. Carboxylate cement—posterior teeth
2. Crown and bridge cement and alloy—posterior teeth
3. I.R.M. (ZnOE and modifiers)—posterior teeth
4. Composite resin (acid etch) and pin (if needed)—anterior teeth
5. Composite and alloy and pin (Class 2) (used as a buildup for crown to be placed later)—posterior teeth
6. Amalgam and pin (Class 2) (used as a buildup for crown to be placed later)—posterior teeth

TECHNIQUES FOR USING VARIOUS MATERIALS
Gutta-percha

Gutta-percha is a rubberlike material commonly packaged in the form of thin sheets. It must be softened by warming and then forced into the cavity preparation. It is used primarily in small restorations such as amalgam, inlay, or gold foil where there is no cusp coverage. Gutta-percha is somewhat soft and will abrade and wash away; therefore, it may be used for only short durations (one to two weeks).

Gutta-percha is fairly easy to apply. A small square of material with a volume slightly greater than the area to be filled is cut from the original sheet. This is grasped in a pair of cotton pliers and very gently warmed over a flame until it is softened throughout (Fig. 12-1). Overheating will cause the gutta-percha to burn. The material is hot enough when it begins to slump. Grasp the

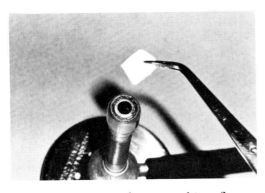

Fig. 12-1. Gutta-percha warmed in a flame.

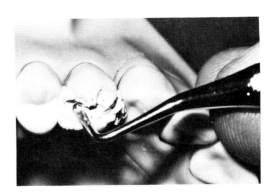

Fig. 12-3. Forcing gutta-percha into the prepared cavity.

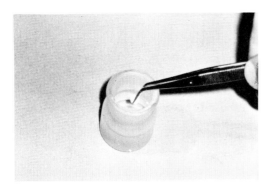

Fig. 12-2. Gutta-percha rolled into a ball and dipped into eucalyptol.

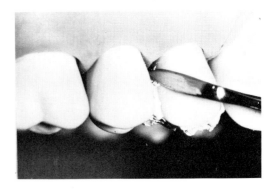

Fig. 12-4. Excess is trimmed away.

warmed gutta-percha in the fingers, roll it into a ball, and dip the ball into a bottle of eucalyptol using cotton pliers (Fig. 12-2). While the gutta-percha is still soft, it is carried to the preparation and forced into the cavity using an amalgam condenser (Fig. 12-3). Caution must be used when placing the material that it is not so hot as to overheat and injure the pulp. The excess gutta-percha found interproximally is removed with a warmed Hollenback carver (Fig. 12-4). The heated end of a plastic instrument can be used to shape the occlusal anatomy (Fig. 12-5). The temporary restoration should provide a smooth comfortable surface that will not irritate or chafe the patient's mouth (Fig. 12-6). The gutta-percha must be dipped into eucalyptol (a solvent for gutta-percha) before placing it in the preparation to form a hermetic seal. If this is not done, it will leak around the margins and tooth sensitivity will result.

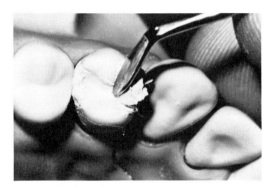

Fig. 12-5. Heated plastic instrument is used to shape the occlusal surface.

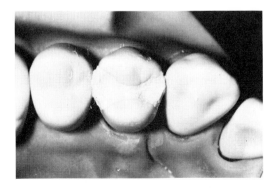

Fig. 12-6. Completed temporary restoration.

Zinc oxide–eugenol cement

Zinc oxide–eugenol cement is supplied as a pastelike material or as a powder or liquid that can be used alone for rather short-duration temporary restorations (up to one week). It is also used as a cementing medium for aluminum shell and acrylic temporary restorations, which will be described later.

Since the material is rather weak after it has set, it may be reinforced to a limited extent using cotton fibers. Zinc oxide and eugenol may be used in similar situations as those described for gutta-percha. It is also limited to restorations that do not involve cusp reduction.

The material is mixed as directed by the manufacturer, and while mixing, cotton fibers may be incorporated into the mix. The material should be placed into a wet cavity with a plastic instrument and the excess material quickly removed. The surface is smoothed with a moistened cotton pellet and contoured to provide proper occlusion and comfort. The set material may be easily shaped using a round bur at slow speeds.

Crown and bridge cement

Unlike the materials previously described, crown and bridge cement should not be used in preparations that have been finished; it is difficult to remove without damage to the preparation. It may be used on a patient who has rampant caries where the initial therapy is to control the decay process. Once the decay has been removed, the necessary cavity liner or base is placed. Retentive undercuts are formed to hold in the cement. The cement is mixed according to the manufacturer's directions, inserted into the cavity, contoured, and smoothed. This material may be used for relatively long periods of time (up to eight or more months). It may be used in areas of occlusion, if necessary, without too much of a problem. Its main limitation to the duration of use is that it tends to wash out or wear away with time. It should be used only for such time as needed until more definitive restorative measures can be employed.

Aluminum shells

Aluminum shell temporary restorations are indicated for temporary maintenance of teeth when there has been cusp reduction. They may be used for durations of about one month or more, the main limitation being that the temporary cementing media often break loose and the aluminum shell may fall off. If the shell has not worn through or been distorted beyond repair, it may be recemented with a fresh mix of temporary cement.

Aluminum shells are supplied in an assortment of sizes. Select a size that will fit over the tooth and yet provide proximal contact (Fig. 12-7). The shell will usually be longer than necessary. Using crown and bridge scissors, trim off enough metal (Fig. 12-8) to allow the shell to extend just beyond the gingival margin of the preparation. If the gingival margin extends around the tooth, the metal should be trimmed (festooned) to follow the height of tissue just within the dental sulcus but

must *not* impinge on soft tissue. This may require trying the shell on the tooth several times to check the extension of the metal. To aid in orienting the shell in the same direction each time, a mark can be scratched on the buccal surface.

With the shell in place, crease the occlusal surface in a mesiodistal direction with the end of a plastic instrument or burnisher (Fig. 12-9). This will initially establish the occlusal form of the temporary restoration. Have the patient close. The aluminum should be soft enough to be further shaped by the opposing tooth (Fig. 12-10). Clinically, care must be taken at this point to assure that the metal of the gingiva is not overextended

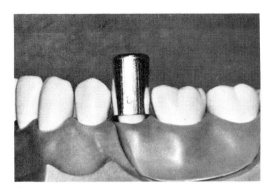

Fig. 12-7. Select the proper size aluminum shell.

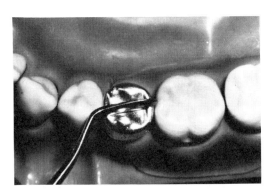

Fig. 12-9. Shape (crease) the occlusal surface.

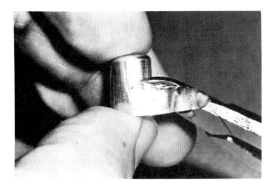

Fig. 12-8. Trim off excess length.

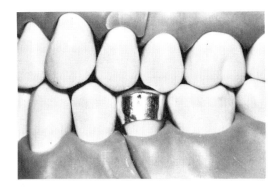

Fig. 12-10. Check extension of the aluminum shell.

(Fig. 12-10). If this occurs and the patient is allowed to close, the gingival attachment may be stripped. Overextension is usually evident by the tissue blanching where there is excess length of metal impinging on the tissue. The occlusal surface should now allow the remaining posterior teeth to come into full occlusal contact. The occlusal form is purely a functional shape and not usually a thing of beauty (Fig. 12-11).

A window may be cut on the buccal and lingual surface where the tooth surface has been left untouched. This does produce a slightly more esthetic temporary restoration, although an acrylic temporary restoration would be a better choice if esthetics are important. The outline of the window is scribed with a pointed instrument (Fig. 12-12) and trimmed with a pair of small curved scissors. A white rubber wheel is used to smooth the burred edge of the temporary restoration to prevent cheek or tongue irritation (Fig. 12-13).

The margins of the temporary restoration are sealed to the tooth with burnishers or the end of a plastic instrument when the temporary restoration is cemented to the tooth (Fig. 12-14). Any calcium hydroxide or zinc oxide–eugenol cement can be used to cement this temporary restoration to the tooth.

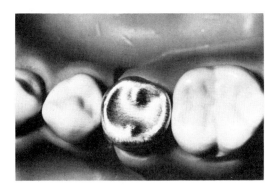

Fig. 12-11. Occlusal form.

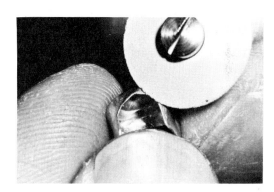

Fig. 12-13. Smooth the edges.

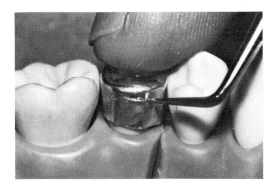

Fig. 12-12. Scribe outline to be removed.

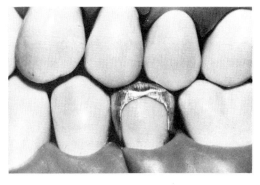

Fig 12-14. Margins sealed to tooth.

Custom-made acrylic

Acrylic temporary restorations can be used successfully only for preparations designed to receive a cast restorative material (gold inlays, crowns, and bridges). If there are any mechanical undercuts in a preparation, it is very difficult, if not impossible, to remove the acrylic material once it has set without damaging the preparation. A temporary material that is easy to remove without damaging the preparation is necessary for amalgam preparations. Acrylic temporary restorations are very useful if a temporary restoration is needed for a prolonged period of time or where esthetics is necessary. They may be used to protect the tooth and provide function for several months to a year. Because the acrylic material will not seal to the tooth by itself, it must be made, contoured, and finally cemented to the tooth with a zinc oxide–eugenol or a calcium hydroxide cementing medium.

Acrylic temporary alginate impression technique

ARMAMENTARIUM

Impression tray
Acrylic (tooth-colored)
Hemostat
Small paint brush
Cotton pliers
Soft rubber abrasive wheel
Pumice
Whiting
Bard Parker No. 15 scalpel
No. 6 round bur
Petrolatum jelly
Separating disk
Acrylic bur
Mixing bowl and spatula
Alginate
Gold knife
Rag wheel
Dappen dish

1 Before beginning the tooth preparation, take an alginate impression of the teeth in the area of the tooth that will require a temporary restoration (Fig. 12-15). To accurately reposition the impression during the fabrication of the temporary restoration, the impression must include several teeth on each side of the tooth to be prepared. It there are irregularities in tooth form caused by fracture, caries, and so forth, these should be filled in with utility or other soft wax before the impression is taken.

2 If study casts are available, the involved tooth can be reshaped in wax. Soak the model for a minute or two and lubricate it with soap and then take an alginate impression of the involved area on the study model.

3 Wrap the impression in a wet paper towel and set it aside until it is time to make the acrylic temporary restoration.

4 After the tooth is prepared and the impression is taken for fabricating the casting, any undercuts remaining should be blocked out with calcium hydroxide cement to prevent locking the acrylic on the tooth. Lightly coat the prepared tooth and adjacent area with petrolatum jelly to help prevent acrylic from sticking to the tooth. The prepared tooth should not be dried but allowed to remain wet with saliva.

5 Trim away excess peripheral or vestibular alginate from the impression with a scalpel (Fig. 12-15) and remove any interproximal alginate to allow greater visibility when reseating the impression.

6 Warm the impression in hot water to accelerate the setting time of the acrylic.

7 Select the proper color of cold cure acrylic and mix to a heavy fluid consistency in a dappen dish. Carefully pour mixed acrylic into the depression of the tooth requiring the temporary restoration. Avoid trapping air bubbles since these will leave voids in the temporary restoration.

8 Allow the acrylic to reach a soft doughy consistency and then seat the impression back in the mouth. Care must be used to accurately reposition the impression on the teeth. If it is forced down on the teeth too hard, the occlusal surface of the temporary restoration will be thin and distorted (Fig. 12-16) and will not be in occlusion. If the impression tray is not seated far enough, the temporary restoration will be elongated and high in occlusion (Fig. 12-16).

9 Allow the impression to remain in place one to three minutes until it reaches a rubbery consistency. If some excess acrylic is visible around the edge of the seated impression, it can be tested from time to time to determine when it is set.

10 Remove the impression. The temporary restoration will usually remain on the tooth. If the temporary material is still in the impression:
　a. Carefully reseat the impression and allow it to set completely.
　b. Tease the temporary material out of impression and allow the acrylic to harden on the tooth.

If the temporary material remains on the tooth, quickly scrape any thin scrylic away from the margins of the preparation using a sharp carver; depending on the consistency of the acrylic, it may be necessary to pinch off the excess to avoid tearing the temporary material (Fig. 12-17).

Excess acrylic will generally be located interproximally and, if allowed to remain and harden, can lock the temporary material on the tooth. This should be removed or reshaped with a sharp gold knife (Fig. 12-18).

11 Gently loosen the temporary material from the preparation with the carving instrument before it has completely set and then reseat it on the tooth. This will help assure that it will not become locked in the preparation when it has completely set.

12 While the acrylic is still soft, have the patient close into centric occlusion to reshape it.

13 Occasionally the acrylic will be completely set when the impression is removed. When this occurs, it may be difficult to remove it from the tooth. Usually the major area holding the temporary restoration in place is the excess acrylic in the gingival embrasures. In any case, remove as much excess flashing as may be on the adjacent teeth and around the preparation. A gold knife may be required to trim away the excess in the gingival embrasures.

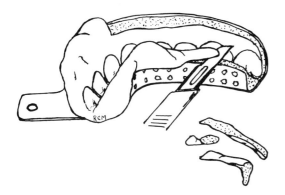

Fig. 12-15. Trimming excess from alginate impression.

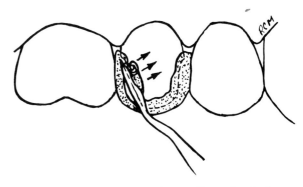

Fig. 12-17. Carving or pinching off acrylic flashing.

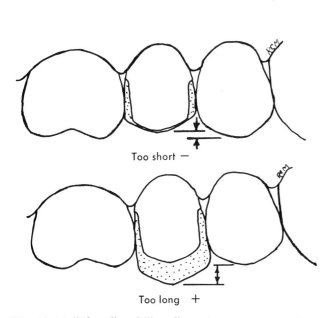

Fig. 12-16. "Short" and "long" acrylic patterns resulting from placing the alginate matrix too firmly or not completely seating it.

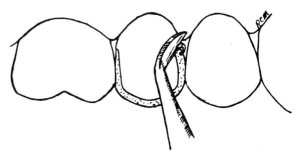

Fig. 12-18. Gold knife used to remove interproximal excess.

When satisfied that the excess has been removed sufficiently to remove the temporary restoration, take a straight chisel and, engaging it interproximally away from margins of the preparation (Fig. 12-19), lightly tap the chisel with the mallet in an occlusal direction. If an adequate thickness of acrylic is exposed to engage the temporary restoration, a pair of hemostats can be used to loosen and remove it.

14 When the acrylic has completely set and the temporary restoration is removed, excess flashing (Fig. 12-20) and recontouring can be done with a $^{7}/_{8}$-inch separating disk and/or acrylic bur (Fig. 12-21).

It is often possible to see the location of the finish line of the preparation on the temporary material since the acrylic usually will extend beyond the margin of the preparation into the gingival sulcus (Fig. 12-21). This line can be marked with a sharp pencil to serve as a guide to prevent overtrimming.

15 Voids or deficiencies at the margins can be repaired by adding acrylic with a small paint brush to pick up powder and monomer located in separate dappen dishes. Fill voids (Fig. 12-22) and allow the temporary restoration to remain on the tooth until the additional acrylic has set. After it has set, trim away any excess and adjust contours.

16 Check the occlusion and make any adjustments with a large round bur or fissure bur and restore the occlusal anatomy.

17 Smooth the temporary restoration with a soft rubber wheel and polish it with a wet rag wheel on a lathe first using pumice and then whiting.

18 The temporary restoration should be rinsed and dried and may be cemented with zinc oxide and eugenol or calcium hydroxide.

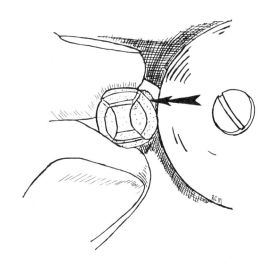

Fig. 12-21. Disk used to remove marginal flashing.

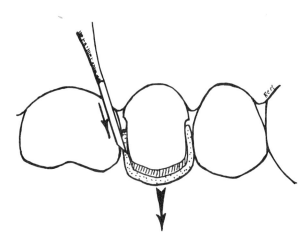

Fig. 12-19. Chisel used to remove the temporary restoration.

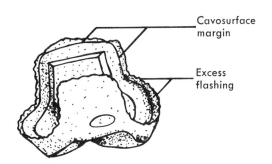

Fig. 12-20. Detail of an unfinished acrylic temporary restoration.

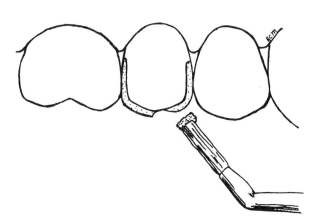

Fig. 12-22. Brush used to add to a deficiency.

One variation of the alginate impression of the tooth that will require a temporary restoration prior to cutting the preparation. The patient's occlusion is checked. The tray is tried on to check the fit. Reference points are selected to allow proper repositioning of the teeth during the impression procedure (Fig. 12-23).

Alginate is mixed and a small amount is wiped into the occlusal detail of the tooth (Fig. 12-24). The remaining alginate is loaded into the tray and an impression is taken (Fig. 12-25). The impression is stored in a wet paper towel. The cavity preparation is then completed (Fig. 12-26). The occlusal clearance is checked to assure adequate thickness of gold in the areas of occlusion (Fig. 12-27). A thin area of acrylic in an occlusal contact will weaken the temporary material. Excess alginate is trimmed from the impression to allow replacement in the mouth. Moisture is blown from the impression to prevent contamination of the acrylic.

The acrylic may be mixed in a dappen dish and poured into the impression or it may be mixed in the impression of the tooth. With an eyedropper,

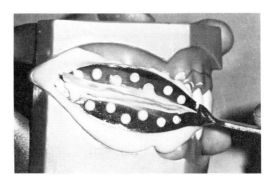

Fig. 12-25. Check-Bite impression tray and alginate in place.

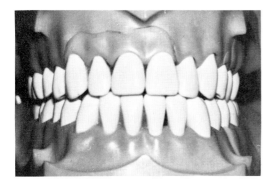

Fig. 12-23. Check occlusal reference points.

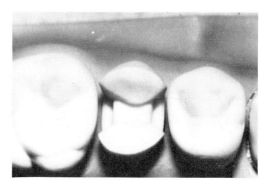

Fig. 12-26. Completed cavity preparation.

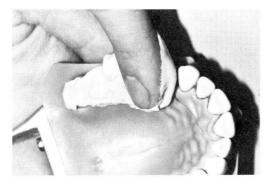

Fig. 12-24. Wiping a small amount of alginate onto the occlusal surface of the unprepared teeth.

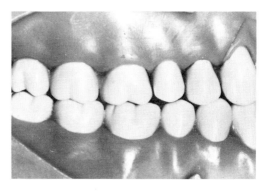

Fig. 12-27. Check the occlusal clearance.

place one drop of monomer in the proper area of the impression (Fig. 12-28). Place enough powder to absorb the monomer (Fig. 12-29). Add more monomer and powder until there is enough acrylic present to make the temporary restoration. Monomer and powder are added in small increments to prevent the excess acrylic from flowing into the impression of the adjacent teeth. Reseat the impression and have the patient close down so the teeth are back in their original position in the impression.

Allow the acrylic to set to a rubbery consistency, remove the impression, and using a Hollenback carver clear the gingival embrasures (Fig. 12-30) and excess acrylic flashing. Tease the temporary material off before it hardens to be sure it will not lock onto the tooth. Replace the tempo-

rary material on the tooth and allow the acrylic to set. When set, it is removed and excess marginal flashing and contour are corrected using a separating disk (Fig. 12-31). Place the temporary restoration back on the tooth and check for submarginal areas or voids with an explorer (Fig. 12-32). An submarginal areas can be corrected by painting on acrylic in these areas (Fig. 12-33).

The temporary restoration is smoothed with a white rubber wheel (Fig. 12-34). A round bur can be used to define the occlusal anatomy (Fig. 12-35), and a soft brush wheel can be used with pumice and whiting to polish the acrylic (Fig. 12-36). The occlusion is checked with marking paper and adjusted if necessary (Fig. 12-37). Usually very little adjustment is necessary with this technique if done properly.

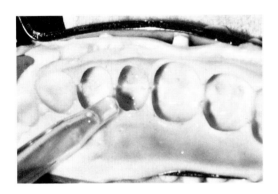

Fig. 12-28. Place acrylic monomer into the tooth impression.

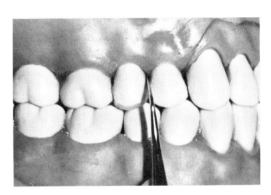

Fig. 12-30. Use a carver to clear the embrasure areas.

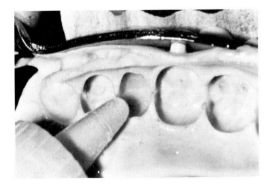

Fig. 12-29. Fill the impression with sufficient powder to form the temporary restoration.

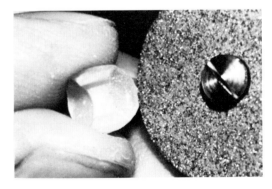

Fig. 12-31. Remove flashing using a disk.

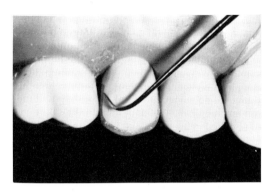

Fig. 12-32. Check for possible deficiencies.

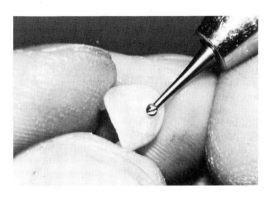

Fig. 12-35. Round bur is used to define the occlusal anatomy.

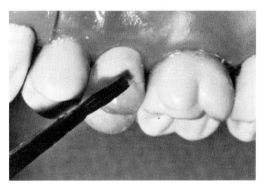

Fig. 12-33. Paint acrylic into deficiencies.

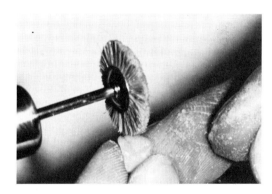

Fig. 12-36. Polish with pumice and whiting.

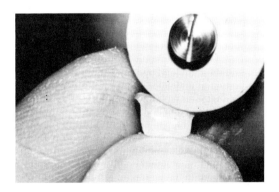

Fig. 12-34. Smooth with a rubber wheel.

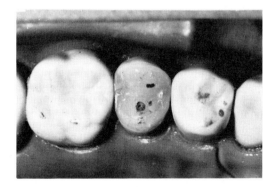

Fig. 12-37. Check the occlusion.

CHAPTER 13

RESINS

Two types of resins are in general use in restorative dentistry: acrylic resins and so-called composite resins. Each type possesses distinct advantages and disadvantages, and their use must be selected in accordance with these characteristics and the restorative functions to be demanded of them.

Use of acrylic resin has been somewhat controversial since its introduction, and its advantages and disadvantages had to be compared largely with those of silicate cement (Chapter 8). Since the development of composite resins, however, use of silicate cements and acrylic resins seems to be declining rapidly in favor of the newer materials.

Acrylic resin

Acrylic resins (polymethyl methacrylate) possess several advantages: (1) they have a high level of esthetic compatibility, (2) they accept a high-luster finish, and (3) they are easy to place. In fact their ease of placement and initial appearance tends to invite their use in unwarranted situations.

Their disadvantages are chiefly as follows: (1) a high modulus of elasticity, (2) a high coefficient of thermal expansion relative to tooth structure, and (3) softness or lack of resistance to abrasion. These factors preclude their recommended use in large areas and/or when the material will be subjected to stress. Their use in restorative dentistry has been largely displaced by filled resins.

Cavity preparations

Cavity preparations for acrylic resins are much the same as those outlined for composite or filled resins, which follow later in this chapter. Retention areas should be emphasized, however, because of their thermal coeffiencient of expansion and elasticity.

Insertion

The material should be managed following the manufacturer's directions. The mechanics of insertion are generally similar to those for other tooth-colored restorative materials described later. However, acrylic resins in current use are quite thin when mixed in bulk and are quite easily flowed into prepared cavities.

NEALON TECHNIQUE

A brush method of placing acrylic resin into prepared cavities advocated by Nealon[1] had the advantage of minimizing shrinkage during polymerization. It is used when a matrix is difficult to use, such as for Class 5 cavities.

The technique employs a fine sable brush and two dappen dishes. (Additional dappen dishes may be used if desired to minimize "contamination" of the monomer as the material is placed.) Place the monomer (liquid) and polymer (powder) in separate dishes. Moisten the brush slightly with monomer and touch it lightly to the polymer to form a small bead on the tip of the brush. Then touch it to a cavity wall. Wipe the brush clean (use a separate dish of monomer if desired) and place another increment of material (monomer and polymer) as described. Small increments are thus placed to build the material to the desired contour.

Finishing

Finishing acrylic restorations is generally the same as described for composite resins. However, they are comparatively soft, thereby demanding special caution. Final finishing for acrylic is achieved by polishing with flour of pumice and a soft rubber cup, followed by a high-shine powder such as tin oxide.

188

Composite resins

The generally used term *composite* is derived from the use of glass, silica, or tricalcium phosphate fillers contained in a resin compound of some type of epoxide molecule. The fillers make up approximately 75% to 80% of the compound by weight.

Composite resins have been widely accepted in place of silicate cements and acrylic resins.

The main advantages of composite resins are their relatively similar coefficient of thermal expansion to tooth structure, their strength, and their resistance to abrasion. The latter characteristic, however, is only of advantage compared to silicate cement and acrylic. Clinically, loss of the material in many cases is evident over a period of time.

Disadvantages of composite resisns include the following: (1) the finished surface is rough, (2) they are subject to wear, and (3) they may abrade opposing surfaces if placed in functional occlusion. Their use for Class 2 restorations is highly questionable and should be elected only as a compromise to metal restorations when esthetics is a critical factor.

Indications and contraindications

1. Composite resins are indicated where the surfaces to be restored are readily visible, esthetics thereby being a primary factor. Composite resins properly placed and finished may be nearly invisible to the untrained eye.
2. Gold foil is superior to composite resins in surface smoothness and marginal adaptation and is therefore preferred when there is limited extension onto the labial surface in Class 3 restorations, or when the restoration will be in extensive contact with soft tissue, such as in Class 5 restorations.
3. Composites may be used instead of gold foil if cost is a limiting factor.
4. Composite restorations are clinically superior to silicate cement in that they are insoluble in oral fluids, unaffected by mouth breathing, less irritating to the pulp, and much more resistant to abrasion.
5. Composite resins are affected less by temperature extremes, polymerization shrinkage, and abrasion than unfilled resins. Because composite resins are compounds of both fillers and resin, they are more difficult to polish than either resin or silicate restorations.

6. Composite resins may serve effectively as temporary Class 4 restorations, especially where the incisal angle is fractured or otherwise involved.
7. Composite resins can be used as a temporary material in anterior and posterior teeth, where esthetics is a major factor, until a more permanent restoration can be placed.
8. Composite resins have been suggested for use in Class 2 cavities; however, at the present time it is recommended that this use be limited to nonfunctioning surfaces where esthetics is the determining factor because:
   a. It is difficult to insert the material so that the cavity is completely filled. Voids may occur in retentive areas or at some area along the margin. These are very difficult to detect and correct when the restoration is in a posterior tooth.
   b. Composite resin does not corrode, as amalgam does, to completely seal the cavity. However, acid etching greatly improves marginal seal.
   c. A matrix does not allow consistently satisfactory contact or contour. With a separator in place, access may be impaired.
   d. Gingival overhangs are far more difficult to detect and remove with composite resin than with amalgam. After insertion, excess amalgam can be readily removed. The composite sets rapidly and there is danger of chipping an excessive amount away, leaving an open margin. In the awkward instrument position necessary to gain access to the overhang, it is difficult to safely direct the force required to remove it.
   e. It is virtually impossible to restore proper occlusion using composite resin in extensive restorations. Additionally, the material is abrasive to opposing surfaces. Rough surfaces are also aggravating to patients.
   f. Many commercially available composites are radiopaque. The others are not readily detectable on x-ray films and are difficult to distinguish from tooth structure visually. This further complicates the removal of gingival overhangs.
9. The translucency of the materials makes them especially esthetic when used to restore access for endodontic teeth.

10. Composite resins are used successfully for building up preparations (foundations) for crowns.

Materials

Composite resins are generally supplied as a system consisting of two pastes or a powder and liquid. One part serves as a catalyst and the other as a universal base. A mixing pad and plastic or wooden disposable spatulas are generally included. Tinting pastes are available in various shades of brown, yellow, gray, and white, any one of which may be used in place or in combination with the regular universal base. Regardless of which paste or combination is used, the proper amount of catalyst paste must always be mixed with the universal or shaded base paste to allow for proper polymerization.

Shade selection

To a degree, the universal paste will assume the natural tooth color owing to its translucency.

Before the dam is placed, select the proper shade. (After the dam is placed, the tooth dehydrates and is not an accurate representation of the natural tooth color.)

1. The universal paste will be the one of choice in most cases where the cavity margins do not extend beyond the labial and lingual line angles of the tooth. If the lingual margin is on the lingual surface rather than the proximal, the darkness of the oral cavity will be transmitted through, causing the restoration to appear dark. Therefore, in such cases, the white-shaded paste should be used.
2. Although shading of the material is entirely empirical, some guidelines may be helpful.
   a. The tinting pastes are more opaque and should be used only where the tooth has a definite yellow, white, brown, or gray cast.
   b. In large restorations, where both labial and lingual enamel has been removed, a tinting paste such as white or yellow may be used to limit translucency and maintain natural color.

CLASS 3 COMPOSITE RESIN RESTORATIONS
Guidelines for cavity preparations

1 A rubber dam is essential in securing and maintaining the operating field. Resins may remain rubbery if contaminated with moisture during the setting period.

2 Decay dictates the extent of the preparation; therefore, considerable variation is found in outline forms.

3 Keep the cavity preparation as small as possible. These areas are normally not exposed to the forces of occlusion. In such circumstances some undermined enamel may be retained if not decalcified.

4 If possible, maintain the labial or lingual wall, depending on the extent of decay. This contributes greatly to the final esthetic result.

5 Adequate access for instrumentation, filling, and finishing procedures must be present. If access to the decay is limited, a separator should be placed before the preparation is begun to minimize destruction of tooth structure and to prevent nicking the adjacent tooth.

6 The contact area is maintained unless involved with decay.

7 The labial and lingual walls are made in one plane.

8 Margins should be smooth with no loose enamel prisms. (See Fig. 13-9.)

9 The cavosurface margins must provide for bulk of filling material. Do not place cavosurface bevels because this would leave a thin, friable flashing of resin.

10 Retention is formed between the incisal and gingival walls by establishing shallow undercuts with a round bur or hand instrument. (See Figs. 13-3 to 13-5.)

11 Clinically, when the preparation is complete, a thin layer of calcium hydroxide* should be placed on the axial wall in the area nearest the pulp if the preparation is deep. Retentive areas and margins must be kept free of base material. If the cavity is very shallow, a base is unnecessary.

12 If the contact area is involved, a separator should be placed if a wedge will not provide adequate separation so that proper contour may be restored.

---

*NOTE: Composites are compatible with calcium hydroxide but may not set completely if in contact with zinc oxide and eugenol or cavity varnish.

Cavity preparation, labial approach

ARMAMENTARIUM

6½-2½-9 hoe
Wedelstaedt chisel
Round burs, Nos. ½, 1, 2, and 3
Calcium hydroxide

1 Select the composite material and shade.

2 Place a rubber dam. Use a separator if it will enhance conservatism.

3 Break into the carious area with a 6½-2½-9 hoe (Figs. 13-1 and 13-2) or small round bur.

4 With a No. 2 round bur establish the desired outline by removing the bulk of weak enamel.

5 If sufficient retention form has not been created by the removal of caries, use a smaller bur (No. ½ or 1) to place slight retentive areas in the gingival dentin toward the lingual wall (Fig. 13-3), toward the labial wall (Fig. 13-4), and in the incisal area (Fig. 13-5).

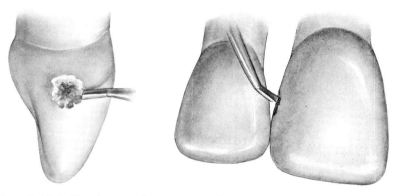

Figs. 13-1 and **13-2.** Break into the cavity with a 6½-2½-9 hoe (or small Wedelstaedt chisel).

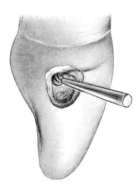
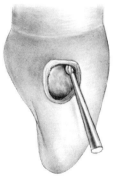
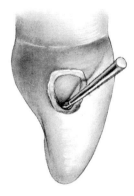

Fig. 13-3. After the caries is removed completely and enamel walls are outlined, place lingual retention with a small round bur.

Fig. 13-4. Establish labial retention.

Fig. 13-5. Place incisal retention.

COMMENT: *Retention for composite resin need be only relatively slight.*

6 The dentin should be covered with a thin layer of calcium hydroxide if the axial wall is near the pulp (Fig. 13-6). A recommended practice is the placement of a coat of calcium hydroxide on the axial wall in deeper cavities.

7 Plane the labial wall using a $6^{1}/_{2}$-$2^{1}/_{2}$-9 hoe (Fig. 13-7). Cavosurface margins must be right angles. A direct thrust movement with the instrument may be used. It should also be moved incisogingivally, planing with the sides of the cutting blade. Large cavities may be planed with Wedelstaedt chisels.

8 Plane the gingival wall with a combination thrust and dragging (hoe) action (Fig. 13-8) and the lingual and incisal walls with similar movements (Fig. 13-9).

Insertion

Most manufacturers supply excellent instructions for management of their composite materials. They should be adhered to closely. Throughout the mixing and placement procedure, time limits are critical.

ARMAMENTARIUM

Celluloid or mylar strip
Plastic instrument or composite syringe
Mixing pad or device provided
Spatula

1 Place a celluloid or mylar strip between the teeth (Fig. 13-10, *A*). The strip may be contoured by drawing it under tension over a blunt instrument such as the end of a mirror handle.

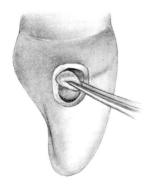

Fig. 13-6. Line the cavity.

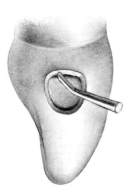

Fig. 13-8. Plane the gingival wall.

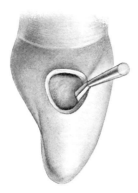

Fig. 13-7. Plane the labial wall with a $6^{1}/_{2}$-$2^{1}/_{2}$-9 hoe.

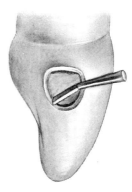

Fig. 13-9. Plane the lingual and incisal walls.

COMMENT: *The hardness of the set material is such that finishing is greatly enhanced if only one cavity is filled at a time. Finishing time can normally be kept to a minimum if meticulous care is taken to place and hold the strip during setting—a relatively difficult thing to do if two cavities are loaded simultaneously.*

2 Place a wood wedge at the gingival area (Fig. 13-10, *B* and *C*) to stabilize the strip, to provide some separation, and to avoid creation of excess gingival flashing.

3 Mix the material following the manufacturer's directions.

4 Using a plastic instrument small enough to enter the cavity, place an increment of the mixed material into the cavity (Fig. 13-10, *A*), usually

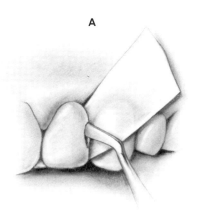

first into the labial retention area (Fig. 15-2). Then force an additional mass toward the axial wall and lingually into the lingual retention (Fig. 15-3). The peculiar viscosity of composite resin demands that it be thoroughly spread over all cavosurface angles.

5 Additional composite is then forced into the incisal area (Fig. 15-4).

6 Sufficient bulk is now placed into the cavity to force the material over the lingual margin and to build the contour to slight excess. To achieve the best adaptation insertion should be completed within thirty seconds following mixing (one minute from start of mix).

COMMENT: *Composite resins are somewhat unusual compared with dental cements. They are sticky and somewhat difficult to force in place. Rather than relying on the strip to force the material over the lingual margin, the material must be forced over the margin with the instrument.*

7 Holding the lingual end of the strip firmly against the lingual surface of the tooth, tighten it firmly around the tooth to form the desired contour. The strip must not be drawn too tight because a deficient contour may result.

8 Hold the strip absolutely still or secure the two ends of the strip with a matrix clip until fully set (Fig. 13-10, *C*). Check the set using a piece of excess material as an indicator.

9 At the end of the desired setting time the strip and wedge may be removed.

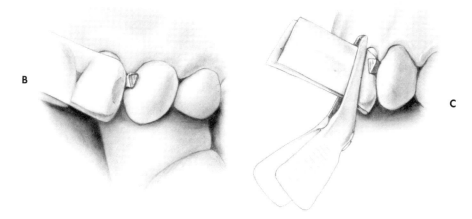

Fig. 13-10. Insertion of composite resin into a prepared Class 3 cavity. **A,** Matrix strip and wedge in place (held on the lingual surface) and increments of the material placed using a plastic instrument. **B,** With the cavity loaded, the strip is drawn tightly around the tooth. **C,** A clip or finger tension is used to hold the strip during setting.

Insertion using a syringe

Because of the critical aspect of the working time of composite resins and their peculiar consistency, use of a syringe is highly recommended (Fig. 13-11). One manufacturer supplies the material in capsules, which provide for injection of the composite into cavities.

Placement of composite resin in increments invites entrapment of air bubbles and, if working time of the material is exceeded, a "layered" or "marbled" appearance of the finished resin may be produced.

The syringe tips must be checked to avoid split ends. The tip allows relatively easy insertion into lingually prepared cavities. As the material is injected, a pumping action may be used to direct the material into undercut areas and over cavo-surface margins.

Finishing

Several minutes (at least five) are normally allowed after the initial set of the material before finishing is begun.

ARMAMENTARIUM

Gold knife
Wedelstaedt chisel
Finishing disks and mandrel
Finishing strips
Finishing burs

1 Use a relatively large twelve-bladed finishing bur to reduce excess bulk if present. Great care must be taken not to cut into enamel. Diamond points produce a rougher surface.

2 With rotary finishing disks (fine or extra-fine garnet) reduce the flashing around the margins buccally and lingually. Keep a continuous stream of air on the area while disking.

3 Very sharp cutting instruments (gold knife, Wedelstaedt chisel, or a scalpel) may be used to reduce flashing. Take great care not to cut toward the restoration because pieces of the composite may be broken out inside the cavosurface angle. Always cut in a direction away from the center of the restoration and remove only very small pieces at a time.

4 Use abrasive finishing strips to finish the removal of flashing and to contour the surface. A separator should be used if there is danger of undercontouring the surface.

COMMENT: *Some operators recommend the use of wax or other lubricant on abrasive disks and strips during final finishing. This is of questionable value, but it may be helpful to reduce the speed of finishing if increased caution is of value.*

Do not polish with a rubber cup and polishing paste. The resin will be removed from between the filler particles leaving them exposed, which results in increased roughness of the surface.

Lingual placement and finishing. Lingual placement of composite materials is somewhat more difficult than the employment of labial access. It preserves labial enamel, thus eliminating the lack of esthetic harmony that develops from staining or color change of composite materials.

Cavity preparation

ARMAMENTARIUM

Small enamel hatchet
Small round burs and contra-angle (high-speed)
Mouth mirror
Wedelstaedt chisel
Gold knife
Disks and mandrel
Finishing strips
Explorer

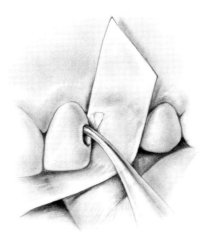

Fig. 13-11. Composite resin is injected into the prepared cavity using a syringe.

1 Select the desired material and shade.

2 Place a rubber dam. Consider possible advantages of separation.

3 Using a small round bur enter the carious area from the lingual aspect (Fig. 13-12). Outline the cavity.

4 Retain the labial wall. Plane the enamel (Fig. 13-13) using Jeffery hatchets or other appropriate instruments.

5 Use a $\frac{1}{4}$ or $\frac{1}{2}$ bur to establish incisal (Fig. 13-14) and gingival retention (Fig. 13-15).

6 Check adequacy of retention with an explorer (Figs. 13-16 and 13-17).

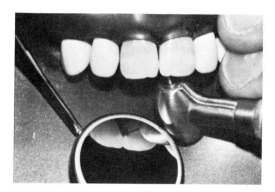

Fig. 13-12. Outline the cavity with a small round bur.

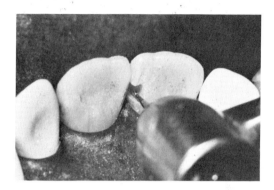

Fig. 13-15. Gingival retention.

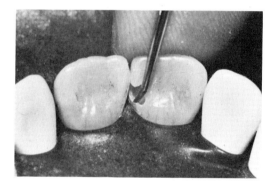

Fig. 13-13. Plane enamel.

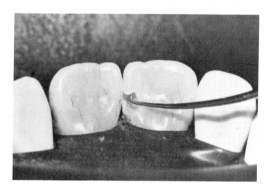

Fig. 13-16. Check incisal retention.

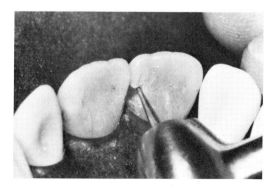

Fig. 13-14. Incisal retention.

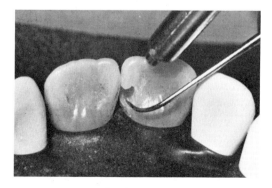

Fig. 13-17. Check gingival retention.

7 When the preparation is in all respects completed (Fig. 13-18), consider the possible advantage of pulp protection and place it if indicated.

8 Place a matrix band between the teeth (Fig. 13-19).

9 Place a separator if the contact area is included in the preparation and separation cannot be achieved using the wedge (Fig. 13-20).

10 Inject the mixed resin material.

11 After the material is thoroughly set, remove the matrix.

12 Using a sharp instrument, cautiously remove excess flashing (Figs. 13-21 and 13-22).

13 Using a sharp twelve-bladed finishing bur, reduce the resin to the proper contour (Fig. 13-23).

14 Lightly finish the surface with small disks (Fig. 13-24). Use a heavy stream of air.

15 Being very careful to retain contour, use strips to finish the remaining proximal surface (Fig. 13-25). Note the wedge to achieve separation.

16 If needed, remove gingival flashing using a gold knife and complete the finish with a strip.

17 Carefully check all margins for flashing and evaluate the contour of the completed restoration (Fig. 13-26).

18 The completed restoration will not be visible from the labial view if the labial wall was retained (Fig. 13-27).

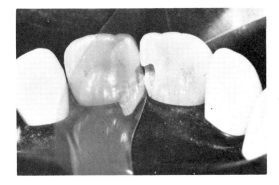

Fig. 13-19. Matrix strip between teeth.

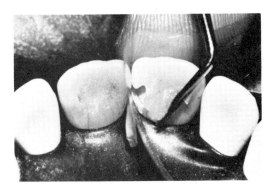

Fig. 13-20. Wedge in place.

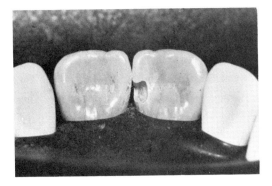

Fig. 13-18. Completed cavity preparation.

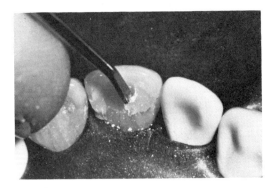

Fig. 13-21. Removal of excess using chisel.

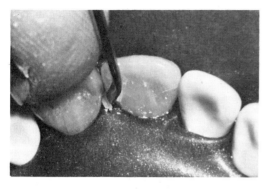

Fig. 13-22. Removal of proximal excess using a gold knife.

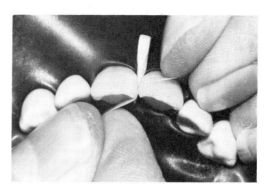

Fig. 13-25. Wedge (separate) and use a finishing strip.

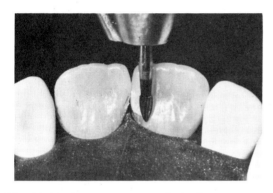

Fig. 13-23. Contour using carbide finishing bur.

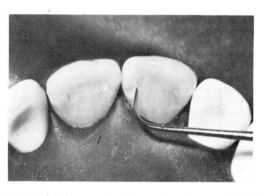

Fig. 13-26. Check completed margins for possible flashing or voids.

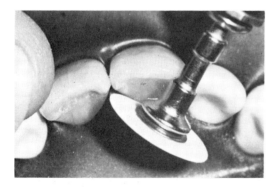

Fig. 13-24. Finish using disk where access permits.

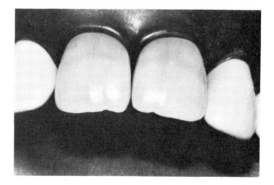

Fig. 13-27. Completed restoration.

CLASS 4 COMPOSITE RESIN RESTORATIONS

Because of the relatively higher strength compared with the tooth-colored resin or cement materials, composite resins may be used to restore broken angles of anterior teeth.

Cavity preparation

The missing angle often presents a problem for the operator to create retention in the incisal area. Retention may be achieved by an undercut in the incisal area (Fig. 13-28, *A*), by the addition of a lingual dovetail, or by the use of pins (Fig. 13-28, *B*). Acid etching of enamel walls is now routinely recommended.

Gingival retention should be somewhat accentuated, although use of pins as shown is to be avoided.

Insertion

Insertion of the material is generally similar to that outlined for Class 3 cavities, inserting it either in increments or with a syringe. A plastic crown form may be cut to aid control of the material; however, the objective may be achieved using a strip in most cases.

The strip should be wedged at its gingival edge and held around the tooth in a manner certain not to result in an undercontoured surface. It is better to overbuild the lingual area (the most difficult area to control) and reduce the excess bulk to the desired contour using abrasive rotary instruments.

CLASS 5 COMPOSITE RESIN RESTORATIONS

Outline form for all resin or cement restorations should be extended only to include the involved area. Areas of erosion occur in teeth subjected to severe stress in addition to other factors, and unless predisposing factors are corrected, relatively early failure of such restorations may be expected.

Cavity preparation

ARMAMENTARIUM

No. 170 (171) or 57 (58) bur
No. 34 or 35 bur
No. ½ or 1 round bur

1 Select the composite shade for the involved tooth (Fig. 13-29).

2 Place a rubber dam and a No. 212 clamp.

3 Outline the cavity using a No. 57 (58) bur (Fig. 13-30). (An inverted cone bur in a straight handpiece may be used to remove bulk.) The walls must be smooth, and cavosurface angles must be right angles.

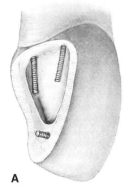
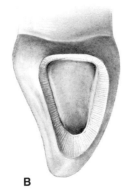

A   **B**

Fig. 13-28. Class 4 composite resin cavity preparation. **A,** With pins. **B,** Normal type.

4 Smooth the axial wall. It should be convex in harmony with the surface of the tooth. An inverted cone bur at low speed may be used to finish this area.

5 Place a retentive groove along the gingivoaxial and incisoaxial line angles (Fig. 13-31), using a No. ½ or 1 round bur (Fig. 13-32).

6 Line the cavity, if necessary, with calcium hydroxide.

7 Plane the enamel walls with a Wedelstaedt chisel (Fig. 13-33).

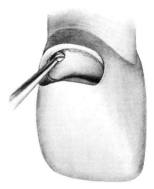

Fig. 13-31. Place a slight retentive undercut groove with a small round bur in the gingival dentin.

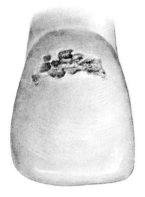

Fig. 13-29. Class 5 carious lesion.

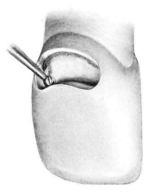

Fig. 13-32. Place slight retentive areas on each end of the incisal wall in dentin, using a small round bur.

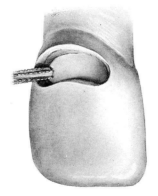

Fig. 13-30. Establish the outline with a No. 57 (58) bur.

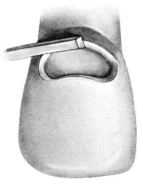

Fig. 13-33. Plane the enamel walls with a contrabevel Wedelstaedt chisel.

Insertion

Various factors may be employed in the insertion of composite resin into prepared Class 5 cavities (Fig. 13-34). The material may be placed into the cavity in increments using a plastic instrument (Fig. 13-35), or it may be injected using a syringe. (Access normally makes the syringe of little advantage.) The excess material is removed by drawing it off toward the margins, great care being taken not to open the margins on the opposite side of the cavity. After the desired contour is achieved, a protective layer of wax may be placed to protect the material from the air.

Finishing

Skillfully placed Class 5 resin restorations should require a minimum or no finishing. However, even the most adept operator must usually resort to abrasive materials to reduce excess contour.

The large twelve-bladed burs and abrasive disks are used cautiously to finish Class 5 composite restorations, as for Class 3 composite restorations. Great care must be observed not to cut into tooth structure, most especially in gingival areas.

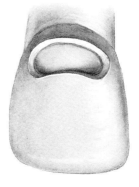

Fig. 13-34. Completed cavity.

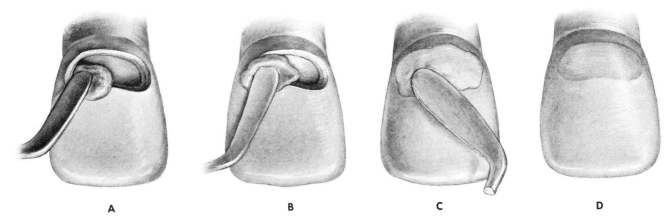

| A | B | C | D |

Fig. 13-35. Class 5 composite resin insertion. **A,** Place a small mass of material in one of the incisal retention areas. **B,** Force an additional quantity of resin into one end of the gingival retention. **C,** After the entire cavity is overfilled, remove most of the excess, cover it with catalyst, and begin working the Gregg 4 and 5 carver with a surfboardlike action toward the margins. **D,** Completed restoration.

Acid etch retention

Buenecore[2] has described the concept of etching enamel to retain acrylic resin. The same principle may be employed to effectively retain composite resin. It is particularly helpful when used to restore broken anterior teeth of younger patients, one advantage being that removal of dentin to create retention is unnecessary or may be minimal.

Restoration of anterior teeth presents the rather obvious problem of esthetics. This problem has been solved, to some extent, by the use of restorative materials, such as unfilled resins, silicate cement, and more recently, filled resins (composite resins).

Porcelain jacket crowns and ceramo-metal crowns can always be used to restore anterior teeth where there has been severe tooth breakdown. Crowns can solve the problem of maintaining esthetics as well as function, but they necessitate removal of much tooth structure and can create problems such as irritation to the pulp owing to removal of most of the outer protective and insulating enamel in addition to possible induction of periodontal disease. In children, crowns or composites are temporary restorations at best because of the incomplete stage of eruption and the height of gingival tissue.

Composite resins work well to restore rather obvious Class 3 lesions, but in the treatment of Class 4 problems, such as fractured incisors or incisors that have lost incisal angles owing to extensive decay or trauma, the difficulty of obtaining adequate retention of the restoration becomes evident. Without the incisal angle it used to be difficult to retain a composite resin unless pins were used or reductions were made to create retention (lingual dovetails). Young patients with large immature pulp chambers and incomplete root formation may not be able to tolerate the use of retentive pins because of possible pulp trauma. If the patient is an adult and the pulp has receded sufficiently, a pin can sometimes be placed at the incisal aspect to help hold in the restoration. When the use of pins is contraindicated, another means is available to gain additional retention for Class 4 restorations. The enamel surrounding the lesion can be specially prepared by acid etching to produce a mechanical bond to retain a composite resin. A combination of pin and acid etch retention may be used where the occlusion is particularly heavy and retention is minimal.

Indications

1. Where there is incisal angle involvement owing to trauma, caries, or developmental defects and the extent of the restoration is minimal and function is limited.
2. Young teeth
3. Developmental abnormalities in young teeth requiring attention because of esthetics:
   a. Severe enamel mottling
   b. Hypocalcified enamel owing to caries

Contraindications

1. Presence of heavy abrading occlusal contacts, such as deep overbite relationships, contraindicates acid etch retention.
2. It is not necessary for Class 3 restorations where conventional retention is adequate, although studies have been made indicating the use of elastic liners to obtain a better marginal seal, minimizing leakage owing to thermal dimensional changes and shrinkage owing to polymerization.
3. It is not necessary in deciduous teeth. Acid etching has little effect on increasing retention. Deciduous enamel is aprismatic to a depth of 25 microns. Removal of this outer enamel layer and roughening the surface may produce enough retention to adequately support a restoration.

BIOMECHANICAL PRINCIPLES

Enamel may be etched using a 30% to 50% orthophosphoric acid solution. The result is a surface that has numerous minute irregularities in the enamel that provide the retentive surface area (Fig. 13-36). If the resin material comes into close

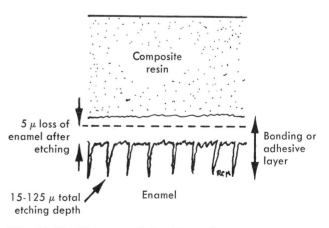

Fig. 13-36. Diagram of the biomechanical aspects of acid etch retention.

contact and enters these irregularities, the retention of the material will usually be strong enough and requires no additional tooth preparation other than caries removal when present. Scanning electron microscope studies have shown that etching of enamel causes a surface enamel loss of approximately 5 microns, whereas the depth of etching varies from 15 to 125 microns.[3] Lee[4] found the bond strength to be approximately 600 to 900 psi on bovine enamel. In a separate study, Laswell[5] found the tensile strength to be up to 2,000 psi. In comparing the bond strength of acid-etched restorations with the diametral tensile strength of most composites, which is about 7,000 psi, it is possible to see that the retention to enamel is the weakest area of this restoration.

Fig. 13-37 shows a photomicrograph (SEM) of dentin that has been "cleaned" by acid etching, thus destroying the protoplasmic processes. Fig. 13-38 illustrates sealant tags that have entered the open unprotected dentinal tubuli.

Creation of mechanical retention by etching is illustrated in Fig. 13-39. Fig. 13-40 illustrates etched enamel on a bevel that crossed the plane of enamel prisms.

Intimate contact of the resin and tooth is of great importance. The surface should actually be "wet" by the resin. A thick pastelike material, such as conventional composite, does not allow

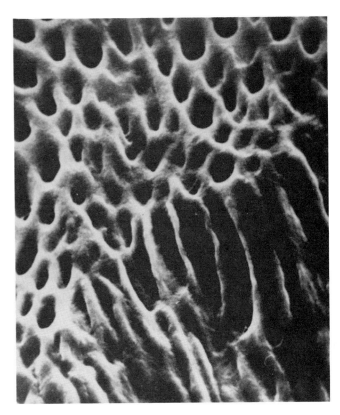

Fig. 13-37. Photomicrograph (SEM) of etched dentin (X660). (From Lorton, L., and Brady, J. : Criteria for successful composite restorations, Gen. Dent. May-June, 1981.)

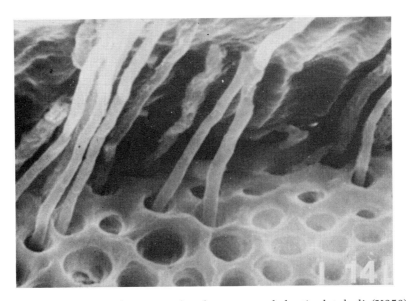

Fig. 13-38. SEM showing sealant tags that have entered dentinal tubuli (X850). (From Lorton, L., and Brady, J.: Criteria for successful composite restorations, Gen Dent. May-June, 1981.)

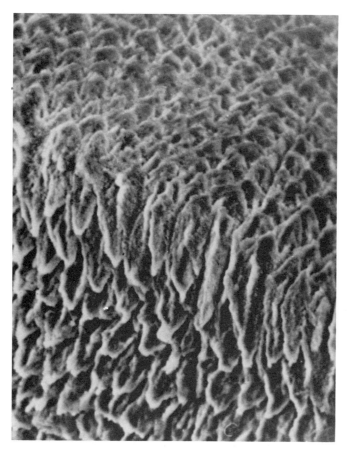

Fig. 13-39. SEM of etched enamel (X600). (From Lorton, L., and Brady J.: Criteria for successful composite restorations, Gen. Dent. May-June, 1981.)

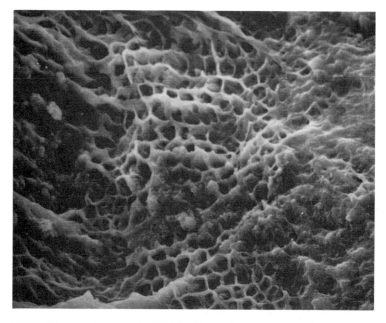

Fig. 13-40. SEM of beveled enamel (X850). (From Lorton, L., and Brady, J.: Criteria for successful composite restorations, Gen. Dent. May-June, 1981.)

this intimate tooth-material contact that is necessary for retention. There are two solutions to this problem:

1. A composite resin that can be mixed thin enough to actually wet and adapt to the tooth surface during insertion (An example of this type is a *powder-liquid type* of composite where the cementing can be varied.)
2. The use of an *intermediary bonding material* to wet and adapt to the etched surface (The actual restoration is a conventional composite resin placed over a liquid two-part adhesive.)

Each of the preceding acid etch methods requires similar preparation of the tooth surface before application of the restorative material. Each type of bonding system has advantages and disadvantages.

The powder-liquid system uses a fairly convenient method of mixing and applying the composite resin in one step. The disadvantage is that the material has proportionately less filler because of the consistency of mix necessary to adapt to the tooth. It tends to pick up stains more readily and wear down faster than conventional resins.

The intermediary bonding agent is actually a liquid resin that comes in two parts that are mixed and coated on the etched enamel surface. A conventional composite resin is then mixed and must be applied to the region requiring restoration before the bonding agent sets. This procedure requires rather hasty mixing and application of both composite and bonding material before either has begun to set. This is difficult to do single-handedly; with an assistant there is no problem. The advantage of this intermediate bonding system is that a conventional resin may be used that is much harder than the powder-liquid resin. These restorations do not wear down as rapidly nor collect stains as readily.

Procedure

1 Examine the color or shade characteristics of the tooth so the appropriate modification of shade can be made. If the tooth is checked for a shade after rubber dam application, the shade may be inaccurate because of tooth desiccation. A desiccated tooth has an increased opacity and whiter than natural tooth coloration. Within a few hours after rubber dam removal, the tooth will rehydrate and again assume its normal coloration.

2 Anesthesia may or may not be necessary for this procedure, depending on the extent of the res-toration. If anesthesia is required, it may be administered first. A shade may be selected while waiting for it to take effect.

3 Rubber dam isolation is necessary for this procedure as for most other restorative operations. Control against saliva, moisture, or other contaminants is critical to the objectives of this procedure.

4 Before attempting to etch the enamel, the surface should be thoroughly cleaned using a water-pumice paste and rubber cup. (Glycerin or oil-based prophy paste may prevent effective etching of the enamel and should not be used.) The tooth should be rinsed and dried.

5 If caries is present, it is removed along with any weak enamel. If the restoration is in an area of heavy stress, it may be necessary to provide additional retention by using undercuts and/or placement of a pin. The cavosurface margin should be beveled to provide greater surface area to increase retention. A long bevel at the margin also allows the composite color to blend with the remaining tooth structure.

6 If considerable dentin is exposed and the pulp is near, measures should be taken for protection from the acid etchant. Calcium hydroxide should be placed over the areas approximating the pulp. Varnish can be placed over the adjacent teeth for protection from the action of the acid. The enamel walls are freshened using hand instruments to remove any varnish that may have covered them. Finishing burs may also be used if access permits.

7 A cotton pellet is soaked with the etchant and applied to the enamel margins. Allow the acid to remain for one minute, then rinse for at least two minutes and dry the preparation. The etched enamel will appear chalky white. If not, repeat the application of acid until the dried surface has the desired appearance. However, guard against overetching. Overetching produces a chalky disorganized surface that creates loss of mechanical retention. (Because of its structure, retention is not enhanced by acid etching of dentin.)

8 Flush the tooth again with water spray to remove any traces of acid. Phillips[6] recommends two minutes of irrigation to thoroughly remove all traces of the acid.

9 Thoroughly dry the tooth with oil-free *dry* air for 30 seconds.

10 Celluloid crown forms cut to fit over the fractured area of the tooth work well to confine the composite resin to the preparation. The composite resin is mixed and the crown form filled.

Place a small amount of resin material over the preparation and seat the crown form over the tooth and hold until set. When a crown form is not available, a plastic matrix strip works fine. The plastic strip is looped around the tooth and passed through both proximal contacts. After the resin material is applied to the preparation, the ends of the matrix are pulled together and held with a slight tension to prevent the excess material from accumulating in the interproximal embrasures where it is difficult to remove.

11 If an intermediary bonding agent is used, it is mixed and applied to the preparation. The composite restorative material should be mixed and inserted into the preparation before the bonding agent sets in order to get good retention.

12 Standard finishing procedures can be used to contour and smooth the restoration once the composite has set. Gross excess contour can be quickly removed with disks or an extra fine tapered diamond bur and water spray. Care must be used not to undercontour or remove any adjacent enamel when finishing these restorations. This is very difficult since the restoration blends very closely with the existing tooth structure.

REFERENCES

1. Nealon, F. H.: Acrylic restorations by the operative non-pressure procedure, J. Prosthet, Dent. **2**:513, 1952.
2. Buenecore, M. G., Matsui, A., and Gwinnett, A. J.: Penetration of resin dental materials into enamel surfaces with reference to bonding, Arch. Oral Biol. **13**:61, 1968.
3. Ibsen, R. L., and Neville, K.: Adhesive restorative dentistry, Philadelphia, 1974, W. B. Saunders Co.
4. Lee, B. D., Phillips, R. W., and Swartz, M. J.: The influence of phosphoric acid on retention of acrylic resin to bovine enamel, J. Am. Dent. Assoc. **82**:1381, 1971.
5. Laswell, H. R., Welk, D. A., and Regenos, J. W.: Attachment of resin restorations to acid pretreated enamel, J. Am. Dent. Assoc. **82**:558, 1971.
6. Phillips, R. W.: Personal communication.

CHAPTER 14

DIRECT GOLD PROCEDURES

Cohesive golds used to restore teeth include gold foil, mat gold, and powdered gold. Each has different characteristics and must be handled accordingly.

Although it is not our purpose here to discuss the history or physical aspects of materials, it should be noted that no other restorative material has demonstrated the longevity possible with gold foil. Modern techniques allow the placement of inconspicuous gold restorations with less effort than required by older methods.

Since the development of powdered gold, several terms have come into use to denote pure gold; *direct gold, compacted gold,* and so forth are in common use. The term *cohesive* seems uniformly appropriate since it denotes the physical property common to all the forms of pure gold that makes its use possible in operative dentistry.

The frequently heard comments to the effect that placement of gold foil is unduly traumatic to oral tissues reflect lack of judgment and skill in its use. It is used successfully in children. This is not to infer, however, that anyone not highly skilled in its use should place cohesive gold restorations in young people. These materials require practice and experience to gain the consistent proficiency required to properly utilize their desirable properties. Beginners should, therefore, confine their cohesive gold operations to mature teeth requiring relatively simple restorations.

Gold is one of the most inert metals known. Pure gold resists oxidation and most other forms of chemical attack. When in a highly purified state, it has the capability of welding to itself on contact. This property is utilized in dentistry to produce the finest dental restorations yet known. Used where indicated and placed with skill, direct restorative gold restorations provide the best seal to a cavity margin. In addition to its marginal adaptation and seal, these restorations can be highly polished. When correctly contoured in gingival areas and highly polished, the tissue response is far superior to any other restorative material now in use.

Storage

It is essential that cohesive golds be stored away from materials such as rubber since sulfur compounds or other contaminants may render it permanently noncohesive.

A box divided into sections is commonly used to make readily available a small quantity of each type of gold while operating. Larger quantities should be stored in sealed bottles. A pellet of cotton dipped in concentrated aqua ammonia should be placed in each container.

Annealing

The term *anneal* as applied to cohesive gold restorations actually refers to a process of *degassing,* the heating of the gold to drive off gases occluded to its surface, and has nothing to do with changing its hardness. When manufactured, golds are rendered noncohesive by being subjected to an atmosphere of ammonia. This treatment prevents the pieces of gold from sticking to each other and from occluding harmful gases that might render them permanently noncohesive. Driving off the layer of gas molecules allows the gold to be welded cold.

Pure golds may be annealed (degassed) by passing each piece through a clean alcohol flame or by heating them on an electric annealer. Flame annealing should be done with an alcohol lamp with a clean wick, adjusted to produce a clear, light blue flame about $3/4$ inch in height. Chemically pure methyl or ethyl alcohol should be used for fuel. The piece of gold is picked up with a small, sharp instrument (made from an old explorer or a piece of iridioplatinum wire) and passed through the hottest part of the flame at a rate that will cause the edges of the gold to glow slightly. Do not overanneal since the gold may be melted in spots or made brittle. It is helpful to use a piece of black cardboard behind the flame so that the flame and the desired glow of the gold may be easily seen.

The advantages of using the alcohol flame for annealing are uniformity, flexibility, and the immediate availability of the gold. The operator is free to call for any size piece or type of gold he may desire at a given moment. Use of an electric annealer requires judgment in estimating the amounts of gold needed for an operation, with the inevitable surplus remaining when the operation is completed. Also, a danger exists of overannealing with an electric annealer if the operator is not careful to use the gold within a reasonable period of time. Overannealing may cause the foil to become somewhat "wiry" or harsh, losing its soft workability.

One great advantage of the electric annealer is that it enables an operator to work alone. He must, however, anticipate the time when he will need the gold since it usually requires eight to ten minutes to anneal.

Methods of condensing

Cohesive golds may be condensed into prepared cavities by (1) hand pressure, (2) hand malleting, (3) an automatic condenser, (4) a pneumatic condenser, or (5) an electronic condenser.

Density and other characteristics of restorations placed by the various methods will unquestionably vary from one operator to another and from one operative situation to another. The restoration of teeth varies so much from one situation to another, each cavity, tooth, and patient being different, that skill and judgment of the operator are the final factors in determining the preferred method. Operators should acquaint themselves with all the methods and receive instruction from a master of each before they judge for themselves which methods they will use.

Use of a particular method in the techniques described is not to imply that other methods of condensation are inferior.

Several factors must be considered regarding the quality or type of condensation to be used or even whether cohesive gold will be used at all. Some of these are (1) age of the patient (by itself not a conclusive factor since gold may be advan-

tageously placed in recently erupted permanent teeth), (2) accessibility of the cavity, (3) depth and size of the cavity, (4) requirements of the procedure, (5) characteristics of the material, (6) condition of the periodontium, (7) temperament of the patient, (8) temperament of the operator, and (9) ability of the operator.

The following comments are offered only as a basis for comparison and are not intended to be complete evaluations.

Hand pressure

Hand pressure is used to condense gold foil mainly in areas of incisal retention in Class 3 foil restorations. Its use is not recommended generally for gold foil, but it is recommended for placement of mat gold and powdered gold. Hand condensation applies pressure for a relatively long period each time the condenser is thrust against the gold. This may subject the periodontal membrane to stress, whereas rapid, light blows applied by malleting should not create the same cumulative effect on the supporting tissues.

Hand malleting

Hand malleting is widely used and possesses the advantages of (1) freedom of the operator to quickly change instruments, (2) freedom from having to adjust an instrument, (3) not requiring the application of pressure to activate the condensing action, and (4) providing the operator with a better "feel" of the material as it is placed than is generally possible with other methods.

Contrary to a popular misconception, most assistants can be quickly trained to hand mallet and usually will greatly enjoy this active participation in operating. The mallet should be very loosely held in the assistant's left hand (right when assisting left-handed operators) and the condenser rhythmically tapped with light but positive blows. The operator may quickly perceive the need for increased or decreased intensity and instruct the assistant accordingly. It is important that the operator step the condenser in rhythm with the malleting, placing the point on the surface of the gold before it is malleted. It can be uncomfortable to the patient if the condenser is struck while off the surface of the gold.

The procedure used while hand malleting is as follows. The assistant places an annealed piece of gold as directed by the operator and then immediately anneals the next piece of gold. By this time the operator will have oriented the first gold, and the malleting is performed while the assistant holds the next piece of annealed gold. When the first gold is condensed, the assistant, signaled by the operator, immediately places the gold being held and anneals another piece. This procedure is very quickly carried out, and the sequence proceeds throughout the placement of the restoration, thus allowing the operator to watch the operation at all times.

Automatic condenser

The automatic condenser (S. S. White) is one method that allows the operator to work alone. It is adjustable, and when pressed to the gold, spring tension is established and released, applying the condensing blow. A common shortcoming on the part of operators using instruments activated by pressure is that of tipping or rolling the condenser as pressure is applied. Dentists should scrupulously train themselves to apply this force in direct line with the desired line of force to keep the surface of the gold smooth as it is stepped.

Pneumatic condenser

The pneumatic (Hollenback*) condenser has the advantage of a contra-angle as well as the straight handpiece for condensing gold. This allows placement of cohesive golds in normally inaccessible places. It is adjustable for intensity and speed and allows the operator to work alone.

Electronic condenser

Electronic mallets possess the advantages noted for the pneumatic condenser but can deliver condensing blows at very high frequencies.

---

*Cleveland Dental Manufacturing Co., Cleveland, Ohio.

Principles of condensing

Regardless of the condensing methods used, several mechanical factors should be considered, the main ones being (1) condenser point size, (2) amount of force, (3) stepping, and (4) line of force.

Size of condenser point

The condenser point should be small to minimize the amount of pressure or force necessary to condense the gold under it. Generally to be preferred are points not over 1 mm. in diameter for gold foil, but slightly larger for powdered and mat gold. They must be serrated and sharp.

Amount of force

The force or pressure used should be the smallest amount possible to thoroughly condense the gold.

Stepping

Stepping, the process of moving the condenser point systematically over the surface of the gold as it is condensed, requires painstaking discipline of a beginner. Only by proper stepping can a dense restoration be placed in the minimun amount of time. Without proper stepping, porosity is certain to occur and proper finishing made difficult or impossible.

To properly step the condenser point as foil is condensed, after a condensing force has been applied the point is moved only enough so that the next area condensed will overlap the first (Fig. 14-1). As each step is thus condensed, a row of steps is created. The next row of steps must partly overlap the first, and successive rows of steps are created so that every particle of gold will have received a condensing force.

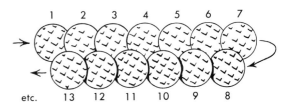

Fig. 14-1. Stepping, as utilized in condensing cohesive gold.

Beginners should practice thoroughly stepping each piece of gold before adding another. With experience will come the skill of condensing the main body of each added piece, the edges of which may be condensed during the condensation of a subsequent addition. This skill, however, can never be acquired until the discipline of proper stepping is mastered.

Line of force

The process of placing gold foil restorations is an exacting procedure, and less experienced operators may be somewhat likely to develop a state of tension that may cause them to overlook the essential factor of proper line of force during condensation. Surely this is one of the greatest reasons for loosening restorations during their placement.

In Class 5 restorations line of force may be less critical than in Class 3 procedures, but it is important nonetheless. The axis of the condenser (Ferrier No. 1, 2, or 3) should be kept perpendicular to the surface of the area of foil being condensed. As one of the peripheral walls is approached, the condenser should be tilted slightly, bisecting the angle (Fig. 14-2), to condense the foil toward it.

In placing Class 3 gold foil restorations the long axis of the condenser handle must be held in a direction that will always drive the foil toward the tooth being restored and generally toward the axial wall. The points used for condensing the bulk of gold in Class 3 cavities (Ferrier Nos. 4, 5, and 7) have angled points for the main purpose of reaching around the adjacent tooth. The bulk of condensation during most Class 3 procedures should be in a direction parallel with the long axis of the tooth but slightly inclined toward the axial wall or into the tooth being restored.

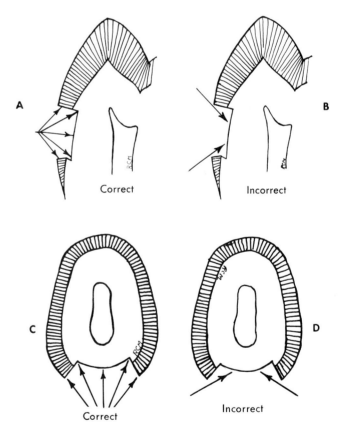

Fig. 14-2. A to **D,** Correct and incorrect lines of force to condense gold in Class 5 cavities.

Gold foil

Gold foil as a dental restorative material is supplied in commercially manufactured pellets of various sizes (cylinders), ropes, and sheets.

The advantages of manufactured cylinders are their ready availability and uniformity. Rope foil, although possessing the same advantages, has the disadvantage of having to be cut into pellets, the action tending to condense the cut edges.

Many operators prefer hand-rolled pellets and cylinders because they can be made to personal preference.

Hand-prepared foil

Rolling pellets and cylinders from sheet gold (usually No. 4 foil) is a simple procedure, and once trained, most assistants can roll a quantity of pellets in a short time.

Numbers to designate sizes of pellets or cylinders indicate the fraction of a sheet of gold foil from which it has been cut (Fig. 14-3). For example, a $^1/_{16}$ pellet is one sixteenth of the 4-inch sheet. Pellets rarely exceed, $^1/_{16}$, and the most commonly used size is the $^1/_{64}$. Cylinders are commonly used in $^1/_8$ or $^1/_{16}$ sizes.

Hand-rolled pellets are normally annealed when placed. Hand-rolled cylinders are often termed "soft" or noncohesive gold since they are not generally annealed for use.

Hands must be absolutely clean and dry for the following procedures. Wiping the hands with alcohol may be helpful in removing moisture and oils that might contaminate the gold.

Rolling pellets

1 Spread a clean towel.

2 With a ruler and pencil prepare a grid on the first sheet of paper in the book, outlining the size of pellets to be rolled. (Observe the margins of the book beyond the gold.) It is efficient to rule the entire grid the size of $^1/_{64}$. Other sizes may then be cut as desired. For example, double a $^1/_{64}$ size to make a $^1/_{32}$ size (Fig. 14-3).

3 Place paper clips on the sides of the book to keep it intact while cutting.

4 Cut a few sections of the book, allowing the cut sections to fall on the towel (Fig. 14-4). The entire thickness of the book should be cut to avoid losing control of it.

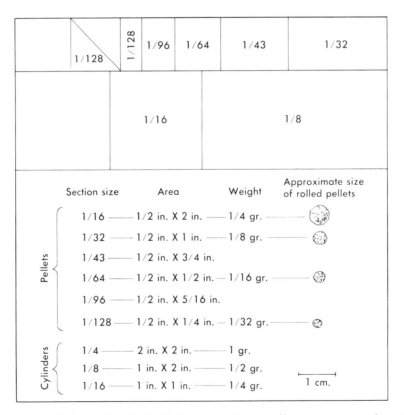

Fig. 14-3. Four-inch sheet of gold divided into sections to illustrate sizes to be rolled into cylinders or pellets and sizes of rolled pellets.

5 Pick up a section of gold with cotton pliers (Fig. 14-5), grasping it gently in the center, which will cup it.

6 Holding the gold lightly with the thumb and forefinger of one hand, fold each corner toward the center with cotton pliers (Figs. 14-6 and 14-7).

7 Gently roll the gold (Fig. 14-8) into a round pellet. It must not be too compact but firm enough to hold its shape. Fig. 14-3 shows average sizes of rolled pellets.

8 Place the pellet in a container with a cotton pellet soaked in ammonia.

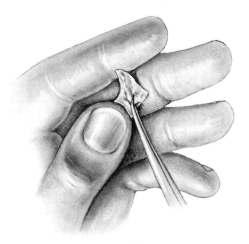

Fig. 14-6. Place gold in left hand.

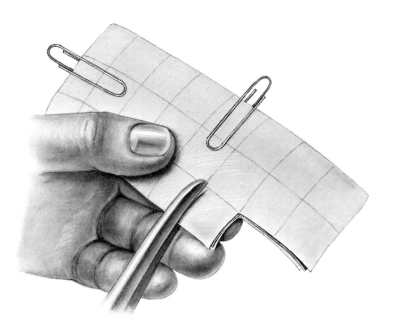

Fig. 14-4. Cut foil into sections of desired size (sheet marked for $^1/_{64}$ size).

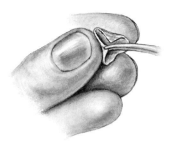

Fig. 14-7. Fold corners in.

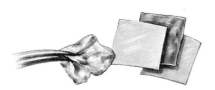

Fig. 14-5. Pick up section of gold with cotton pliers.

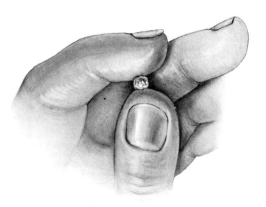

Fig. 14-8. Roll into pellet.

Rolling cylinders

1 Spread a clean towel.

2 Rule the book of foil for the size of cylinders desired (Fig. 14-3).

3 Place paper clips on two or three sides of the book.

4 With sharp scissors cut a few sections of gold, allowing them to fall on the towel.

5 Place a strip of gold flat on the towel (Fig. 14-9).

6 Using a thin spatula, fold the gold lengthwise, roughly in thirds. It is helpful to push the underlying towel toward the spatula to make the fold (Fig. 14-10). In making the second fold, keep the freed edge of the foil short of the other edge so that succeeding folds will place it inside the cylinder.

7 Fold the strip enough times to obtain the desired width, usually 1.5 to 2 mm.

8 Place the strip on the heel of the hand, holding about half the strip with the little finger (Fig. 14-11).

9 With a jeweler's broach or the end cut off the eye of a large sewing needle, press the free end of the strip into the palm of the hand to engage it and roll it into a cylinder (Fig. 14-12).

10 Carefully slide the cylinder off the broach (Fig. 14-13) and gently pinch its ends with cotton pliers to prevent its unrolling and to make the ends uniform (Fig. 14-14).

11 Place the cylinder in a container with a small cotton pellet soaked in ammonia. When handling cylinders, always use cotton pliers and pick them up endwise to avoid flattening them (Fig. 14-14).

Laminated foil

Laminated gold foil, as suggested by Stebner,[1] is created by folding an entire sheet of foil, in the same manner as is done for cylinders (Figs. 14-9 and 14-10), to a width of about 3 mm., which creates a strip of thirty-two thicknesses of gold. The strip is then cut into triangles or convenient lengths that may be utilized to lay over margins during placement of foil or on axial walls to build bulk rapidly. The main advantage is use of the technique to protect the cavosurface enamel during condensation.

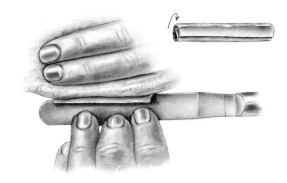

Fig. 14-10. Fold the upper third of the gold downward, short of the bottom edge. Fold enough times to create a strip 1 to 1.5 mm. wide.

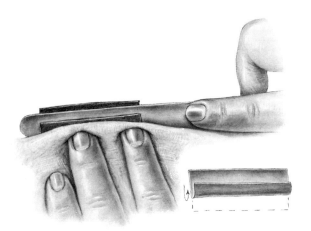

Fig. 14-9. Using a thin spatula, fold over a third of the section of gold.

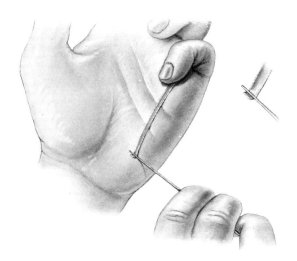

Fig. 14-11. Hold the strip in the left hand.

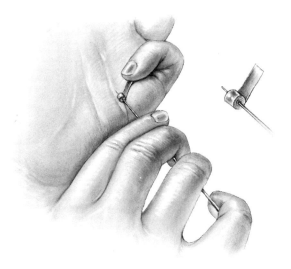

Fig. 14-12. Roll the cylinder with a jeweler's broach (or open-eyed darning needle).

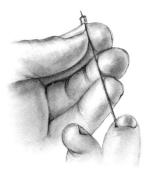

Fig. 14-13. Slip the cylinder off the broach.

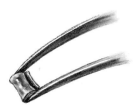

Fig. 14-14. Flatten the cylinder ends to keep the cylinder from unrolling.

Class 1 gold foil restorations

Class 1 cavity preparations for cohesive gold are similar to those for amalgam in that the same general steps are followed. However, the completed cavity preparation is different allowing more tooth structure to be conserved because it is not necessary to create 90-degree cavosurface margins. In fact, they may be slightly beveled. Thus the cavity walls are not undercut except slightly in some areas of dentin to create retention.

MAXILLARY PREMOLAR
Cavity preparation (Fig. 14-15)

ARMAMENTARIUM

No. 170 bur
No. 169L bur

1 Enter the tooth on the mesial side of the distal pit with the No. 170 bur until it enters dentin. Extend the distal wall buccally and lingually only enough to include caries and the deepest parts of sharp developmental grooves. In making this preparation do not tip the handpiece from side to side since no undercuts are created at this time.

2 Extend the cut mesially through the central grooves. Width of the cut need only be enough to accommodate a small condensing point.

3 Extend the mesial wall buccally and lingually to include caries and sharp developmental grooves.

4 With a No. 169L bur sharpen the line angles joining each of the four walls, thus slightly extending the preparation to include the developmental grooves. When this is done, tilt the tip of the bur just slightly and establish very small undercuts in dentin buccally and lingually in the point angles.

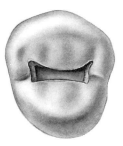

Fig. 14-15. Class 1 gold foil cavity preparation in a maxillary premolar.

5 Apply cavity varnish and very lightly plane the cavosurface margins, creating a slight bevel on the cavosurface angle with a No. 169L bur.

Insertion

ARMAMENTARIUM

Ferrier No. 4 condenser
Holding instrument

1 Place a ¹/₃₂ gold pellet in the distal part of the cavity. Use a straight condenser (or pigtail holder) as a holding instrument. Condense the foil with a Ferrier No. 4 (7) condenser, first into the linguodistal retention, then across into distobuccal retention. If this does not provide sufficient bulk of gold to ensure that it is securely locked, insert another pellet or two while still using the holding instrument.

2 Remove the holding instrument and condense additional pellets of gold. The angle of the plugger should be directed toward the distal wall, slightly lingually when condensing gold adjacent to the lingual wall and slightly buccally when condensing to the buccal wall. The foil is thus built up first to the distal cavosurface margin.

3 The mesial portion of the cavity is then filled to the mesial cavosurface margin.

4 Gold is then built over the lingual margin starting at the distal end, carefully keeping a bulk of gold at all times ahead of the condenser point to avoid chipping the enamel, until it joins the mesial margin already covered.

5 The buccal margin is then covered. If the cavity preparation was conservative, sufficient bulk of foil probably has been placed by this time. If it has not, build the proper contour.

Finishing

See Figs. 14-39 to 14-42 for steps of the Class 2 gold foil restoration that apply to the occlusal area for finishing.

Class 2 gold foil restorations

Gold foil is sometimes indicated for restoration of relatively small Class 2 carious lesions in premolars and the mesial surfaces of molars. As a procedure, it has the distinct advantage of conserving tooth structure while meeting esthetic requirements and extension for prevention.

MAXILLARY PREMOLAR

ARMAMENTARIUM

No. 170 bur
No. 169L bur
Spoon excavator
Binangle chisel
Gingival margin trimmers

Cavity preparation

The occlusal portion of the cavity preparation is that described for the Class 1 preparation (Fig. 14-15).

1 With a No. 170 (169L) bur cut toward the contact area, then buccally and lingually only enough to provide access to make the proximal cut (Fig. 14-16).

2 With the No. 169L bur cut gingivally down the dentinoenamel junction, cutting both enamel and dentin through the carious area to the desired gingival depth (Figs. 14-17 and 14-18).

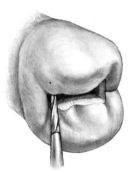

Fig. 14-16. Extension of occlusal cut toward contact area, No. 170 bur.

3 Keeping the occlusal buccolingual extension very narrow, tip the handpiece buccally and lingually to extend the gingival width buccolingually.

4 If after cutting into the enamel at the ends of the proximal cut the enamel does not fall away, use an instrument (spoon) to break it out (Figs. 14-19 and 14-20).

5 Use a binangle chisel (enamel hatchet) to plane the proximal and gingival walls (Fig. 14-21).

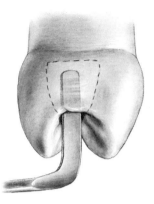

Fig. 14-19. Enamel wall being broken out with a spoon excavator.

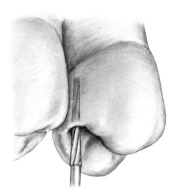

Fig. 14-17. Proximal cut made with No. 169L bur.

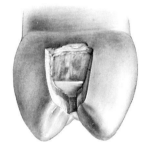

Fig. 14-20. Proximal enamel broken out.

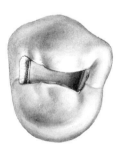

Fig. 14-18. Extension of initial proximal cut.

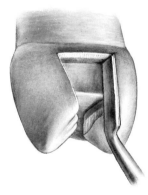

Fig. 14-21. Planing proximal and gingival walls with binangle chisel.

6 The retention areas may be started using a No. 169L bur (Fig. 14-22), but they may be more safely established using only gingival margin trimmers (Fig. 14-23). The binangle chisel may be used to start these areas.

7 Sharpen the gingivoaxial line angle with the gingival margin trimmer (Fig. 14-24).

8 Plane the gingival enamel (Fig. 14-25). A bevel is not necessary, but the enamel must be planed to remove unsupported and loose prisms.

9 If the pulpal floor is rough, it may be smoothed with a 10-4-8 hoe.

10 If a slight occlusal bevel has not been previously established when planing with the binangle chisel (enamel hatchet), it may be planed with a No. 170 bur using slow speed.

The completed cavity is shown in Figs. 14-26 and 14-27.

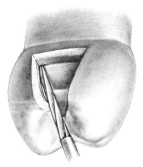

Fig. 14-22. Starting retention areas with No. 169L bur.

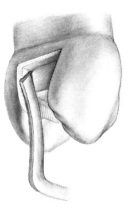

Fig. 14-23. Cutting lingual retention with gingival margin trimmer.

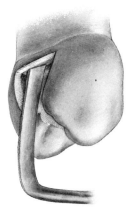

Fig. 14-24. Sharpening gingivoaxial line angle with gingival margin trimmer.

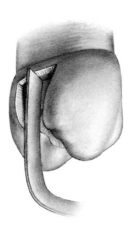

Fig. 14-25. Planing gingival enamel with a gingival margin trimmer.

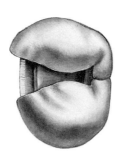

Fig. 14-26. Occlusal view of completed cavity preparation.

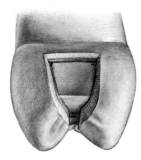

Fig. 14-27. Distal view of completed preparation.

Insertion

ARMAMENTARIUM

Parallelogram condensers
Condensing points as indicated

1 Place a ⅛ or ¼ cylinder of gold foil with one end against the axial wall and force it against the lingual proximal wall with a Ferrier parallelogram (Fig. 14-28).

2 Place another cylinder against the other proximal wall in like manner.

3 Place a ¼ cylinder between the first two (Fig. 14-29).

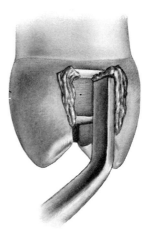

Fig. 14-28. Insertion of gold foil, Class 2 cavity. Placement of buccal and lingual ⅛ or ¼ cylinders.

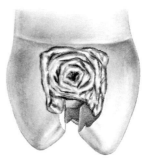

Fig. 14-29. Quarter cylinder is inserted between the first two.

4 Using parallelograms condense all cylinders gingivally (Fig. 14-30).

5 Using a straight parallelogram condenser (Stebner No. 1) or a large bayonet condenser, mallet the soft foil to condense it. Use a line of force toward the axial wall (Fig. 14-31).

6 Using cohesive foil, start to build the occlusal gold along the mesial wall, locking the first gold between the buccal and lingual walls (Fig. 14-32).

7 Continue to build up the gold to the cavosurface angle (Fig. 14-33) proximally, keeping it sloped from the marginal ridge.

8 Build the foil over the occlusoaxial line angle onto the soft foil proximally in the cavity (Fig. 14-34). Care must be exercised at all times to keep the condensing line of force in a direction that will not rock the proximal cylinders out of the cavity.

9 Continue to build up the proximal gold, condensing it against the contact area of the adjacent tooth (Fig. 14-35). Fig. 14-36 shows the buccal view with occlusal gold in place.

10 Complete the desired contour (Fig. 14-37).

11 If access permits, as with MO restorations, a foot condenser, Jeffery No. 19, may be used to contour the proximal gold under the contact area (Fig. 14-38). If this cannot be done, as with DO restorations, this area should be carefully burnished to accomplish the same objective, using a Spratley burnisher or similar instrument. (A foot condenser point in a right-angle condenser is also recommended.)

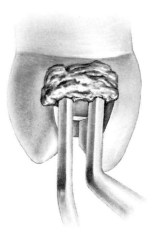

Fig. 14-30. All cylinders are pressed firmly gingivally.

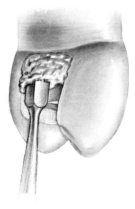

Fig. 14-31. Foil is firmly condensed by malleting.

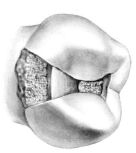

Fig. 14-32. Foil is started in the occlusal portion.

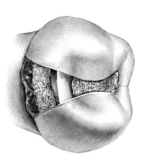

Fig. 14-33. Occlusal foil is built up to the marginal ridge.

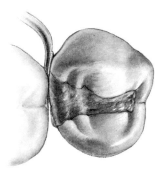

Fig. 14-36. Condensing proximal gold with a foot condenser.

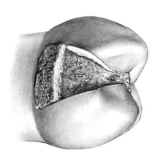

Fig. 14-34. Occlusal gold is extended onto the proximal (soft) gold.

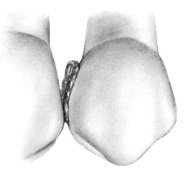

Fig. 14-37. Buccal view after occlusal gold is placed.

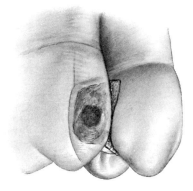

Fig. 14-35. Gold is built occlusally, firmly contacting the adjacent tooth.

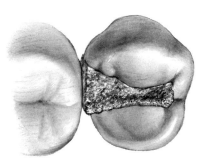

Fig. 14-38. Placement of the foil is complete.

Finishing

ARMAMENTARIUM

Small round finishing burs
Separator
Gordon White saw
Burnishers
Gold files
Linen finishing strips
Gold knife
Finishing disks
Discoid and cleoid carvers
Rubber cup

1 With small stones and round finishing burs (Figs. 14-39 and 14-40) establish the occlusal anatomy and eliminate excess gold from the margins. Rotate all rotary instruments from the center of the restoration toward the margin.

2 Place a separator. Some circumstances may warrant placement of the separator before this time, but it is normally placed after the gold is inserted.

3 Apply sufficient separation to allow passage of a Gordon White saw and/or strips between the contacts.

4 Burnish the gold over the proximal margins using burnishers or dull files (Fig. 14-41).

5 Use a gold knife to carefully eliminate excess gold (Fig. 14-42). The gold knife may be more easily controlled if used as a push instrument instead of using the sharp cutting edge (Fig. 14-85).

6 Finish the proximal margins cautiously, starting with extra fine garnet ³/₈ disks and graduating to finer grits (Fig. 14-43).

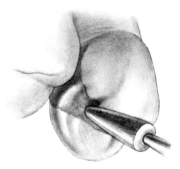

Fig. 14-39. Finishing a Class 2 gold foil restoration. Finger stone to smooth occlusal surface.

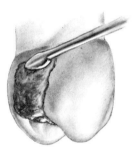

Fig. 14-41. Rhein file to smooth proximal surface.

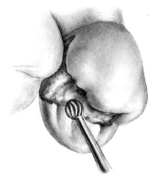

Fig. 14-40. Finishing bur to smooth the margins and rough in occlusal anatomy.

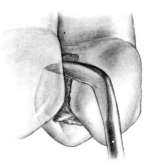

Fig. 14-42. Gold knife to remove excess gold and contour proximal gold.

7 Without reducing the contact area establish the proximal contour, using first a lightning strip and then fine cuttle linen finishing strips (Fig. 14-44).

8 Finish carving and burnishing the occlusal surface with discoid and cleoid carvers (Fig 14-45).

9 Burnish the proximal area.

10 Strip the proximal area with an extra fine cuttle strip.

11 Polish with pumice and high-shine powder, using a small soft rubber cup at slow speed and light pressure (Fig. 14-46).

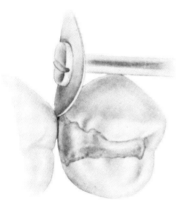

Fig. 14-43. Three-eighth inch finishing disk.

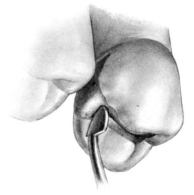

Fig. 14-45. Occlusal anatomy refined with cleoid carver.

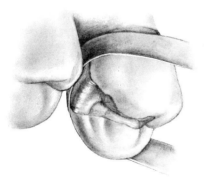

Fig. 14-44. Linen finishing strip on proximal surface.

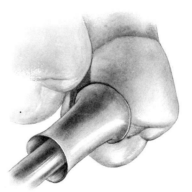

Fig. 14-46. Flour of pumice and high-polishing medium for polishing, using a small rubber cup.

ATYPICAL CLASS 2 GOLD FOIL RESTORATIONS

At least two situations offer opportunities to restore Class 2 caries without making the usual step through the occlusal surface. Both are highly recommended for conservation of tooth structure and esthetics.

MESIAL PLACEMENT, MANDIBULAR FIRST PREMOLARS

The mesial surface of mandibular first premolars often can be conservatively restored with gold foil, thereby preserving the occlusal surface (Fig. 14-47, *A* and *B*). The preparation follows the same basic steps as that for a mandibular Class 3 foil preparation.

MESIAL PLACEMENT, FIRST MOLARS

Carious lesions of first molars can conveniently be restored in children at the time the second deciduous molar is lost, using a technique advocated by Jeffery[2] (Fig. 14-47, *C*). The rapidity with which the second premolars sometimes erupt makes it essential that treatment not be delayed in these cases. It is often advisable to remove the deciduous molar at the same appointment that the foil is placed.

The rubber dam must firmly retract the gingival tissue on the mesial surface of the molar. A molar clamp is placed in a normal position buccolingually and worked gingivally to help ensure this retraction. Several minutes are often required to effect this retraction adequately since it must be accomplished gently but firmly.

Cavity preparation

1 Outline the cavity to proper extension (based on that indicated when second premolar is erupted in place) using an inverted cone bur, No. 34 or 35. A V-shaped diamond disk may be used in a contra-angle handpiece to remove bulk. Use care not to undercut the marginal ridge.

2 Create internal form using a smaller inverted cone bur and hand instruments.

3 Retention form is established using an angle former to sharpen the gingivoaxial line angle. The occlusal retention is placed in the buccal and lingual areas toward the cusps and not at the expense of the marginal ridge. A small inverted cone bur is sometimes adequate. Retentive areas in the gingival, buccal, and lingual point angles need not be created.

4 Varnish the cavity and plane the enamel walls using a Wedelstaedt chisel.

Insertion

Placement of the gold is somewhat similar to that in Class 5 restorations. Noncohesive cylinders may be placed on the buccal and gingival walls as in Class 5 cavities. A bulk of gold is then placed between the linguogingival point angle and the occlusolingual retention area and condensed to wedge it firmly in place while held. When this gold is properly condensed, it should not be necessary to continue holding the gold while the cavity is filled to the desired contour.

Finishing

Finishing will usually be as followed for a Class 5 restoration.

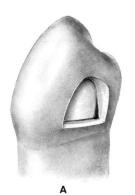 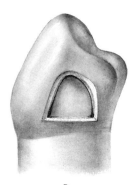 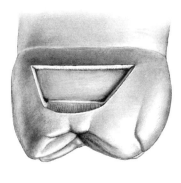

A   B   C

Fig. 14-47. Atypical Class 2 cavity preparations. **A** and **B**, Mesial aspect of mandibular first premolars. **C**, Mesial aspect of maxillary first molar.

Class 3 gold foil restorations
LINGUAL PLACEMENT, MAXILLARY INCISOR

Display of gold has become increasingly objectionable. Gold foil as a restorative material fell into virtual disuse for a time. However, improved techniques, which permit the placement of gold inconspicuously, are increasing its use in restoration of proximal surfaces of anterior teeth.

The following procedure, as developed and taught by Alexander Jeffery,[3] provides an excellent method, easily mastered, to restore carious lesions in maxillary anterior teeth if they are treated before they have destroyed the tooth too far in a labial direction (Fig. 14-48).

Cavity preparation

ARMAMENTARIUM

Ferrier No. 1 separator (modified)
Set of Jeffery cutting instruments or their equivalent

1 Place a rubber dam and Ferrier No. 1 separator (modified). The separator must be placed in a manner that will facilitate instrumentation. It is helpful to rotate it in the direction toward which the instruments will be inserted into the cavity. Stabilize the separator with compound.

2 With a Jeffery No. 2 hatchet, cleave away unsupported enamel (Fig. 14-49).

3 Use a No. 33½ (34) inverted cone bur to establish the lingual outline to the linguogingival line angle (Fig. 14-50).

4 With the No. 33½ (34) bur establish the gingival wall (Fig. 14-51). While establishing the gingival wall, the bulk of the tooth structure to be restored is removed. The labial extension must be very carefully established. It is helpful to use direction vision between the teeth to establish labial extention.

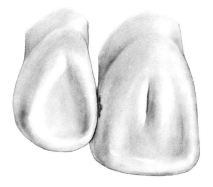

Fig. 14-48. Carious lesion.

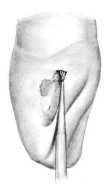

Fig. 14-50. Use a No. 33½ or 34 bur to establish lingual outline and start gingival wall.

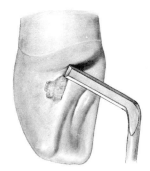

Fig. 14-49. Cleave enamel with Jeffery No. 2 hatchet to enter cavity.

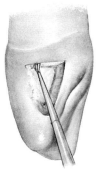

Fig. 14-51. Extend gingival wall.

5 Remove bulk in the incisal retention area with a No. 33½ inverted cone bur (Fig. 14-52). A contra-angle may be helpful in some cases, although it is seldom necessary.

6 Remove a small amount of dentin in the lingual retention area (Fig. 14-53) and then the labial retention area (Fig. 14-54).

7 Use a Jeffery No. 5 offset hatchet to remove bulk from the incisal retention area while sharpening the axioincisal line angle (Fig. 14-55). The axial wall meets the incisal wall in an arcuate retention area, not a sharp point.

8 With a small Wedelstaedt chisel, Jeffery No. 11, plane the lingual wall and bevel the incisal wall (Fig. 14-56).

COMMENT: *One of the most critical parts of this operation is that of removing sufficient tooth structure in the curve of the incisal portion of the lingual wall. This is essential to facilitate use of condensing points in placement of the foil.*

9 Plane the gingival and labial walls with a Jeffery hatchet No. 7 (Fig. 14-57).

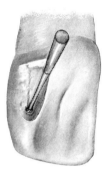

Fig. 14-52. With No. 33½ bur remove incisal bulk.

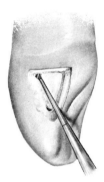

Fig. 14-54. Remove bulk in the labial retention area.

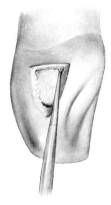

Fig. 14-53. Remove bulk in lingual retention area.

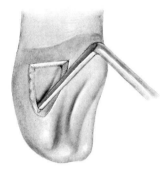

Fig. 14-55. With a Jeffery No. 5 hatchet remove bulk from the incisal area.

10 Using a Jeffery hatchet No. 6 as a hoe, slightly bevel the labial enamel (Fig. 14-58), and as a chisel, plane the labial part of the gingival wall (Fig. 14-59).

11 Create the final incisal retention with a Jeffery No. 10 hatchet (Fig. 14-60). The instrument must be used with a light chopping action to avoid breaking it. The area created must be in the middle of the proximal surface of the tooth, not toward the lingual surface. The incisal portion of the linguoaxial line angle is also sharpened.

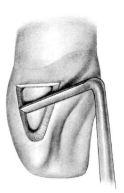

Fig. 14-58. With a Jeffery No. 6 hatchet bevel the labial enamel.

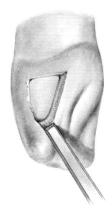

Fig. 14-56. With a small Wedelstaedt chisel (Jeffery No. 11) plane the lingual wall and start the incisal bevel.

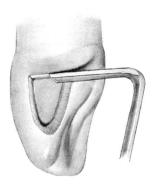

Fig. 14-59. With the No. 6 hatchet plane the labial portion of the gingival enamel.

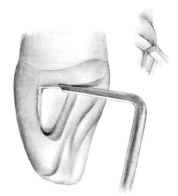

Fig. 14-57. Plane the gingival and labial walls with a Jeffery No. 7 hatchet.

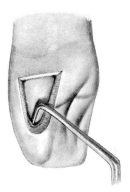

Fig. 14-60. Cut the final incisal retention with a Jeffery No. 10 hatchet.

12 Using a Jeffery No. 9 bayonet angle former, form the lingual retention point (Fig. 14-61). This is created by thrusting the instrument gingivally, planing the dentin of the gingival part of the lingual wall. At the same time the gingivoaxial line angle is sharpened by planing the dentin of the gingival wall, creating an axial slope to provide the gingival retention.

COMMENT: *The labial and lingual retention points should be kept small. They facilitate starting the placement of the foil, the main retentive factors of a Class 3 gold foil restoration being the gingival and incisal walls.*

13 Sharpen the labial retention with a Jeffery No. 5 offset hatchet (Fig. 14-62). Establish the labial portion of the gingival retention by sharpening the labioaxial line angle, creating a slight undercut in the dentin.

14 Place a small convenience point in the labial retention with a No. 33¼ inverted cone bur (Fig. 14-63). About half the depth of the bur head is sufficient.

15 Line the cavity with varnish and lightly replane margins touched by the varnish.

16 Completed cavity preparation (Fig. 14-64).

Insertion

ARMAMENTARIUM

Jeffery condensers or their equivalent

1 Place a ¹/₁₂₈ (¹/₆₄) pellet in the labial convenience point. Force the gold into the convenience point and condense it with two or three blows of the mallet, using a Jeffery No. 12 (Ferrier No. 4) condenser (Fig. 14-65). Use of a holding instrument is unnecessary.

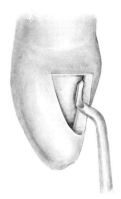

Fig. 14-61. Sharpen the lingual retention with a Jeffery No. 5 angle former and plane the dentin of the gingival wall.

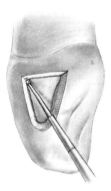

Fig. 14-63. Place a labial convenience point with a No. 33½ bur.

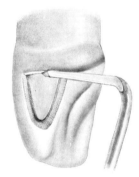

Fig. 14-62. With a Jeffery No. 5 hatchet sharpen the labial retention and sharpen the axiogingival line angle by planing the gingival dentin.

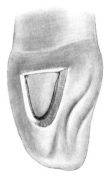

Fig. 14-64. Completed cavity preparation.

2 Place another pellet of gold over the first and condense it (Fig. 14-66). Place the next pellet over the last and along the linguogingival line angle over the cavosurface margin and condense it.

3 Condense additional pellets along the gingivoaxial line angle into the gingival retention (Fig. 14-67).

4 Condense additional pellets into the lingual retention using a Jeffery No. 16 bayonet condenser (Fig. 14-68).

5 With the Jeffery No. 12 condenser (Ferrier No. 4) condense additional foil over the entire gingival wall (Fig. 14-69).

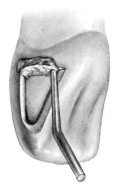

Fig. 14-67. Build gold along axiogingival line angle into lingual retention.

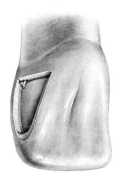

Fig. 14-65. Placement of first piece of gold in labial convenience point.

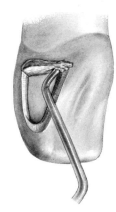

Fig. 14-68. Condense gold in lingual retention with bayonnet condenser (Jeffery No. 16).

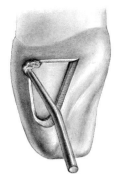

Fig. 14-66. Place additional gold along the labiogingival line angle.

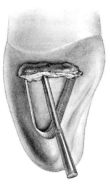

Fig. 14-69. Increase bulk of gold on gingival wall.

6 Use a foot condenser, Jeffery No. 15 (Ferrier No. 12), to condense the foil over the gingival margin (Fig. 14-70).

7 Build the foil incisally, keeping the height of gold over the labial margin higher than over the lingual margin (Fig. 14-71).

8 When the level of the gold approaches the incisal area, use a Jeffery No. 21 condenser with hand pressure to condense gold into the incisal area (Fig. 14-72).

9 Use a Jeffery No. 16 condenser to mallet the gold into the incisal area (Fig. 14-73). Where this is not possible, particular care must be used to hand condense the foil thoroughly. A contra-angle mechanical or electronic condenser may help.

10 Use a Ferrier No. 7 condenser to condense the gold up the labial margin (Fig. 14-74).

COMMENT: *It is essential that gold be scrupulously condensed to the labial margin at all times.*

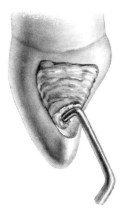

Fig. 14-72. Use a Jeffery No. 21 condenser to condense gold in incisal retention.

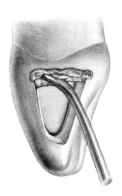

Fig. 14-70. Use a foot condenser along gingival margin.

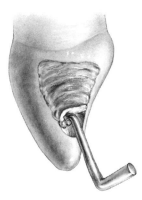

Fig. 14-73. Use a Jeffery No. 16 condenser to condense incisal gold.

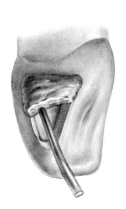

Fig. 14-71. Build up the foil.

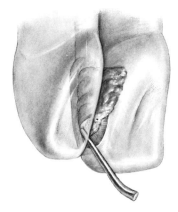

Fig. 14-74. Use a Ferrier No. 7 condenser to ensure condensation of gold up the labial margin.

11 Complete placing the foil with a Jeffery No. 12 (Ferrier No. 4) condenser (Fig. 14-75).

12 Condense the entire surface of the foil with a foot condenser (Ferrier No. 12) (Fig. 14-76).

13 Use a Jeffery No. 19 foot condenser to condense the foil over the labial margin, adding gold if necessary (Fig. 14-114).

Fig. 14-77 includes typical Class 3 lingual foil preparations on different teeth. In general, cavities prepared to restore mesial surfaces should be extended less than those on distal surfaces. Thus the cavities shown in Fig. 14-77, *A, B,* and *E,* are narrower labiolingually than the cavities shown in Fig. 14-64 and Fig. 14-77, *C* and *D.*

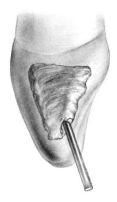

Fig. 14-75. Complete placement of gold.

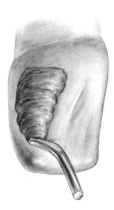

Fig. 14-76. Establish final contour with foot condenser.

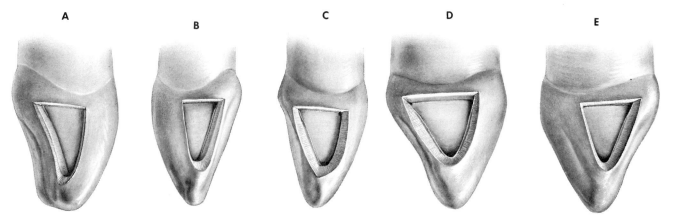

Fig. 4-77. Inconspicuous cavity preparations. **A,** Mesial aspect of maxillary left central incisor. **B,** Mesial aspect of maxillary right lateral incisor. **C,** Distal aspect of maxillary right lateral incisor. **D,** Distal aspect of maxillary right canine. **E,** Mesial aspect of right canine.

Finishing

ARMAMENTARIUM

Gold knife
Gordon White saw
Discoid or cleoid carver
Spratley burnisher or Walls carver
Foot condenser
Finger stone
Finishing disks
Finishing strips

The following steps, although generally executed in the order outlined, will usually be performed as the situation requires and not necessarily in the order described.

1 Pass a gold knife through the contact area if possible (Fig. 14-78). Add a slight amount of separation if necessary. The proximal surface of the gold is burnished with the knife. A Gordon White saw may also be used to open the contact area to facilitate finishing.

2 Burnish the surface of the gold using a cleoid or discoid carver or other suitable burnisher (Spratley burnisher or Walls carver) on the lingual surface (Fig. 14-79) to smooth the surface while also dragging the gold toward the margins. A bedbug file may also be used.

3 Excess gold may be pushed off margin areas using a foot condenser (Fig. 14-80). The condenser is used with a burnishing action applied firmly to the surface of the gold while the condenser is malleted, thus driving off the excess gold.

4 If a stone is used, it must be perfectly true, used at slow speed, and always rotated toward the tooth margin (Fig. 14-81).

5 Disks, ³/₈-inch fine or extra-fine cuttle, are used to establish final contour and a smoother surface (Fig. 14-82). A contra-angle is seldom necessary, especially if the mandrel is extended several millimeters from its normal position in the handpiece. With the index finger of the left hand stretch the rubber dam tightly when disking close to the gingiva. Always use a stream of cold air on the tooth and use very slow speed. Start with fine garnet disks and progress to finer grits.

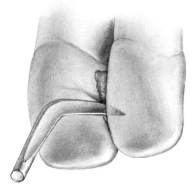

Fig. 14-78. Removal of excess gold and burnishing with gold knife.

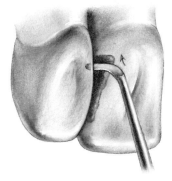

Fig. 14-80. Removal of excess gold in gingival area by malleting with a Ferrier No. 12 foot condenser.

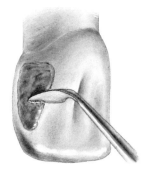

Fig. 14-79. Removal of excess gold with cleoid or discoid carver.

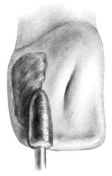

Fig. 14-81. Stone used to contour lingual area.

6 After proper contour is established, pass an extra fine, extra-narrow linen strip over the foil to finish areas not accessible to disks (Figs. 14-83 and 14-84). If the lingual aspect of the strip cannot be easily controlled with the index finger while guiding the strip over the tooth, a cotton roll may help. Use cold air to protect against heating the pulp.

7 A high luster may be created with the use of flour of pumice and a high-polishing agent such as tin oxide. However, an extremely high finish may not be desirable esthetically.

Use of gold knife

The so-called gold knife may be used to accomplish a large portion of finishing of cohesive golds as well as other restorative materials. If a pulling action is used (Fig. 14-85, *A*), very small bits of gold are shaved off in a direction diagonal to the edge of the blade. This is a difficult action to master since large chunks of gold may be removed or the entire restoration may be pried loose unless the instrument is skillfully employed.

The gold knife may be more easily and safely used with a push action (Fig. 14-85, *B*). The excess at the margins may be pushed off with the back of the blade, using a burnishing action.

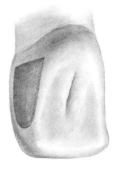

Fig. 14-84. Completed restoration.

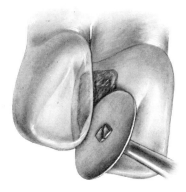

Fig. 14-82. Abrasive disk used to contour and establish smooth surface.

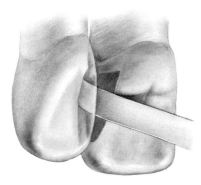

Fig. 14-83. Linen strip used to establish contour and polish.

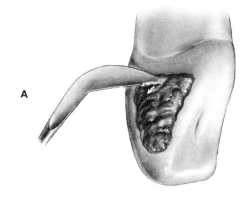

A

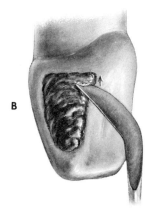

B

Fig. 14-85. Use of gold knife. **A,** Use of pull gold knife. **B,** Use of pull gold knife to remove gold by pushing action.

LABIAL (CONVENTIONAL) PLACEMENT, MAXILLARY INCISOR

Cavity preparation

ARMAMENTARIUM

Ferrier No. 1 separator
6½-2½-9 hoe
No. 33½ bur
Wedelstaedt chisels
Angle formers

1 Place a rubber dam and Ferrier No. 1 separator.

2 Enter the cavity with a 6½-2½-9 hoe (10-4-8 Wedelstaedt). Cleave away undermined enamel (Fig. 14-86). If the cavity is not immediately accessible, make an opening in the enamel with a small round bur.

3 With a No. 33½ (34) inverted cone bur in a straight handpiece remove enough labial enamel to create access and establish the labial portion of the gingival wall and the labioginigval line angle (Fig. 14-87). Using the bur size as a guide to judge depth, remove enough dentin to roughly begin the internal form gingivally and incisally. Remove sufficient bulk lingually to facilitate step 6.

COMMENT: *When establishing the line angles on the gingival wall, rotate the bur in a direction that will tend to carry the cur into the cavity.*

4 With a small contrabevel Wedelstaedt chisel (11½-15-3) establish the labial outline form (Fig. 14-88).

5 Using the same instrument, establish the incisal outline form (Fig. 14-89). An angle former may be used to establish this bevel (Fig. 14-90).

6 Open the lingual aspect of the cavity with the same Wedelstaedt chisel at the incisal area and start to form the lingual wall from the lingual side of the tooth (Fig. 14-91).

7 With the inverted cone bur remove the gingival portion of the lingual enamel, establishing the lingual portion of the gingival wall and creating the linguogingival line angle (Fig. 14-92).

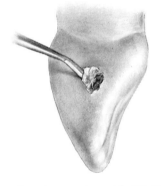

Fig. 14-86. Opening cavity with 6½-2½-9 hoe.

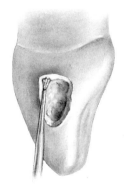

Fig. 14-87. Establishing labial extension and gingival wall.

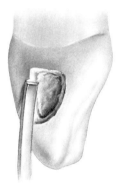

Fig. 14-88. Planing labial wall with Wedelstaedt chisel.

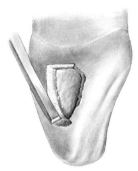

Fig. 14-89. Planing incisal outline with Wedelstaedt chisel.

8 Plane the remainder of the lingual wall with a contrabevel Wedelstaedt chisel (Fig. 14-93).

9 Use a 6$\frac{1}{2}$-2$\frac{1}{2}$-9 hoe to establish the internal (resistance) form. Plane the gingival portion of the labial wall in dentin (Fig. 14-94, *A*). The instrument must be held in a manner that will establish an obtuse line angle joining the enamel wall and the axial wall. While performing this action, at the same time plane the dentin portion of the gingival wall, using the 6$\frac{1}{2}$-2$\frac{1}{2}$-9 as a hoe. A labioaxiogingival point angle is thus established.

10 Establish the middle of the wall with the same instrument, thrusting the instrument toward the axial wall and dragging it incisally and gingivally, planing with the sides of the instrument (Fig. 14-94, *B*).

11 With the 6$\frac{1}{2}$-2$\frac{1}{2}$-9 hoe prepare the incisal area (Fig. 14-94, *C*).

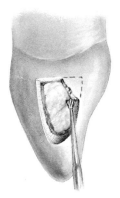

Fig. 14-92. Removal of linguogingival bulk with inverted cone bur.

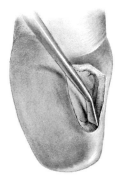

Fig. 14-90. Planing incisal wall with angle former.

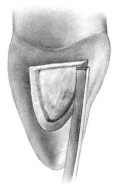

Fig. 14-93. Gingival part of lingual wall planed with Wedelstaedt chisel.

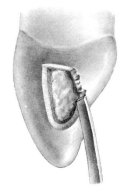

Fig. 14-91. Establishing lingual wall.

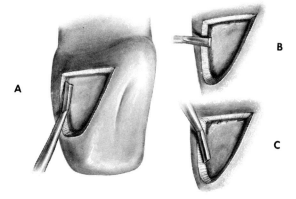

Fig. 14-94. Resistence form of labial wall established with 6$\frac{1}{2}$-2$\frac{1}{2}$-9 hoe. **A,** Planing the gingival portion of the labial walls and the labial portion of the gingival wall. **B,** Planing the middle portion of the labial wall. **C,** Planing the incisal portion of the labial wall and the incisal area.

12 Form the lingual wall. Start at the gingival wall by preparing a linguoaxiogingival point angle. Thrust the instrument gingivally to form the lingual wall, then drag it as a hoe to plane the lingual portion of the gingival wall. Drag the $6^{1}/_{2}$-$2^{1}/_{2}$-9 hoe incisally to complete the lingual wall (Fig. 14-95).

13 Form the incisal wall by joining the lingual and labial walls, using the $6^{1}/_{2}$-$2^{1}/_{2}$-9 hoe with both chisel and hoe actions. The incisal enamel may be reduced somewhat in this area, thus shortening the bevel.

14 Insert the $6^{1}/_{2}$-$2^{1}/_{2}$-9 hoe as shown to establish the lingual point angle (Fig. 14-96).

15 Lightly plane the axial wall with the $6^{1}/_{2}$-$2^{1}/_{2}$-9 hoe (Fig. 14-97). The completed wall will be convex.

COMMENT: *Extreme care must be exercised not to undermine the lingual enamel. The linguoaxial line angle must be obtuse. The internal wall must be established entirely in dentin.*

16 With a small angle former (7-80-$2^{1}/_{2}$-9) cut a retentive point into the labioaxiogingival point angle and at the same time complete the axial slope in the labial part of the dentin of the gingival wall. Usually this step will be performed with the instrument inserted from the labial aspect (Fig. 14-98). However, it may be accomplished from the lingual aspect if the outline of the cavity is extensive enough to permit it (Fig. 14-98). Do not deepen the axial wall.

17 Establish retention form lingually with the same angle former. With the instrument laid in the labial incisal curvature the linguoaxiogingival point angle is sharpened to create a retentive point (Fig. 14-99) to provide gingival retention. This step may also be accomplished with the opposite angle former, with the cutting blade laid flat on the gingival wall and hoe and chisel movements used to establish the desired form (Fig. 14-99).

COMMENT: *Both gingival retention points should be small and should not extend greatly incisally. Their purpose is to facilitate starting the placement of the foil, the main retentive factor in a Class 3 gold foil restoration being the lock between the gingival and incisal walls.*

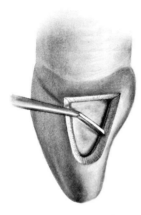

Fig. 14-95. Lingual resistance form established.

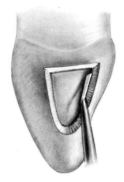

Fig. 14-96. Completion of planing lingual wall and sharpening linguogingival line angle and linguogingivoaxial point angle using the $6^{1}/_{2}$-$2^{1}/_{2}$-9 hoe.

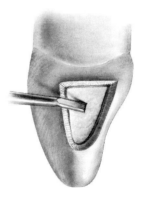

Fig. 14-97. Axial wall smoothed.

18 Form the incisal retention with a 3-1½-18 hatchet, using a chopping action. This area will not be a point but is actually a groove planed in dentin in a labiolingual direction (Fig. 14-100). Do not undermine enamel.

19 Lightly plane the gingival enamel with a 6½-2½-9 hoe to remove short prisms (Fig. 14-101).

20 (Optional) Place a convenience pit in the lingual retention point using a No. 33¼ inverted cone bur. The depth of this pit should be only about half the depth of the bur head (Fig. 14-102).

21 Line the cavity with varnish and lightly replane those margins that may have been touched by the varnish.

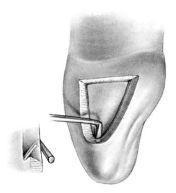

Fig. 14-100. Creation of incisal retention with 3-1½-28 hatchet.

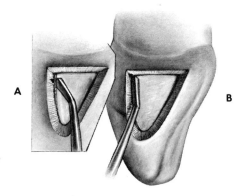

Fig. 14-98. A, Labial retention (optional) being cut from lingual aspect if access permits. **B,** Labial portion of gingival wall (retention form) established with angle former from labial aspect.

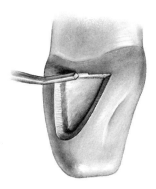

Fig. 14-101. Planing gingival enamel with 6½-2½-9 hoe.

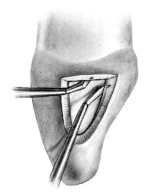

Fig. 14-99. Lingual portion of retentive form cut in gingival wall and lingual retention angle established with angle former.

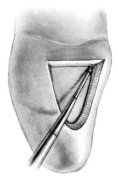

Fig. 14-102. Placement of convenience point with No. 33¼ bur.

Insertion, using holding instrument

ARMAMENTARIUM

Holding instruments
Ferrier No. 4 condenser

1 Place a ¹/₆₄ pellet in the linguogingival line angle. With a curved holding instrument hold the gold firmly against the gingival wall (Fig. 14-103, *A*). The holding instrument must be clear of the retention area. With a Ferrier No. 4 plugger condense the foil into the lingual retention point.

2 Condense another pellet into the lingual retention area, still holding the first gold with the holder (Fig. 14-103, *B*).

3 Condense three or four pellets along the gingivoaxial line angle, then into the labial retention area (Fig. 14-103, *C*). Condense sufficient gold into the labial retention area to ensure total stability. Remove the holder. (Size of the cavity or preference of the operator may require placement of more gold than that described or the used of the holder during the next two steps. Once the gold is firmly tied between the gingival retention points, the holder may be removed.)

Insertion, without holding instrument

ARMAMENTARIUM

Ferrier No. 4 condenser
Jeffery No. 16 condenser
Straight parallelogram
Foot condenser
Ferrier No. 11 condenser
Jeffery No. 19 condenser

1 Place a ¹/₆₄ pellet of foil over the convenience point in the lingual retention area. Press it into place in the convenience point with a Ferrier No. 4 condenser. Mallet the condenser two or three times (Fig. 14-104).

2 Place another ¹/₆₄ pellet in the lingual retention area and mallet it to the first and along the linguogingival line angle.

3 Condense three or four pellets along the gingivoaxial line angle, then into the labial retention point. Condense a couple of pellets into the labial retention area to firmly secure the foil into place (Fig. 14-105). If the cavity preparation is conservative, a Jeffery No. 16 condenser is helpful to condense the foil into the labial retention area (Fig. 14-106).

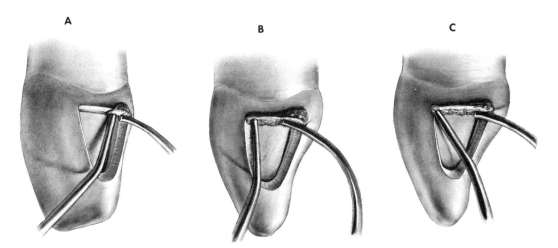

Fig. 14-103. Starting placement of foil when convenience pit is not used. **A,** Pellet of gold placed in lingual retention point and linguogingival line angles, held with holding instrument and condensed with No. 1 condenser. **B,** Additional pellets of gold placed along gingival wall and tied into labial retention area. **C,** Where access allows, foil may be condensed into labial retention with condenser point from lingual aspect.

4 Place additional pellets on the linguogingival shoulder and then over the entire gingival wall. A straight parallelogram can be used to condense the area over the lingual shoulder (Fig. 14-107). The foil should fold firmly over the gingival cavo-surface margin. To be certain it is condensed in his critical area the foil may be lightly condensed along the gingival margin with a Ferrier No. 12 foot plugger (Fig. 14-108).

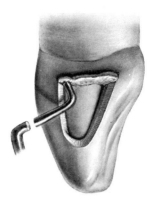

Fig. 14-106. Use of Jeffery No. 16 bayonet condenser point in labial retention.

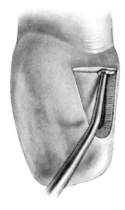

Fig. 14-104. First pellet of gold condensed into convenience pit with No. 1 condenser point.

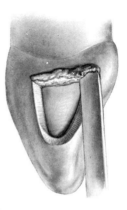

Fig. 14-107. Condensing gold on gingival shoulder using straight parallelogram.

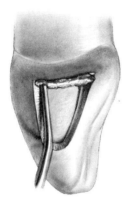

Fig. 14-105. Additional pellets condensed along gingival wall and into labial retention.

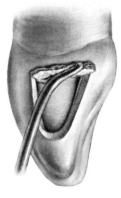

Fig. 14-108. Condensing gold over gingival margin using a Ferrier No. 12 foot condenser.

5 Build the gold incisally, keeping the bulk of the gold higher on the lingual wall than the labial. It is essential to watch the line of force as the foil is condensed (Fig. 14-109). Most cases allow occasional condensation along the lingual side of the tooth.

6 When the level of gold on the lingual margin begins to approach the incisal curve of the preparation, gold is condensed into the incisal retention area. A Ferrier No. 11 plugger is used to condense foil by hand pressure into the retention area (Fig. 14-110). A bayonet plugger, Ferrier No. 8 or Jeffery No. 16, may be used to mallet into this area.

7 When the incisal retention area is filled and condensed and the resistance form filled (Fig. 14-111), begin "making the turn," building the foil up the lingual margin and then over the incisal margin, using a Ferrier No. 4 condenser (Fig. 14-112).

8 Condense foil on over the labial margin and to full contour.

9 Use a foot condenser to condense and contour the entire surface of the gold and to ensure that all margins are covered (Fig. 14-113).

10 Contour the foil below the contact area with a Jeffery No. 19 condenser (Fig. 14-114).

Finishing

See Figs. 14-78 through 14-84 for finishing the gold after inserting.

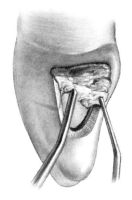

Fig. 14-109. Buildup of bulk of gold.

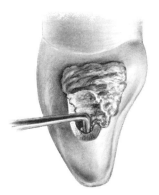

Fig. 14-110. Gold condensed into incisal retention area using a Ferrier No. 11 condenser (Jeffery No. 16 bayonet condenser).

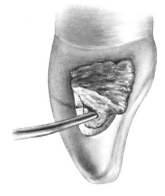

Fig. 14-111. Buildup of bulk of gold in incisal retention area with Ferrier No. 4 condenser.

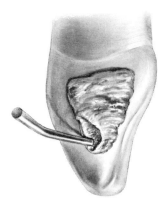

Fig. 14-112. Completing the turn in incisal area.

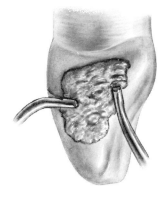

Fig. 14-113. Use of Ferrier No. 12 foot condenser to contour surface.

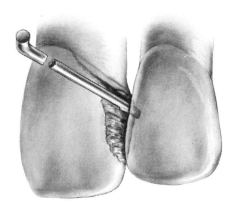

Fig. 14-114. Jeffery No. 19 condenser used between teeth.

LABIAL PLACEMENT, MANDIBULAR INCISOR
Cavity preparation

ARMAMENTARIUM
6½-2½-9 hoe
No 33½ bur
Small Wedelstaedt chisel
Angle formers
3-1½-28 hatchet

1 Break away part of the labial enamel and the carious lesion with a 6½-2½-9 hoe (Fig. 14-115). This may not be practicable in all cases.

2 With a No. 33½ bur in a straight handpiece open the cavity to the desired labial extension (Fig. 14-116) and rough out the carious portion of the cavity to the general lingual extension. Do not overcut the lingual wall.

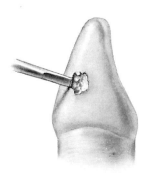

Fig. 14-115. Break away labial enamel into cavity with 6½-2½-9 hoe.

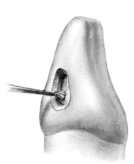

Fig. 14-116. With No. 33½ bur open cavity to labial outline.

3 Create the incisal outline in conjunction with the previous step to provide access to cut the gingival wall.

4 Establish the gingival wall to its proper width buccolingually and to its desired depth (Fig. 14-117). Normally the depth of the cavity does not need to be much deeper than the diameter of the No. 33½ bur. It must be emphasized that the labial extension of the gingival wall needs to be only sufficient to provide access to place the restorative material.

5 Smooth the lingual wall with the end of the No. 33½ bur (Fig. 14-118). The lingual wall should be flat, without bevels, and at approximately a right angle to the pulpal wall.

6 Establish the internal (resistance) form (Fig. 14-119). Use the adjacent tooth as a guide to establish the desired minimal extension (Fig. 14-120).

7 Use a contrabevel Wedelstaedt chisel to plane the gingival portion of the labial wall (Figs. 14-121 and 14-122).

8 With the same Wedelstaedt chisel, plane the remainder of the labial wall and the incisal curve (Fig. 14-123). An angle former may be helpful in reaching the lingual portion of the incisal curve. Do not extend a bevel onto the lingual wall (Fig. 14-124).

9 With a 6½-2½-9 hoe, plane the internal (resistance) form (Fig. 14-125). (See also Fig. 14-94.)

10 Plane the lingual wall with the 6½-2½-9 hoe. (Fig. 14-126).

11 Establish the lingual retention with a small angle former (7-80-2½-9), using both hoe and thrust movements (Fig. 14-127). The lingual portion of the gingival wall is also planed to make the gingival wall retentive.

12 Using a 3-1½-28 or 3-1-32 hatchet, place the labial retention and complete the labial portion of the gingival wall (Fig. 14-128). The completed gingival wall should be flat and meet the axial wall at an acute angle.

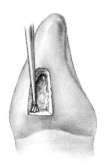

Fig. 14-117. Establish gingival wall with No. 33½ bur.

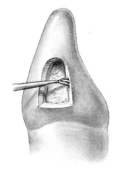

Fig. 14-118. Establish lingual wall.

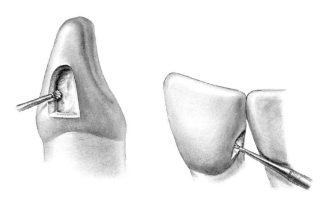

Figs. 14-119 and **14-120.** Start internal (resistance) form.

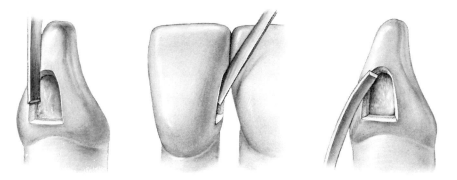

Figs. 14-121 to **14-123.** Plane labial enamel wall and incisal curve with a small Wedelstaedt chisel.

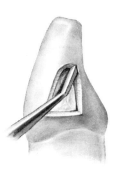

Fig. 14-124. Plane incisal enamel with angle former.

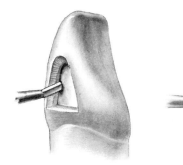

Figs. 14-125 and **14-126.** Plane internal resistance form with a $6\frac{1}{2}$-$2\frac{1}{2}$-9 hoe.

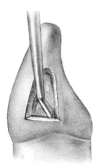

Fig. 14-127. Cut the lingual retention and the lingual portion of the gingival wall with an angle former.

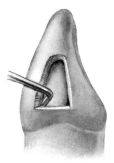

Fig. 14-128. With a 3-$1\frac{1}{2}$-28 or 3-1-32 hatchet plane the labial portion of the gingival wall and place the labial retention.

13 Establish the incisal retention using a 3-1¹/₂-28 hatchet with a chopping action (Fig. 14-129). Care must be taken not to undermine the labial or lingual enamel, nor should the incisal angle by weakened.

14 Bevel the gingival enamel slightly with a 6¹/₂-2¹/₂-9 hoe (Fig. 14-130).

15 Line the cavity with varnish and replane the enamel as appropriate (Fig. 14-131).

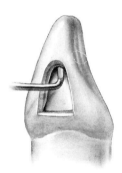

Fig. 14-129. Place the incisal retention using the same instrument.

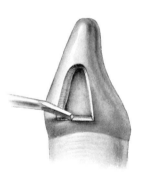

Fig. 14-130. Plane the gingival enamel with a 6¹/₂-2¹/₂-9 hoe.

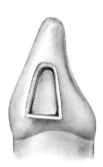

Fig. 14-131. Completed cavity preparation.

Insertion

ARMAMENTARIUM

Holding instrument
Jeffery No. 16 condenser
Ferrier No. 4 condenser
Jeffery No. 19 condenser

If the operator wishes to use a tiny convenience point established with a No. 33¹/₄ bur in the lingual retention area, half the depth of the bur head, starting the foil is made much easier since the requirement for a holding instrument is eliminated. Following is the procedure used with a holding instrument. The same general steps are utilized with either technique.

1 Place a ¹/₆₄ (¹/₁₂₈) pellet in the lingual retention. Force the pellet into the retentive area with a Ferrier No. 4 condenser or its equivalent. Holding a margin of the gold, lightly mallet the gold (Fig. 14-132).

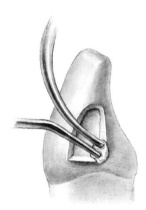

Fig. 14-132. Placement of first pellet.

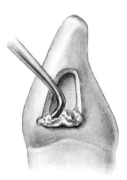

Fig. 14-133. Build across the gingival wall into the labial retention.

2 Add sufficient pellets to build the gold labially along the gingival wall and into the labial retention. Use a Jeffery No. 16 bayonet condenser in the labial area (Fig. 14-133). The holding instrument may now be removed.

3 To protect the lingual wall Stebner[4] recommends using laminated foil laid on the lingual wall (Fig. 14-134) and regular pellets condensed to it (Fig. 14-135).

COMMENT: *Great care must be exercised in condensing foil against the lingual wall. It should not be necessary at any time to use a line of force directly toward the lingual wall. The line of force should be directed primarily toward the gingival wall as the buildup is made.*

4 Build the foil up the lingual wall, into the incisal retentive area (Fig. 14-136), and labially around the incisal curve (Fig. 14-137).

5 Place the remaining foil to the desired contour. A foot plugger may be used to establish final contour as with a Jeffery No. 19 condenser (Fig. 14-138).

Finishing

Finishing is accomplished using the general techniques outlined for the upper Class 3 foil restorations.

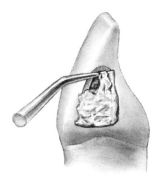

Fig. 14-136. Build up into incisal retention.

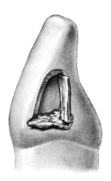

Fig. 14-134. Place a strip of laminated foil on the lingual wall (optional).

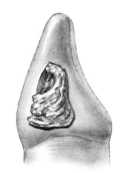

Fig. 14-137. Incisal bulk built up.

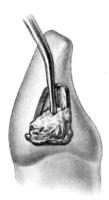

Fig. 14-135. Build up bulk of gold.

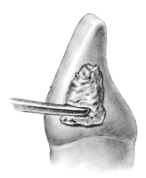

Fig. 14-138. Insertion completed and the surface completed with a Jeffery No. 19 condenser.

Class 4 gold foil restorations

Although few operators seem to utilize gold foil to restore broken angles of anterior teeth, its use is highly recommended if the display of gold is not great. The present inexcusable tendency to go to full coverage in all cases of broken angles is probably prompted by several factors, among them overextended silicate restorations and lack of skill in placement of restorations of a more conservative type.

Fig. 14-139 shows two views of a preparation form advocated by Stebner.[4]

The principles to be borne in mind in preparing a cavity for a Class 4 cohesive gold restoration are generally the following:

1. Emphasize gingival retention.
2. If possible, gain retentive factor such as that shown on the axial walls in Fig. 14-139.
3. Prepare an incisal step as dictated by the needs of the case. That is, do not necessarily extend the preparation across the incisal edge, but slope the incisal wall away from the axial wall to increase stability of the restoration under stress (resistance form) and to form a lock (retention form). The incisal step need not be as extensive as that shown in Fig. 14-139, but it must be of adequate bulk to provide strength.

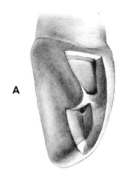

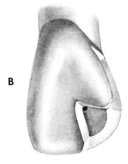

Fig. 14-139. Class 4 gold foil preparation. **A,** Mesiolingual view. **B,** Lingual view.

Class 5 gold foil restorations

Cohesive golds are frequently indicated for the restoration of gingival third lesions. Properly placed, no material provides greater longevity or greater compatibility with tissues of the oral cavity.

Cavity preparation

The same steps as those described in Chapter 7, Figs. 7-42 through 7-50, are followed. Variations are many and generally will fall within the types shown in Figs. 7-51 through 7-56. Curving the occlusal outline is a matter of discretion and is used to conserve tooth structure, especially in maxillary teeth. A curved gingival outline is rarely necessary.

Insertion of gold foil using noncohesive cylinders[5]

ARMAMENTARIUM

Parallelograms
Ferrier No. 1 condenser
Foot condenser

Procedure

The following procedure may seem confusing when first attempted by an operator. The operator may feel somewhat "tangled" in the first steps. However, further experience will prove the procedure's value in terms of time saved and the ease with which enamel margins are protected. Follow these steps after the cavity has been lined with cavity varnish and the margins planed (Fig. 14-140).

1 Place a $\frac{1}{8}$ cylinder with one end against the axial wall and press it firmly against the distal wall using parallelograms (Fig. 14-141). Alternately, one instrument should firmly hold the foil while the other, with as few motions as possible, presses it to the distal wall and wedges it between the retentive walls.

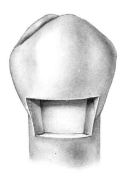

Fig. 14-140. Cavity preparation.

2 Cover the mesial wall with a ⅛ cylinder in the same manner.

3 Place a ⅛ cylinder in the same manner on the gingival wall, wedging it between the mesial and distal cylinders (Fig. 14-142).

4 Flatten a ⅛ cylinder gently with finger pressure and, using a parallelogram as a guide, slide it into place on the occlusal wall between the mesial and distal cylinders. Press it firmly in place, wedging it between the mesial and distal gold (Figs. 14-143 and 14-144).

COMMENT: *W. I. Ferrier, who devised this technique, described the placement of the gingival and occlusal cylinders differently. He placed the cylinder with one end against the wall being covered and forced it in place. The essential factor at this point is not how neat this arrangement looks but that all four peripheral walls are covered with a reasonably uniform bulk of the "soft" foil.*

5 Place a ¹⁄₃₂ annealed pellet on the axial wall at the distal wall and press it in place (Fig. 14-145). Follow it with another ¹⁄₃₂ pellet (and a third if necessary) to provide a bulk of gold that can be firmly wedged against the gingival and occlusal walls. Mallet these pellets, using a No. 1 condenser while holding the mass with a holding instrument (Fig. 14-145). The cohesive foil is thus wedged securely between the two retentive walls. Holding the foil after these pellets are condensed should not be necessary.

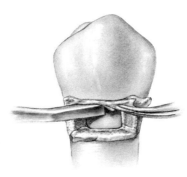

Fig. 14-143. Insertion of occlusal cylinder with cotton pliers, using parallelogram as a guide.

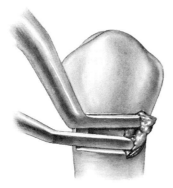

Fig. 14-141. Placement of first cylinder using parallelograms.

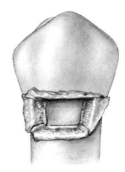

Fig. 14-144. External walls lined with cylinders.

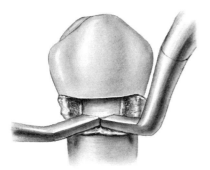

Fig. 14-142. Placement of gingival cylinder.

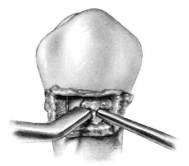

Fig. 14-145. First two or three pellets of gold (¹⁄₆₄ or ¹⁄₃₂) held in place and condensed to wedge gold in place.

6 Add pellets, condensing each in turn to cover the axial wall until sufficient bulk is established to lock all cylinders in place and ensure complete stability (Fig. 14-146).

7 Build up the foil on the distal wall, starting along the distoaxial line angle until the cavosurface margin is reached. The foil may safely be malleted in such a manner that the foil is driven off the margin (pinched off) as it is condensed to the margin. This margin should thus be clearly visible and free of excess while foil within the cavity thoroughly abuts it along its entire length (Fig. 14-147).

8 Build up the gold against the distal wall in the same manner (Fig. 14-148).

9 Condense gold against the gingival wall. Again, be certain all excess gold is removed beyond the margin once the foil is condensed to it (Fig. 14-149).

10 Condense gold against the occlusal wall in the same manner, starting at one end and working the excess gold off as it is condensed along the margin (Figs. 14-150 to 14-152).

11 All that remains is to build up desired contour. At all times keep the surface of the gold smooth and free of pits or depressions, and when gold is condensed beyond the margins, pinch it off (Fig. 14-159). (It is sometimes helpful, when contour is almost complete, to slightly overextend the last few pellets. However, this should be minimal and only for the purpose of ensuring adequate contour. The excess thus created should be capable of quick removal during the finishing steps.)

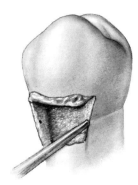

Fig. 14-147. Gold built up distal wall and pinched off over margin.

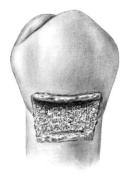

Fig. 14-148. Gold built up mesial wall and excess pinched off over margin.

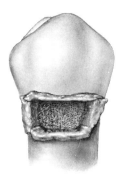

Fig. 14-146. Cohesive gold covering axial wall and holding cylinders in place.

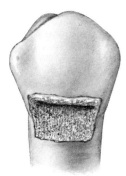

Fig. 14-149. Gingival margin, excess pinched off.

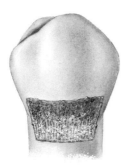

Fig. 14-150. Foil condensed to all margins and excess removed.

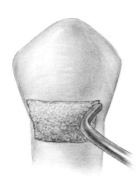

Fig. 14-151. Build to contour and condense with Ferrier No. 12 foot plugger.

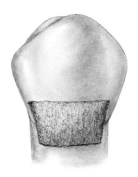

Fig. 14-152. Completed contour.

Insertion of gold foil without cylinders

ARMAMENTARIUM

Ferrier No. 1 condenser
Holding instrument
Foot condenser

Occasionally, especially for smaller cavities, it may be desirable to place the gold without cylinders. Even so, however, maximum margin protection can be attained by placing even one cylinder along the occlusal wall, although it is not illustrated here.

1 Place a $\frac{1}{64}$ ($\frac{1}{32}$) pellet in the distoaxiogingival point angle. Press it lightly in place (Fig. 14-153).

2 Place another $\frac{1}{64}$ ($\frac{1}{32}$) pellet and possibly a third and fourth beside the first toward the occlusal wall and press it lightly in place. Hold one edge with a holding instrument and lightly condense the gold to wedge it firmly (Fig. 14-154).

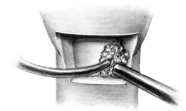

Fig. 14-153. Place a $\frac{1}{64}$ or $\frac{1}{32}$ pellet in a point angle.

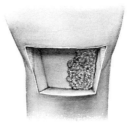

Fig. 14-154. Place another pellet or two along the distoaxial line angle and condense them to wedge the mass between the occlusal (incisal) and gingival walls.

3 Condense additional pellets over these and build the gold toward the mesial wall. When sufficient bulk has been placed, the gold should not need to be held (Fig. 14-155).

COMMENT: *It is important that an adequate quantity of gold be placed as quickly as possible to ensure positive control of it. Thus the first mass of gold is firmly condensed in a manner to wedge it between the occlusal and gingival walls.*

4 When the axial wall is completely covered with a thickness of gold to ensure that it cannot be rocked loose (Fig. 14-155), build the gold up to the distal margin until it is covered (Fig. 14-156).

5 Pinch off the excess along this margin.

6 Build gold up to the mesial margin and pinch off the excess (Fig. 14-157).

7 Build up the gingival gold and pinch off the excess.

8 Build up the occlusal gold, keeping the excess pinched off.

COMMENT: *Protecting the enamel from chipping is not difficult if a bulk of the gold is always ahead of the condenser point. Thus pellets of adequate substance should be used. This does not mean use of large pellets, but they should not be fluffy or loosely rolled.*

9 Build the gold to full contour (Fig. 14-158).

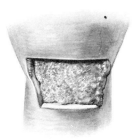

Fig. 14-156. Foil built over distal cavosurface margin.

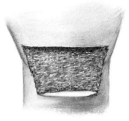

Fig. 14-157. Foil built to mesial and distal margins and excess removed.

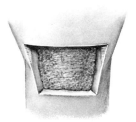

Fig. 14-155. Axial wall covered.

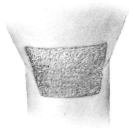

Fig. 14-158. Foil built to gingival and occlusal margins and filled to contour.

Finishing

ARMAMENTARIUM

Foot condenser
Spratley burnishers (Walls carver)
Finishing disks (³/₈ inch)
Gold knife
Wedelstaedt chisel
Gregg 4 and 5 carver
Rubber cup and polishing media

The following steps, although generally executed in the order described, will vary according to the operator's preference.

1 Use a foot condenser to burnish excess off the margins. This is done with firm hand pressure and a burnishing action while the instrument is malleted (Fig. 14-159).

2 Burnish the entire surface of the gold with a Spratley burnisher (Walls carver) (Fig. 14-160). This instrument is excellent for removing gold beyond the margins. A file may be preferred to establish contour.

3 Disk the gold with a ³/₈-inch extra fine cuttle disk (Fig. 14-161). Be certain to keep disks continually in motion to avoid creating flat areas. Keep a stream of cold air on the tooth whenever the disk is in contact with the tooth.

4 Disk with finer grits; as contour is attained the surface is smoothed. Contra-angle handpieces are rarely necessary to finish Class 5 restorations since direct access is usually available. It is helpful, especially when working as shown in Fig. 14-162, to extend the mandrel from the handpiece about ¼ inch.

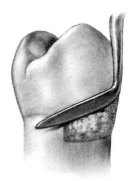

Fig. 14-160. Trim margins and burnish with Spratley burnisher (Ward carver).

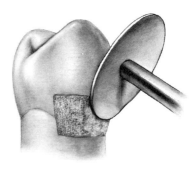

Fig. 14-161. Disk with ³/₈-inch disk.

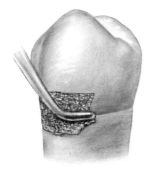

Fig. 14-159. Burnish excess off margins with foot condenser as the instrument is malleted.

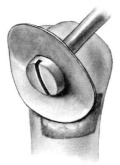

Fig. 14-162. Disk reversed on mandrel to facilitate reaching margins.

5 Trim the excess from the gingival margin. This may be done with a Wedelstaedt chisel, by pushing the gold off with the back of a gold knife blade, or a combination of these methods (Fig. 14-163). It is often effective to lay the blade of the gold knife flat on the jaw of the No. 212 clamp, and using the clamp jaw as a fulcrum, use the side of the tip of the gold knife with light pressure to reduce the excess gold.

COMMENT: *Finishing the gingival margin of a Class 5 restoration is the most critical part of the entire procedure. The utmost care must be exercised to avoid ditching this area. Any discrepancy, whether by overfinishing or underfinishing, may create an irritant to the gingival tissue.*

6 Burnish the surface thoroughly with a blunt burnisher such as a very dull Gregg 4 and 5 carver (Fig. 14-164).

7 Using a small, soft rubber cup at slow speed and light pressure, polish with dry flour of pumice (avoid the cementum!) or Zircate* and finally with a dry, extra fine finishing powder (Fig. 14-165). Polishing with these materials should be accomplished in a few seconds if the preceding steps are meticulously performed.

COMMENT: *Difficulty in seeing a margin is sometimes experienced. It is helpful to shadow the area with a finger. Varying the intensity of the shadow is helpful in evaluating areas that are difficult to see.*

---

*L. D. Caulk Co., Milford, Del.

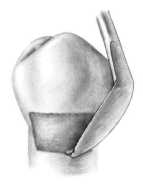

Fig. 14-163. Remove gingival excess with gold knife. (Knife may also be laid flat on clamp jaw and, using the clamp jaw as a fulcrum, used with light pressure to burnish away excess.)

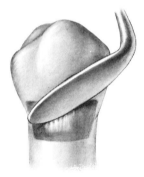

Fig. 14-164. Burnish with blunt burnisher, Gregg 4 and 5 carver.

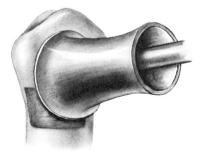

Fig. 14-165. High shine using soft rubber cup, dry pumice, and then fine polish.

Class 6 gold foil restorations

Abraded anterior teeth (Fig. 14-166) and cusps of posterior teeth can frequently be restored with cohesive golds. These restorations become extremely hard in function and afford excellent protection to the teeth.

Cavity preparation

ARMAMENTARIUM

No. 170 bur
No. 33½ bur
Wedelstaedt chisel

1 With a No. 170 bur prepare a lingual and labial wall (Fig. 14-167). Establish these walls close to, but not extended to, the enamel. They must not be undercut, but the line angles should be obtuse (Figs. 14-168 and 14-169).

2 With a No. 33½ bur place small retentive areas in the mesial and distal walls (Fig. 14-168). These may be sharpened with instruments if desired. However, these restorations must be accomplished with a minimum of reduction of tooth structure.

3 Bevel the entire cavosurface angle (Fig. 14-170). Extend the bevel over the enamel.

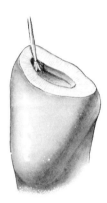

Fig. 14-168. Establish mesial and distal retention areas with No. 33¼ (33½) bur.

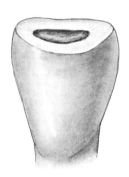

Fig. 14-166. Unprepared cavity.

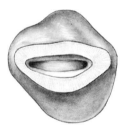

Fig. 14-169. Incisal view.

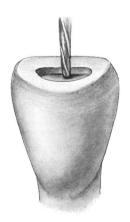

Fig. 14-167. Establish walls with No. 170 bur.

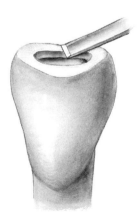

Fig. 14-170. Use Wedelstaedt chisel to bevel all margins.

Insertion

ARMAMENTARIUM

Ferrier No. 1 or No. 4 condenser
Holding instrument

Placement of the gold is simply a matter of condensing a pellet into one of the retention areas and building the gold across into the other one. The remainder of the cavity is then filled, exercising care not to mallet unduly against the lingual wall.

Finishing

Finishing Class 6 cohesive gold restorations is no great task. However, it is important that the sharp edges that frequently exist on these teeth be contoured to protect them from chipping during function (Fig. 14-171). A completed restoration is shown in Fig. 14-172.

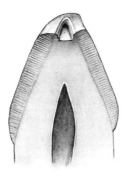

Fig. 14-171. Sectional view of cavity preparation.

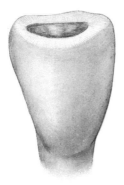

Fig. 14-172. Completed restoration.

Mat gold

Mat or sponge gold finds its greatest use in dentistry in restoring gingival third lesions. It may be used to advantage in extensive cases when the operator wishes to reduce the amount of malleting that might be normally required. It is of great value in cases in which the operator wishes to quickly lock a mass of gold into retentive areas to establish a base on which to build the remaining gold.

It is supplied in strips of various widths so that it can be cut into desired sizes.

Class 5 insertion

1 Cut a piece of mat gold approximately the size of the axial wall. Anneal it as is done with foil, but allow time for the heat to dissipate before placing it in the cavity. A piece of mat gold contains considerably more gold than a foil pellet of comparable volume.

2 Press it into cavity with parallelogram condensers (Fig. 14-173) and condense it into all line and point angles, using a rocking or rolling motion.

COMMENT: *Although it is commonly thought that hand pressure is adequate to condense mat gold, each operator must decide whether the gold is adequately condensed by hand pressure only. Try placing it as described, and then use malleting condensation to compare. It must also be decided whether it is essential that all the gold in a Class 5 restoration be thoroughly condensed.*

3 Place a narrow strip of mat gold along the mesial (or distal) margin. This strip should extend slightly over the cavosurface margin. As it is condensed in place, the excess should be pinched or burnished off with the condenser (Fig. 14-173). Properly executed, this will adequately support and protect the cavosurface enamel during the balance of the procedure.

4 Place and condense a strip along the opposite margin (mesial or distal).

5 Condense a strip in like manner along the gingival margin.

6 Condense a strip along the incisal margin. All margins should now be protected (Fig. 14-173, *D*). Additional pieces of mat gold may be condensed as indicated to build the bulk of the volume of the cavity, care being exercised not to extend the mat gold beyond the margin or to full contour. The restoration is then built to contour (veneered) with cohesive gold and finished by normal foil procedures.

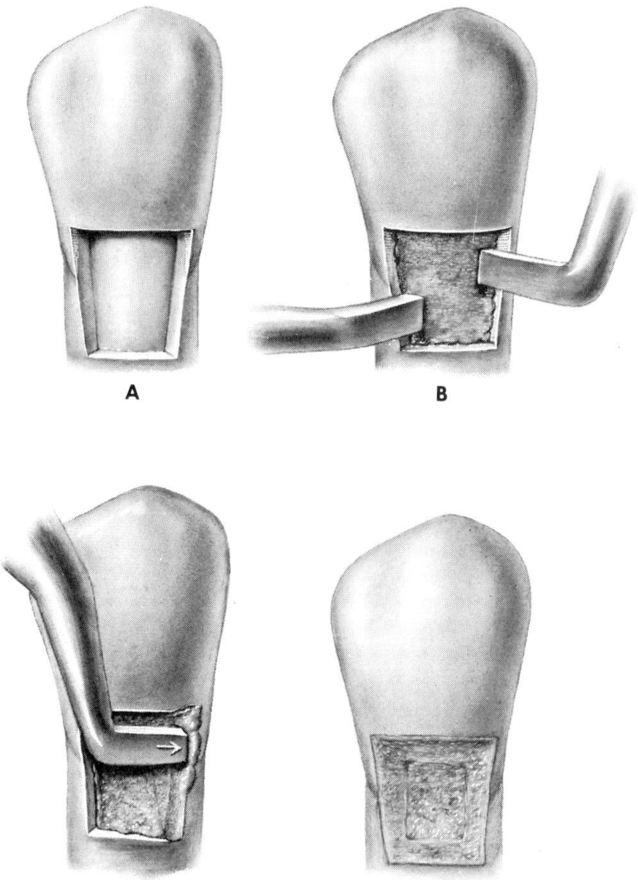

Powdered gold

Powdered gold (Goldent*) is crystalline gold wrapped in gold foil. It is supplied in various sized pieces, each piece containing by weight many times that of a foil pellet of similar size.

Powdered gold is not gold foil and must be used with different skill and technique. It must not be expected, for example, that it can be "wadded" into a cavity to achieve successful results. As with all cohesive golds, it must be methodically and thoroughly condensed as it is placed.

Cavities prepared for powdered gold may be the same as those prepared for gold foil, but with retentive factors slightly increased. Round retention areas are advocated by Baum,[6] although they need not be excessive.

It is not deemed practical to repeat principles and procedures for a material so similar to those already described. Therefore, the following discussion is provided in somewhat abbreviated form as a comparison of the technique, not an evaluation of merits.

Cavity preparations

Cavity preparations should be generally like conventional foil preparations, but long bevels should be avoided and severely sharp internal point angles are not necessary. Slightly rounded retentive areas are preferred by some to facilitate placement of this material.

Annealing

Powdered gold must be thoroughly annealed, preferably a piece at a time over an alcohol flame until it begins to glow slightly, but allowing a longer period at this point than for pellets or foil. It must be allowed to cool for two or three seconds before being placed in the cavity. Overannealing seems to make the gold crystalline and difficult to condense because of lowered plasticity. Underannealing does not create the necessary degree of cohesiveness.

Condensation

Hand pressure with special convex-faced instruments is generally recommended for this material. Malleting condensation may be used and at times may be desirable. A factor that must be emphasized is that of applying adequate force to the condensing point. This material cannot be merely pushed or molded in place and expected to work

Fig. 14-173. Use of mat gold in Class 5 cavity. **A,** Cavity preparation (unusually large). **B,** Strip of mat gold, about the same size as floor of cavity, being condensed in place. **C,** Strip of mat gold laid along margin and condensed; lower portion is shown pinched off over margin. **D,** Strips of mat gold have been condensed along all margins and pinched off, leaving contour to be built up with gold foil or other cohesive gold.

*Morgan Hastings & Co., Philadelphia, Pa.

properly. Condensation should begin on one edge of each piece of gold and each particle forced to the previously placed gold with a rolling or rocking motion, with a simultaneous twisting of the condenser point. A force of 6 to 8 pounds is recommended.

CLASS 3 POWDERED GOLD RESTORATIONS

Cavity preparation

As previously mentioned, the cavities for powdered gold are generally prepared the same as for gold foil, the bevels being held to a minimum and retentive factors slightly emphasized.

Insertion

1 Place and condense a small pellet into the initial retention point, depending on whether labial or lingual placement is being utilized.

2 Lightly place three or four pellets along the gingival floor. Firmly condense these, beginning with the first pellet placed and working toward the opposite retention area. This initial placement should be stabilized with a holding instrument while being condensed. It may then be malleted with a foil condenser if desired.

3 Build the gold incisally, using instruments indicated and hand condensation. Care must be taken to condense the gold meticulously over the margins as it is placed to avoid bridging and creating deficiencies. These defects can be almost impossible to correct later unless the margin is accessible to allow some of the gold to be removed with a small bur.

4 Condense the gold into the incisal retention.

5 Establish the final contour.

Finishing

The same finishing techniques for foil are utilized for powdered gold.

CLASS 2 POWDERED GOLD RESTORATIONS

Cavity preparations are the same as those used for gold foil. Placement of powdered gold may be facilitated by the placement of a matrix band well blocked with a wedge and compound.

Miscellaneous problems
Contaminated surface

If, for whatever cause, gold will not readily cohere when condensed, the surface of the gold already condensed should be thoroughly freshened with a sharp inverted cone bur. The gold surface should then be condensed with a sharp condenser point before adding new gold.

Overcondensing

Inexperienced operators occasionally mention difficulty encountered from "overcondensation." Excessive condensation is not technically possible so should not create a problem other than that of wasted time. It is possible, however, to encounter a degree of difficulty from the use of dull condenser points, which might create a surface appearance that may seem somewhat burnished, or "overcondensed." Gold more readily adheres to a surface condensed with a sharp, serrated condenser.

Adding to a previously placed restoration

It is easy to add to a previously placed foil restoration. Occasionally, usually because of erosion adjacent to the restoration, it is desirable to add to the old gold. It is important that the retentive factor not be destroyed, thereby loosening the restoration. The area to be added is prepared, placing proper outline, resistance, and retentive forms. The surface of the previously placed gold is freshened with a bur and malleted with a sharp condenser. The new gold should readily cohere to the old.

When margins fail to finish

When difficulty is experienced finishing cohesive gold margins, be certain first that the gold is not loose. Second, be certain excess gold is completely removed from the margins. If the cavosurface margins have been chipped during gold placement, burnish the gold into them and complete the finish. Do not try to eliminate chalky margins by disking or using other finishing steps.

"Chalky" margins

"Chalky" margins result from either an underextended cavity preparation (carious area not included) or from improper treatment of the margins during gold placement.

Pitted surface finish

If a surface contains pits or areas that will not polish, burnish thoroughly. If pitting remains, the gold is inadequately condensed. The condition can be improved by using an inverted cone bur to reduce the surface slightly. Mallet the surface with a sharp condenser point, place additional foil, and finish.

Finished restoration appears "black"

Class 3 restorations highly finished may initially appear very dark and conspicuous. They can be improved by finishing with an extra fine strip or pumice rather than by creating a high shine.

Postoperative discomfort

If the retraction of soft tissue has been severe, a gingival dressing is helpful in reducing postoperative pain (Fig. 3-69). If postoperative pain from thermal changes is present, check the occlusion on the tooth and correct it if indicated. Hyperemic pulps associated with Class 5 gold restorations can also occasionally be alleviated by placing a gingival dressing for a few days. Postoperative pain should not occur if placement of the restoration has been carefully executed.

REFERENCES

1. Stebner, C. M.: Table clinic, American Academy of Restorative Dentistry, Feb. 5, 1967, Chicago, Ill.
2. Jeffery, A. W.: Gold foil filling, description of special technique, J. Am. Dent. Assoc. **34**:593, 1947.
3. Jeffery, A. W.: Invisible Class III gold foil restorations, J. Am. Dent. Assoc. **54**:1, 1957.
4. Stebner, C. M.: Personal communication, Feb. 1967.
5. Ferrier, W. I.: Gold foil operations, 1959, University of Washington Press, Seattle, Wash.
6. Baum, L.: Gold foil (filling golds) in dental practice, Dent. Clin. North Am., p. 199, March, 1965.

CHAPTER 15

DENTAL CEMENT RESTORATIONS

Cements for dental purpose may be grouped into four categories: (1) complete restorations, (2) treatment of deep lesions, (3) temporary protection or short-term restorations, and (4) to retain castings and ceramic restorations.

Cement restorations

Cements are used to restore teeth when colors of other materials may be objectionable and mechanical and economic factors do not warrant use of more time-consuming procedures. They are not normally indicated for extensive restorations, where they will be subjectecd to stress, when mouth breathing is a problem, or in mouths in which for other reasons they are durable for only short periods of time.

SILICATE CEMENT

Silicate restorations usually survive for relatively few years, but they are useful when carefully placed in young persons to control caries-produced lesions until use of a material of a more durable nature is indicated. In selected cases they may provide several years of service before being replaced. It must be recognized that silicate cement is soluble in the oral cavity. This dissolution, although gradual, requires the dentist to make judgments as to when silicate cement restorations should be replaced. Because of their fluoride content, silicate cements have the advantage of inhibiting recurrent caries.

Class 3 silicate restorations

It is not desirable to extend cavity preparations for silicate restorations further than is essential to (1) properly manipulate the material and (2) include the carious lesion. Enamel, unless it is thin or otherwise defective, should be retained even though it may be undermined by caries. All carious material must be thoroughly removed, of course. Use of a rubber dam is essential for proper control of the operative field, and placement of a separator is sometimes desirable to increase access so that sound enamel may be preserved.

Cavity preparation

Cavity preparation for proximal silicate restorations is generally the same as described for Class 3 composite resin restorations (Chapter 13, Figs. 13-1 through 13-9).

Insertion

Most manufacturers supply excellent instructions for handling their silicate cements. These directions should be closely observed. Throughout the mixing and placement procedure, time limits are critical. Emphasis must be placed on rapid, vigorous mixing, skillful placement, and adequate setting time before placement is completed. Thin mixes are not desirable; on the other hand, excessively heavy mixes, even though they can be inserted into the cavity, are not desirable because they do not produce a strong material.

ARMAMENTARIUM

Celluloid strip
Plastic instrument
Glass slab and stainless steel spatula
Silicate cement
Cocoa butter or petrolatum jelly
Lacquer

1 Place a celluloid strip between the teeth (Fig. 15-1).

2 Mix the cement according to the manufacturer's directions.

3 With a plastic instrument small enough to enter the prepared cavity, place a small mass of cement into the cavity, usually into the labial retention area (Fig. 15-2). Then force an additional mass toward the axial wall and lingually into the lingual retention area (Fig. 15-3).

4 Additional cement is then forced into the incisal area (Fig. 15-4).

5 Sufficient bulk is now placed into the cavity to force cement over the lingual margin and build the contour to excess.

6 Holding the lingual end of the strip, tighten it firmly around the surface of the tooth being restored. It is sometimes possible, by "rocking" the strip, to force considerable excess cement beyond the margins of the restoration; however, great care must be used not to pull the strip too tight, which will result in a deficient contour (Fig. 15-5).

7 A wood wedge placed between the strip and the adjacent tooth is sometimes helpful in establishing gingival contour and lessening gingival excess or flash (Fig. 13-10).

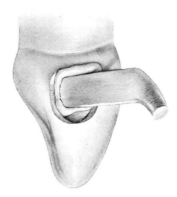

Fig. 15-3. Additional cement forced into the lingual retention.

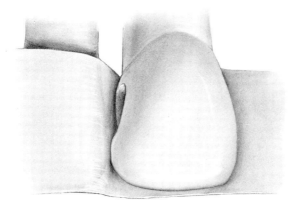

Fig. 15-1. Matrix around teeth.

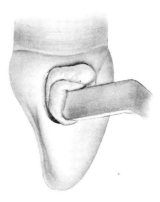

Fig. 15-4. Cement forced into incisal retention.

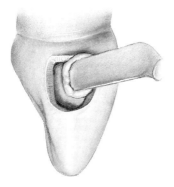

Fig. 15-2. Insertion of first mass of the mix into labial retentive area.

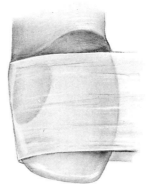

Fig. 15-5. After sufficient bulk is placed, draw the band tightly around the area being restored.

8 Roll a piece of the unused mix into a stick or rod for testing to determine when the cement is set. When the rod breaks cleanly, the strip may be removed.

9 Cover the silicate immediately with petrolatum jelly or cocoa butter and do not disturb it for several minutes, preferably fifteen minutes.

Finishing

Technically, it is desirable to allow an interval of at least twenty-four hours to elapse before performing the final finish on a silicate cement restoration. Although few operators seem to observe this precaution, it must not be overlooked if maximum longevity of the restoration is to be obtained by permitting the gelation process to proceed undisturbed.

The ideal silicate is one that requires no finishing, having been contoured by its matrix as it was placed. Flashing over the margins, however, is inevitable and must be removed.

ARMAMENTARIUM

Finishing disk
Gold knife
Wedelstaedt chisels
Finishing strips
Cocoa butter
Lacquer

1 With an extra fine cuttle disk coated with cocoa butter, running at very slow speed and with light pressure, remove the excess silicate on the labial and lingual surfaces. To break this excess away will frequently remove a portion of the silicate below the margin, so great caution must be used. However, an instrument (gold knife or Wedelstaedt chisel) may be used to push off gingival excess not immediately adjacent to the margin if carefully done.

2 With a lubricated finishing strip slowly remove the remaining excess and establish the proper contour.

3 Wipe off the lubricant and apply a coat of lacquer or varnish prior to removal of the dam.

Class 5 silicate restorations

As with all silicate restorations, the outline of the cavity should be extended to include only the involved area. Areas of erosion occur in teeth subject to severe stress, and the predisposing factors, if not corrected, will lead to relatively early failure of cement restorations in such cases.

Cavity preparation

ARMAMENTARIUM

No. 57 (58) or 170 (171) bur
No. 1 round bur

1 Select the shade of silicate.
2 Place a rubber dam and SSW No. 212 clamp.
3 If a matrix is to be used, it should be made at this time.
4 Create the cavity outline using a No. 57 (58) bur (Fig. 13-30). An inverted cone bur is often useful to remove bulk. The cavity should be extended to include only the involved area, walls should be smooth, and the cavosurface margin must be a right angle.
5 Place a retentive groove along the gingival (Fig. 13-31) and incisal walls, using a No. 1 round bur (Fig. 13-32).
6 Line the cavity with varnish.
7 Plane the enamel walls with a Wedelstaedt chisel (Fig. 13-33).

Insertion

Two general procedures may be followed to insert Class 5 silicates: one utilizes a matrix, and the second is the so-called iron-in technique.

MATRIX TECHNIQUE

Prior to preparing the cavity make a compound impression of the area being restored. The compound may be carried in a metal tray contoured to the tooth as for a gingival porcelain inlay (Figs. 16-13 to 16-17).

1 The defects of the tooth are built to contour with wax and lightly coated with cocoa butter.
2 The compound is warmed, pressed in place, and chilled.
3 The cocoa butter is thoroughly removed from the tooth and the cavity prepared.
4 Overfill the cavity. The cement should be inserted into the cavity, starting in one corner and forced from this starting point into all angles so that bubbles are not trapped.
5 Press the compound matrix (a thin coat of cocoa butter has been left on it) firmly in place and hold it until the silicate is set.

"IRON-IN" OR "IRON ON" TECHNIQUE

Clinical experience and research indicate that the "iron-in" procedure provides highly acceptable results.[1] It has the advantages of easily establishing contour and reducing or eliminating finishing time.

1 Fill the cavity, starting at one corner (Fig. 13-35).

2 Place a second portion of the mix into the cavity and force it into the opposing gingival corner (Fig. 13-35), then into the remaining retentive areas, filling the cavity to excess (Fig. 13-35).

3 Establish contour to excess, and carefully pinch off the excess beyond the margins with a Gregg No. 4 or 5 carver, using a burnishing, surfboardlike action (Fig. 13-35).

4 Cover the silicate with a small amount of lubricant (cocoa butter or petrolatum jelly), and keep it covered throughout the remaining procedure.

5 Move the blade of the instrument, surfboard style, from the center of the restoration toward the margins, working the excess toward the margins and pinching it off. Continue to contour the restoration in this fashion. If properly done, a "skin" or film seems to form on the surface. Continue a light burnishing action until the cement is set. As gelation occurs, use less and less force until the desired contour is achieved and no excess extends over the margins. Properly executed, the silicate should require very little or no finishing.

The "iron-in" technique may be applied to Class 3 restorations, where access permits, generally as follows:

1. Lightly lubricate a matrix strip and place it between the teeth. (Remove any colored printed matter from the strip as it may color the silicate.)
2. Fill the cavity.
3. Draw the strip out labially.
4. With a Gregg carver proceed to iron the silicate as described for the Class 5 restoration.

Finishing

Placing a finish on a Class 5 silicate restoration is simply a matter of judicious use of abrasive disks, starting, for example, with extra fine cuttle and finishing with fine sand. The disks must be run very slowly and kept lubricated.

SILICOPHOSPHATE CEMENT

Used as a restorative material, silicophosphate cement should be handled in the same manner as any siliceous cement. Cavity preparations are the same as have been described, and the mixing technique, although it is a hybrid cement, should follow manufacturer's directions with emphasis placed on rapid and vigorous mixing.

Silicophosphates are less translucent but less irritating and less soluble than silicate cements and are recommended where minimally displayed.

REFERENCE
1. Mitchem, J. C.: Validity of laboratory tests in predicting clinical behavior of silicate cement, J. Prosthst. Dent. **18**:168, 1967.

CHAPTER 16

PORCELAIN INLAYS

Porcelain inlays are extremely durable in the oral cavity, being insoluble. They are highly thermal resistant, duplicate to a great degree the appearance of tooth enamel, and are highly resistant to recurrent caries. Their disadvantages are the relatively intricate laboratory procedures involved in their fabrication, and they occasionally develop a visible cement line at their margins over a period of time. Silicate cement, of course, will usually develop somewhat the same discoloration over its entire surface while it is destroyed over a shorter period of time.

It is unfortunate that despite the wide usage of porcelain for full crowns, it is not employed extensively in the operative field for inlays. Its advantages make it extremely desirable as a restorative material. Its main disadvantage is its relative complexity of fabrication. Porcelain's lack of popularity for inlays is unwarranted.

Class 3 porcelain inlay

The cavity preparation for a porcelain inlay for a Class 3 restoration must not be extended incisally more than necessary because of the danger of weakening the incisal angle. Extension should be adequate to include the area of the lesion and provide access for insertion of the inlay. Insertion may be from the lingual or labial aspect.

Large Class 3 inlays are not generally indicated if they are inserted from the labial aspect and extend lingually to the degree that they may be displaced by occlusal force.

LINGUAL PLACEMENT
Cavity preparation

ARMAMENTARIUM

No. 170 (171) bur
Jeffery hatchet

1 Select the desired porcelain shade.
2 Place a rubber dam and a Ferrier separator. Slightly separate the teeth.
3 Enter the cavity with a No. 170 bur, removing all caries. Establish outline form, creating opposing grooves incisally and gingivally and a line of draw that enables the completed inlay to be inserted into the prepared cavity (Fig. 16-1).

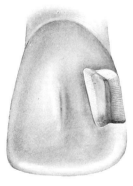

Fig. 16-1. Typical Class 3 porcelain inlay cavity preparation, lingual insertion.

4 Extend the cavity labially only far enough to place the margin in sound tooth structure.

5 Plane the margins with a Jeffery No. 7 hatchet. All margins must be as near right angles as possible.

LABIAL INSERTION

Cavity preparation

ARMAMENTARIUM

No. 170 (171, 700, 701) bur
Wedelstaedt chisel

1 Select the desired porcelain shade.

2 Place a rubber dam and Ferrier separator. Slightly separate the teeth.

3 Open the cavity with a No. 170 bur. Establish outline form and opposing grooves incisally and gingivally.

4 Extend the cavity lingually to sound enamel.

5 Plane the walls with a small Wedelstaedt chisel. If the lingual margin is extended well onto the lingual surface, an angle former (or gingival margin trimmer) may be used to plane the lingual wall. All peripheral walls should meet the tooth surface at right angles (Fig. 16-2).

IMPRESSION TECHNIQUE

Elastic impression materials enable the operator to produce accurate dies of prepared cavities for porcelain inlays. An extremely hard die is essential to the best technique. Hydrocolloid may be used but does not permit creation of other than a stone die, which will not withstand swaging.

Rubber or silicone impression materials are desirable because they permit copper or silver plating or may be poured in Kryptex* to form extremely hard dies that easily withstand swaging during the laboratory procedures.

ARMAMENTARIUM

Modeling compound
Perforated brass tray material
Impression material (rubber or silicone)
Plastic instrument

1 Soften a small amount of modeling compound and press in place on the teeth on the opposite side from which the cavity has been prepared.

2 Remove the compound and trim away a small amount in the area that meets the margin of the prepared cavity (Fig. 16-3). The compound is to act only as a stop to prevent impression material from flowing past the prepared margin, which makes it difficult to remove the impression when set.

---

*S. S. White Co., Philadelphia, Pa.

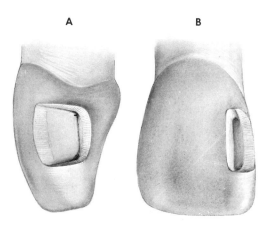

Fig. 16-2. Labial Class 3 porcelain inlay cavity preparation. **A,** Mesiolabial view. **B,** Labial view.

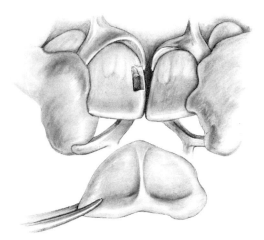

Fig. 16-3. Compound stop formed and trimmed between the teeth to allow impression material to show just past the margin.

3 Cut a strip of perforated brass stock to lay over the surface of the tooth being restored and the one adjacent (Fig. 16-4). A tray of quick-setting acrylic may also be used with rubber cement adhesive.

4 Mix the impression material and introduce it into the cavity with a plastic instrument while the compound stop is held in place. A syringe may be helpful, of course, but is usually not necessary.

5 Load a mound of impression material on the tray and place it over the two teeth. Allow the impression to set thoroughly.

6 Remove the impression and examine it for detail (Fig. 16-5). Two impressions are recommended.

7 Mix a syrupy mix of Kryptex die material (Figs. 16-18 to 16-20), and with a small sable hair brush paint the Kryptex over the impression and build up a small mound adequate to serve as a base.

8 When the die has set thoroughly, separate it from the impression and trim the excess (Fig. 16-6).

The remainder of the procedures performed in the laboratory are as described under the section relating to Class 5 procedures (Figs. 16-21 to 16-28).

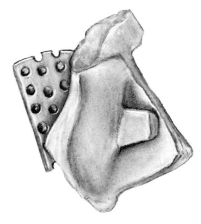

Fig. 16-5. Impression of the prepared cavity.

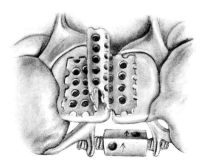

Fig. 16-4. Tray formed from perforated tray stock.

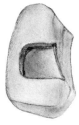

Fig. 16-6. Trimmed die.

Class 4 gold-porcelain inlay[1]

Broken incisal angles present perplexing problems if a display of gold is objectionable in an anterior tooth. Fusing porcelain to gold has become a widely accepted procedure for full crowns and has possibilities for Class 4 inlays.

The following procedure has relatively limited applications but is included for the benefit of experienced ceramists. It has the distinct advantage of not requiring reduction of the entire crown for a full-coverage restoration.

Cavity preparation

The cavity is prepared much as for a Class 4 gold inlay. Margins that are to be finished in gold may be beveled, and the porcelain margin is finished with a right cavosurface angle.

ARMAMENTARIUM

Torpedo-shaped diamond point (small wheel stone)
No. 34 or 35 bur
No. 169L (170) bur
White finishing stone
Angle former or gingival margin trimmer

1 Select the shade of porcelain.

2 Place a rubber dam.

3 As for the Class 4 gold inlay, make an incisal cut with the torpedo-shaped diamond point (Fig. 10-30) and place an incisal step with an inverted cone bur (Fig. 10-31).

4 With a No. 169L (170) bur prepare the proximal box (Fig. 10-32). For this procedure the labial margin is of necessity extended; otherwise a gold restoration would suffice.

5 Plane the labial proximal wall with a binangle or Wedelstaedt chisel, establishing a right-angle cavosurface margin. The proximal wall should meet the gingival wall in a curve (Fig 10-33).

6 Bevel the lingual margins with a No. 170 bur (Fig. 10-34).

7 Bevel the lingual half or two thirds of the gingival margin, using an angle former (Fig. 10-35) or gingival margin trimmer. Leave the labial half or third of the margin at right angles for the porcelain (Fig. 16-7).

8 Using a No. 169L bur, place the incisal pinhole about 2 mm. deep. Then place the gingival pinholes (Fig. 10-37). The labial pin may be omitted if pins of adequate strength can be created for the other two.

9 Disk the labial proximal wall. Be careful to leave a sharp line on the incisal edge at the point where the incisal gold will meet the incisal porcelain in the completed restoration (Fig. 16-7).

IMPRESSION TECHNIQUE

The impression is taken as for a gold inlay, using materials of the operator's choice. Rubber or silicone may be used to fabricate a Kryptex die since an extremely hard die is preferable. A hydrocolloid impression is also desirable to allow the Kryptex die to be mounted in it and the remaining teeth poured to provide an index to establish proper contact on the completed restoration.

Laboratory procedure

1 Wax a pattern for the gold inlay (Fig. 16-8). Extend the wax labially only to the end of the gingival margin, then to the mesioincisal angle, leaving 1.5 to 2 mm. of the labial proximal wall un-

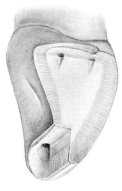

Fig. 16-7. Typical preparation for a Class 4 gold-porcelain inlay.

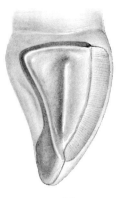

Fig. 16-8. Gold casting.

covered. Wax the lingual contour as appropriate and establish sharp finish lines in the wax where the gold will abut the finished porcelain.

Place a "rib" or ridge on the proximal aspect of the wax pattern that will support the porcelain.

COMMENT: *It may be easier to wax the entire lingual surface of the restoration, thereby requiring only the labial portion of the inlay to be built up in porcelain. However, two factors must be considered. First, the completed porcelain seems of better color and more brilliant if not backed by gold. Second, occlusal function on gold used for ceramic procedures is not desirable. The gold is soft and flows, ultimately resulting in fracture of the porcelain. Whenever possible, it is preferred to place the porcelain in occlusion rather than the gold.*

2 Cast and finish the inlay according to proper procedures for ceramic gold.

3 Block out the undercuts on the die below the gingival margin with modeling compound (Fig. 16-9).

4 Adapt a platinum matrix from 0.00075-inch platinum foil (Fig. 16-9). Extend the platinum well beyond the margins of the inlay and die.

5 With a sharp knife cut the platinum away from the areas of the pinholes (Fig. 16-9).

6 Place the gold inlay over the matrix on the die.

7 Place droplets of sticky wax along the margin of the inlay to attach it to the platinum matrix (Fig. 16-10).

8 Place droplets of porcelain between the drops of sticky wax (Fig. 16-10).

9 Remove the assembled inlay and matrix and place it on a bed of silex powder on a firing tray. It must be placed in a manner that will not permit the inlay to shift on the matrix while the wax is burned out and the porcelain fused.

10 Fire the assembly in a furnace to fuse the porcelain droplets.

11 Place the assembly back on the die and reburnish the platinum to the margins on the die.

12 The firing procedure is basically the same as that for building up a porcelain crown on a bold base. The opaque porcelain must not extend labially beyond the gold casting.

As the porcelain is built up and fired, it will shrink toward the gold casting, drawing the platinum away from the labial margin. A method of controlling this is to place a thin layer of wax on the proximal platinum after the opaque has been fired and the matrix readapted. The porcelain is

then placed and fired. The void thus created may then be filled and fired.

Possibly a better method is that of building the porcelain on the proximal walls and inlay and scoring it deeply to divide it so that it will shrink in opposite directions, the final buildup filling the void.

A variation of the foregoing is that of investing the gold-platinum assembly in an investment for firing. The droplets of porcelain are not placed to fuse the casting and matrix together when using this method. The disadvantage of this technique is that it cannot be tried on the die for adjusting the contact.

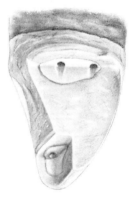

Fig. 16-9. Platinum matrix (0.00075 inch) with undercut blocked out below the gingival margins.

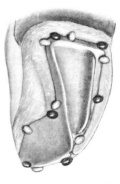

Fig. 16-10. Droplets of sticky wax (dark) used to retain the matrix and the casting together. The white droplets are porcelain that will, when fixed, lock the matrix and casting together.

13 After the porcelain has been properly contoured and glazed the porcelain droplets are ground off, the platinum matrix removed, and the gold polished (Fig. 16-11).

After the inlay has been tried on the tooth it should be gold plated. This can be done with a Caulk gold plating kit.* To facilitate plating by this method it is essential that the inlay be thoroughly cleaned, using an ultrasonic cleaning unit. Conventional pickling and cleaning do not allow the gold to accept the plating adequately.

Placing the inlay in the tooth without gold plating creates a dark halo in the area of the relatively dark gold used for porcelain-gold procedures.

CEMENTATION

Cementation of these inlays is similar to that for all porcelain inlays, silicophosphate cement being preferred.

---

*L. D. Caulk Co., Milford, Del.

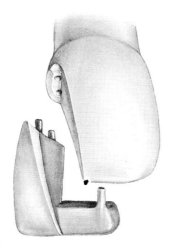

Fig. 16-11. Completed inlay.

Class 5 porcelain inlay

Class 5 porcelain inlays find their greatest use in maxillary anterior teeth and premolars. They are extremely durable.

Cavity preparation

The cavity preparation is basically the same as that for a gold inlay, but without bevels.

ARMAMENTARIUM
No. 170 (171) or 57 (58) bur
Wedelstaedt chisel
6½-2½-9 hoe

1 Select the shade of porcelain.

2 Place a rubber dam and a No. 212 clamp stabilized with modeling compound.

3 Prepare the cavity with a tapered fissure bur (No. 170 or 171). The outline must include all defective enamel. The outline may vary, but the peripheral walls must be smooth and without sharp line angles (Fig. 16-12) except for the axial line angles, which must be sharp but slightly obtuse. The occlusal (incisal) and gingival walls should diverge slightly. The cavosurface margins must be sharp and at right angles to the tooth surface. Depth of the cavity should be about 1.5 mm. and not over 2 mm. (Fig. 16-12).

4 Plane the cavity walls with a small Wedelstaedt chisel and/or a 6½-2½-9 hoe.

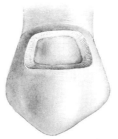

Fig. 16-12. Typical Class 5 cavity preparation for a porcelain inlay.

IMPRESSION TECHNIQUES

A variety of materials may be used, each having advantages and disadvantages. Rubber and silicone impressions may be plated or may be poured in Kryptex die material. Compound also serves these same desirable qualities but is less time consuming.

Compound impressions

ARMAMENTARIUM

Metal stock, brass or aluminum strips
Crown and bridge shears
Contouring pliers

1 With the crown and bridge shears shape one end of a stiff metal strip (Fig. 16-13) so that it may be contoured to roughly approximate the surface of the tooth surrounding the prepared cavity.

2 Contour the end of the metal strip with contouring pliers to the area being operated on (Fig. 16-14). Both ends of the tray may be prepared to obtain two impressions.

3 Moisten the prepared cavity with saliva.

4 Place a small mound of red stick compound on the prepared tray. Warm the compound and shape to a point (Fig. 16-15). While it is still fluid, quickly press the compound into the wet cavity and chill while holding it perfectly stable (Fig. 16-16). Chilling may be with air and wet cotton rolls.

5 Remove the impression from the cavity and inspect for sharpness of detail (Fig. 16-17).

6 Repeat for a second impression.

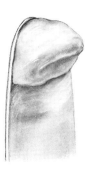

Fig. 16-15. Compound warmed and formed on the tray.

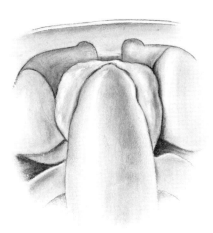

Fig. 16-16. Impression on the tooth.

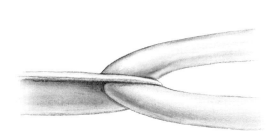

Fig. 16-13. Contouring a metal impression tray.

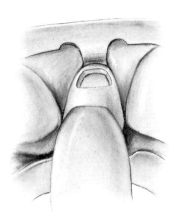

Fig. 16-14. Tray size and shape must approximate that of the prepared cavity.

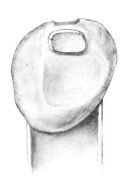

Fig. 16-17. Completed impression.

Rubber or silicone impression

ARMAMENTARIUM

Perforated tray stock
Contouring pliers
Crown and bridge shears
Plastic instrument

1 Cut a strip of perforated tray stock to the contour of the facial area of the cavity.

2 Contour the end of the strip using contouring pliers.

3 Mix the impression material.

4 With a plastic instrument fill the cavity to avoid trapping air.

5 Load a mound of the impression material onto the tray and press it into place over the cavity. The tray must be held perfectly stable during the setting process.

6 After the impression has set thoroughly (about ten minutes) remove and inspect it for detail.

MAKING THE DIE
Kryptex die

1 Place ten to twelve drops of Kryptex liquid on a chilled glass slab. Place about half a cupful of Kryptex powder on the other half of the slab.

2 Introduce about half of the powder into the liquid. Use a folding action and whip (beat) thoroughly to mix the powder into the liquid. Quickly add additional amounts of powder until a thick, syrupy consistency is obtained. A proper consistency will allow a string of the mix to follow the spatula as it is raised from the slab. The string should break quickly and fall back into the mix and disappear. Mixing should take about one minute.

3 With a fine sable hair brush paint the mix into the impression to avoid trapping air (Fig. 16-18). Place a mound of the mix over the painted impression. The die should extend about 3 mm. beyond the margins of the cavity and be about 5 mm. thick to ensure adequate strength (Fig. 16-19).

4 After the Kryptex is thoroughly set (about forty-five minutes) separate it from the impression (immerse the compound in 130° F. water for ten to fifteen seconds). Tenacious compound may be removed with chloroform and cotton.

5 Trim the die to approximate the tooth contour, using mounted stones and preserving the prepared margins (Fig. 16-20). The facial surface of the die must slope in all directions away from the cavity, and the size of the die should be reduced to within 3 to 4 mm. of the cavity.

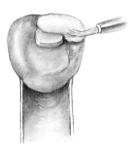

Fig. 16-18. Painting Kryptex on the impression.

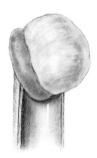

Fig. 16-19. Poured die.

Fig. 16-20. Completed die.

Plated dies

Excellent dies may be created by copper or silver plating. To do this follow the manufacturer's directions for plating. When the plating is complete, fill the plated impression with quick-setting acrylic. The impression and die are then separated. The remaining steps are the same as those for the Kryptex die.

MOUNTING THE DIE

ARMAMENTARIUM

Trimmed die
Swager cup
Compound
Wax spatula
Knife

1 The trimmed die is mounted on a swager cup using red compound. The compound must be seared (luted) to the cup to stabilize it. Add to the first layer a small mound in the center of the cup to approximate the size of the die base.

2 Seat the die into the soft compound, and with a wax spatula seal the compound to the die, making the mound smooth and continuous with the facial surface of the die surrounding the prepared cavity (Fig. 16-21). The surface of the die should be mounted well above (5 mm.) the face of the cup and domed evenly.

3 With a sharp knife carve the compound to the desired contour. Flat areas will assist in stabilizing the platinum matrix so that it will seat positively each time it is returned to the die (Fig. 16-22). The area around the dome should be flat and must meet the margins of the dome at a sharp line. The brim thus created on the platinum matrix serves to reinforce the dome to prevent it from warping, much the same as a man's hat brim supports the crown to maintain its shape. The dome should be reasonably hemispherical to give strength to the platinum matrix so that it will not warp as it is fired.

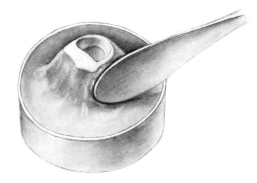

Fig. 16-21. Smoothing compound around the die on a swaging cup.

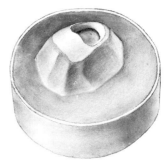

Fig. 16-22. Compound carved to desired contour.

PLATINUM MATRIX

ARMAMENTARIUM

0.00075-inch platinum foil
Swager
Mounted die in cup
Hammer
Burnishing instrument
Gas-air torch
Crown and bridge shears
Cotton

1 Cut a piece of 0.00075-inch platinum foil to cover the die and dome area on the compound. It should extend onto the flat area completely around the dome.

2 Center the piece of foil over the die and press it onto the die with the index finger. While firmly holding the foil in place, burnish the remainder of the foil over the crown portion.

3 Use a sharp blade to make four cuts in the cavity portion of the matrix (Fig. 16-23). Terminate these cuts about 0.5 mm. from the cavity margins.

4 Press the four flaps down into the cavity.

5 Place a pellet of cotton approximately the size of the cavity into the cavity. Place the mounting into the swager and hit the plunger sharply.

The swager (Fig. 16-24) has two major parts, a cylinder and a plunger. Approximately ³/₄ inch of modeling clay is placed in the end of the cylinder under the plunger. Over the modeling clay is a disk of rubber dam material to protect the platinum matrix as it is swaged. The rubber dam disk must be replaced occasionally to keep the platinum clean.

6 Remove the cup from the swager. The swaged matrix should appear extremely sharp in every detail. Cut a small piece of platinum foil to fit the interior of the cavity. This may be done by lightly pressing a piece of foil over the cavity in the die to indicate its outline. Carefully cut out this outline.

7 Carefully place this piece of foil in the cavity. Place a cotton pellet over it and push it into place.

8 Place the cup in the swager and rap the plunger firmly.

9 Remove the cup from the swager and examine the matrix. Slide a very thin blade under the edge of the matrix to start its removal. If the patch has stuck in the swager, carefully remove it with cotton pliers and replace it in the die.

10 Remove the platinum matrix from the die and sweat it with a gas-air torch. The platinum should be heated white hot, cooled, and replaced

on the die. Carefully burnish out all wrinkles in the cavity. A blunt wood point may be helpful for this. Reswage and burnish about three times, each time sweating the foil in the torch flame to ensure that it is well adapted (Fig. 16-25).

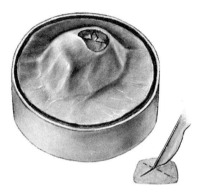

Fig. 16-23. Cuts made in cavity portion of the platinum matrix.

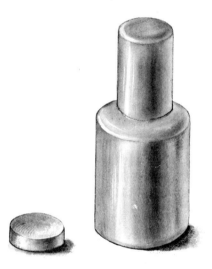

Fig. 16-24. Platinum matrix swager and swaging cup.

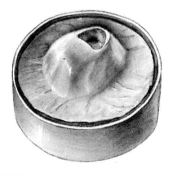

Fig. 16-25. Completed platinum matrix.

PORCELAIN MANIPULATION

ARMAMENTARIUM

Porcelain, usually gingival portion of shade selected
Mounted matrix
Small, sable artist's brush
Firing try
Glass slab
Porcelain knife
Distilled water

1 Place a supply of porcelain on a glass slab and add several drops of distilled water.

2 Make a thin mix of porcelain and water and carry a small amount of the mix to the floor of the matrix using a small, artist's sable brush (Fig. 16-26). Use a vibrating action when placing the porcelain.

3 Add additional amounts of the mix until level with the cavity margins. Do not overfill. Remove any porcelain that extends beyond the margins. Condensing the porcelain is a skill that is difficult to describe. The addition of water and vibration of various types may be used as well as a technique of "whipping" with a brush. However, with practice the porcelain can be placed quite rapidly using the method described. Use care not to disturb the underlying porcelain as additions are vibrated into place with the brush.

For large inlays or for difficulty encountered with shrinkage or warping when the case is fired, it is suggested that the first buildup be scored from each corner of the cavity, forming an X. This will allow the shrinkage to occur without pulling the matrix out of shape.

4 Remove the matrix from the swaging cup and place it on a firing tray. Place the tray on the edge of the furnace in a location that will be warm enough to dry it without boiling the water, which would disrupt the condensation.

5 When thoroughly dry, the tray may be placed into the hot furnace.

6 Elevate the temperature to firing temperature for the first bake.

7 Remove the tray from the muffle, place it on an asbestos base (a coil of asbestos as supplied for inlay investment will do), and cover it with a heavy glass tumbler. Allow it to cool to room temperature.

8 Return the matrix to the swaging cup and reswage.

9 Make appropriate additions to the first bake, slightly overfilling the cavity, but do not allow the porcelain to extend beyond the margins. Remove any excess powder with the brush.

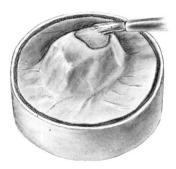

Fig. 16-26. Porcelain buildup.

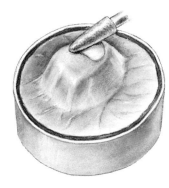

Fig. 16-27. Grinding surface of the porcelain.

10 Fire the porcelain as before, dry it, place it into the muffle between 1200° and 1500° F., and take it out at 2050° F.

11 When the surface of the porcelain has reached its desired contour (or if contour is excessive), it must be stoned to finish it properly (Fig. 16-27). Using a smooth diamond point (torpedo, wheel, or whatever shape the operator prefers), reduce the surface carefully to proper contour. Use plenty of water, washing the porcelain completely clean occasionally. The final contour must be smoothly ground and finished exactly flush with the platinum matrix at the margins.

Should characterization of the surface be desired, this may be done using a knife-edged separating disk. Sharpen it on a diamond instrument. Then place slight mesiodistal grooves as desired to break up the light on the surface of the finished inlay (Fig. 16-28).

12 Clean the porcelain thoroughly prior to firing. An ultrasonic cleaner is of great value to the ceramist for this purpose.

13 For the final bake fire to 2150° F. Observe all the precautions noted previously relating to placement of the inlay in the muffle and removal to avoid crazing.

REMOVAL OF THE PLATINUM MATRIX

1 Dip the matrix in water.

2 Cut the corners to the inlay with scissors and carefully peel the platinum from first the margins and then the rest of the inlay.

3 A sharp-pointed instrument may be helpful to scrape off any obstinate particles. An inverted cone carbide bur may also be used, but avoid the use of steel burs or stones.

CEMENTATION

ARMAMENTARIUM

Silicophosphate cement (Fluorothin) and liquid
Glass slab
Stainless steel or agate spatula
Wheel bur No. 11 (12)
Knife-edged separating disk
Cavity varnish
Cotton pliers and cotton
Plastic instrument

1 Place the rubber dam and No. 212 clamp.

2 Remove the temporary material.

3 Thoroughly clean the prepared cavity.

4 Using the wheel bur No. 11 (12), groove the occlusal and gingival walls. This should be slight and placed in dentin (Fig. 16-29).

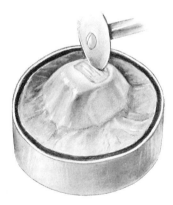

Fig. 16-28. Adding characterizing grooves.

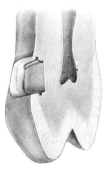

Fig. 16-29. Cross section of the prepared cavity showing properly placed retention grooves.

5 Groove the occlusal and gingival walls of the inlay using a small, knife-edged separating disk (Fig. 16-30).

6 Paint the internal form of the cavity with cavity varnish, but avoid the margins.

7 Mix the silicophosphate cement to a creamy consistency as described for the die. Beat it well.

8 With a plastic instrument carry a small portion of the cement into the cavity, starting at one corner and filling it to avoid trapping air.

9 Cover the internal surfaces of the inlay with cement and insert it into the cavity. Use a vibratory motion to seat it, and hold it with an orangewood stick until thoroughly set (Fig. 16-31). It is advisable to cover the area with a protective coat of lubricant (cocoa butter or petrolatum jelly) while setting.

COMMENT: *For cementation of all-ceramic restorations the white or gray shades are recommended. White, being completely neutral, will neither add nor detract from the shade of the porcelain, which should match the tooth. Occasionally a restoration will appear more harmonious if cemented with a gray shade, also neutral, which lends a graying effect that is sometimes desirable.*

REFERENCE

1. Howard, W. W.: Porcelain fused to gold for Class IV inlays, J. Prosthet. Dent. **13**:761, 1963.

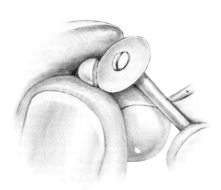

Fig. 16-30. Grooving the inlay.

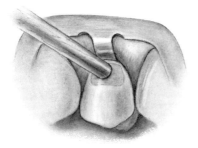

Fig. 16-31. Completed inlay held in place with an orangewood stick during cementation.

GLOSSARY

The following terms are generally defined only as they are used in the field of operative dentistry. Appropriate sections of the text should be read for greater clarity and detail.

abrasion An area of wear on a tooth. Also the process of grinding or wearing away of tooth structure by means of abrasive materials or devices, possibly in conjunction with improper toothbrushing technique or bruxism.

abrasive A material or device capable of removing a substance. In dentistry, refers to cutting or wearing away of tooth structure or restorative materials, or shaping and polishing by means of disks, stones, pumice, or other materials and devices.

access The opening made in a tooth to reach a cavity. Also the space necessary to allow instrumentation and vision to properly treat a lesion in a tooth.

acrylic resin See *resin—acrylic resin.*

adaptation Conformation of a material or device to a particular requirement or situation—for example, the conformation or approximation of a restorative material to the walls of a prepared cavity, or the placement of a matrix band on a tooth to create proper contour of the surface of the completed restoration.

adjustment of occlusion Recontouring the functional surfaces of a tooth or teeth to improve function.

airbrasive technique A process of cavity preparation by means of fine aluminum oxide particles, carried by a high-velocity stream of carbon dioxide gas.

alloy The product of the fusion of two or more metals that are mutually soluble in a liquid state.

    amalgam alloy An alloy, one of the metals of which is mercury.

    dental gold alloy An alloy, the principal metal of which is gold; used to restore teeth.

    silver alloy An alloy used for amalgam restorations, the principal ingredient of which is silver. Also a slang term used to designate silver amalgam.

amalgam An alloy, one of the metals of which is mercury.

    copper amalgam An alloy of which the principal metal is copper and one of the metals is mercury.

    dental amalgam An amalgam used in dentistry to restore teeth or to fabricate laboratory dies.

    silver amalgam An alloy of which the principal metal is silver and one of the metals is mercury.

amalgam squeeze cloth A piece of fabric used to wring or squeeze excess mercury from a plastic mix of amalgam.

amalgamation The process of trituration or the mixing of alloy or metal particles with mercury to make amalgam.

amalgamator Normally, a powered mechanical device for amalgamation. The alloy and mercury may, however, be amalgamated by means of a manually operated mortar and pestle.

angle The intersection or junction of two or more lines (point angle) or two planes (line angle).

    cavosurface angle Commonly referred to as the prepared cavity margin, it is the angle formed by the junction of the peripheral walls of the prepared cavity and the surface of the tooth.

    line angle An angle formed by the junction of two walls in a prepared cavity.

    point angle The junction or intersection of three walls or three line angles in a prepared cavity.

angle former One of a series of monangle paired cutting instruments, the cutting edge forming an acute angle with the long axis of the blade.

    bayonet angle former One of a series of binangle paired cutting instruments, the blade of which is approximately parallel with the handle and the cutting edge of which forms an acute angle with the long axis of the blade.

anneal To soften a metal by controlled heating and cooling.

    annealing of cohesive gold The process of degassing pure gold to allow it to be cold-welded. In this case the term does not refer to softening of the metal.

anterior Located forward of.

    anterior teeth The incisors and canines (cuspids).

applicator A device used for placement of a solution or medication. It may be a cotton pledget or swab, a metal loop or rod, or it may be made of wood.

approximal Next to or adjacent to.

attachment, epithelial See *epithelial attachment.*

attrition Wearing away of tooth structure by means of friction; abrasion.

autopolymerization Self-curing.

axiopulpal line angle The line angle formed by the junction of the axial and pulpal walls of a prepared cavity.

base Usually a layer of material interposed between a metal restoration and dentin in that portion of a prepared cavity that may be near the dental pulp. It may also be for the purpose of blocking out an undercut in a prepared cavity but generally is used to provide protection for the dental pulp by providing insulation and/or medication.

bayonet A binangled hand instrument, the blade or nib of which is generally parallel with the handle. See also *angle former—bayonet angle former*, and *condenser—bayonet condenser*.

bevel The inclination or placement of one plane relative to another, other than at an angle of 90 degrees. On a cutting instrument, refers to the plane established relative to the long axis of the blade to create a sharp edge. In a prepared cavity, refers to the cut made at a cavosurface angle that establishes an angle greater than 90 degrees to the peripheral cavity wall and cuts obliquely across enamel prisms.

    cavosurface bevel (as above).

    contrabevel On a cutting instrument, a reverse bevel or bevel placed on the side of the cutting blade opposite that which is customary; usually on the inside of the blade or one the side nearest the handle.

binangle An instrument with two bends in its shank.

bruxism* An involuntary clenching of the teeth associated with forceful lateral or protrusive jaw movements; results in rubbing, gritting, or grinding together of the teeth.

buccal Situated toward or in relation to the cheek.

bur A rotary cutting instrument with steel blades, which form the cutting head.

    carbide bur A bur the head of which is made of tungsten carbide steel.

    crosscut bur A bur that has cuts in its blades at right angles to its long axis.

    end-cutting bur A bur with cutting blades only on its end.

    excavating bur A general term used, especially by G. V. Black, to designate a bur used to reduce or remove tooth structure during cavity preparation procedures.

    finishing bur A bur with blades closer together than cutting burs, for use in finishing metallic restorations. Special finishing burs are also designed for finishing resin restorations.

    inverted cone bur A bur with a head shaped like a cone, with the larger end away from the shank.

    round bur A bur with a ball-shaped head.

    straight fissure bur A bur with a cylindrically shaped head, the blades of which are not crosscut.

    tapered fissure bur A bur that is similar to a straight fissure bur except that the head is slightly tapered toward the end away from the shank, and the end is at a right angle to the shank. May be plain fissure or crosscut.

burnish To rub with a burnisher to reform, harden, or stretch metal.

burnisher An instrument with blunt edges used to work harden and polish gold restorations; also used to burnish gold to cavosurface margins. Burnishers are of various forms. Some—for example, those that are convex in form—are used to burnish metal matrix bands to the desired contour.

burnout The phase of a lost wax casting procedure during which the wax or plastic pattern in the mold (investment) is burned away or eliminated.

canal, pulp See *pulp, dental—pulp canal*.

canine See *cuspid*.

capping, pulp A material or materials placed over an exposed dental pulp, normally interposed between remaining tooth structure and the outer restorative material. Also the procedure or act of placing a pulp cap.

    direct pulp capping Placement of a material on an exposed dental pulp.

    indirect pulp capping A procedure in which material is placed near the pulp over carious dentin if actual exposure of the pulp is anticipated. The pulp is thus afforded an opportunity to calcify in the area of the carious exposure. The treatment material and residual caries are removed at a later time. Sometimes called *remineralization*.

caries A disease of the hard or calcified tissues of teeth, characterized by demineralization of the inorganic substance and destruction of the organic substance.

carious Affected or altered by caries.

carver An instrument used to shape restorative materials or wax.

carving *v.* Shaping or forming.
    n. An object that has been shaped or formed—for example, a wax carving.

cast *n.* Reproduction of a form.
    v. To reproduce a form—for example, to throw molten gold alloy into a mold in the process of fabricating a gold alloy restoration.

casting machine A device or mechanical apparatus used to insert molten metal into a mold.

    air pressure vacuum casting machine A casting machine that uses compressed air to force the molten metal into the mold.

    centrifugal casting machine A casting machine that uses centrifugal force to press the molten metal into the mold.

    vacuum casting machine A casting machine that uses vacuum to force the molten metal into the mold.

*Boucher, C. O., editor: Current clinical dental terminology, 2, ed. St. Louis, 1974, The C. V. Mosby Co.

cavity Generally denotes a carious lesion in a tooth.

cavity classification A system or arrangement of cavities into groups according to similar characteristics or requirements for instrumentation.

anatomic cavity classification The system that designates the location of the cavity or prepared cavity according to the surfaces of the tooth in which the cavity exists or in which the restoration will be placed.

Black's cavity classification A system devised by G. V. Black to designate locations and types of carious lesions.

cavity floor An improper term used to designate the pulpal wall of a prepared cavity.

cavity lining or **liner** A material placed on the walls of a prepared cavity to seal dentinal tubules and decrease microleakage.

cavity toilet See *toilet of cavity.*

cavity varnish See *varnish, cavity.*

cavity wall One of the component walls of a prepared cavity.

complex cavity A prepared cavity that involves three or more surfaces of a tooth—for example, MOD.

compound cavity A cavity that involves two surfaces of a tooth—for example, DO.

fissure cavity See *cavity—pit and fissure cavity.*

gingival cavity A cavity in the gingival third of the clinical crown of a tooth.

pit and fissure cavity A cavity located in a developmental defect such as an anatomical pit or fissure in the anamel of a tooth.

prepared cavity The preparation established in a tooth to receive and retain a restoration.

proximal cavity A cavity located in a surface of a tooth that contacts or faces another tooth in the same arch.

pulp cavity The space within a tooth enclosed by dentin and containing the dental pulp.

simple cavity A cavity in only one surface of a tooth.

cavosurface angle See *angle—cavosurface angle.*

cavosurface bevel See *bevel—cavosurface bevel.*

cement Any of many materials used for various purposes such as luting cast restorations in prepared cavities, capping pulps, forming cavity bases, or serving as temporary restorations, or it may be used as the overall restorative material

cement base Cement placed in the deep portion of a prepared cavity to serve as thermal insulation.

cement dressing An application of a cement to soft tissues postoperatively for its analgesic and protective properties. Such a cement usually contains some or all of the following ingredients: zinc oxide, eugenol, tannic acid, rosin, zinc stearate, mineral oil, and asbestos fibers.

cement line The exposed cement between the restorative material (gold, porcelain, plastic) and tooth structure.

copper cement Cement, one of the ingredients of which is copper oxide.

silicate cement A relatively hard, somewhat translucent, tooth-colored cement used primarily to restore anterior teeth. Sometimes referred to as *synthetic porcelain* (undesirable) or *porcelain* (improper). Supplied as powder (acid-soluble glass prepared by fusion of SiO_2, CaO, Al_2O_3, and so forth with fluoride flux) and liquid (buffered solution of phosphoric acid).

silicophosphate cement A mixture of silicate and zinc phosphate cements. Used as a restorative material (less translucent than silicate) and luting agent.

zinc phosphate cement A relatively hard cement used for cement bases, for luting cast restorations and orthodontic bands, and as a temporary restorative material. Supplied as powder (calcined zinc oxide and magnesium oxide) and liquid (buffered phosphoric acid solution).

cementation The procedure of cementing a restoration or appliance in place, to lute or attach it in or to a tooth.

cementoenamel junction See *junction—cementoenamel junction.*

cementoproximal Pertaining to the area of cementum on a proximal surface of a clinical crown of a tooth.

cementum A specialized, calcified connective tissue that covers the surface of the root of a tooth.

cervical Relating to the cementoenamel junction (cervical line) of a tooth.

cervical line See *junction—cementoenamel junction.*

chamber, pulp See *pulp, dental—pulp chamber.*

chamfer A type of finish line established in some preparations to receive cast restorations. It is characterized by a smooth outward curve from the axial wall to the cavosurface margin.

channel A hole prepared to receive a pin as part of a restoration.

chisel Any of several types of hand cutting instruments used to cleave enamel and plane enamel and dentin. Its blade is beveled on its end on only one side to establish the cutting edge.

bibevel chisel A chisel, usually very small, with its blade sharpened on both sides of its end to create its cutting edge.

binangle chisel A chisel with two bends in its shank.

contrabevel chisel A chisel with the bevel on the end of its blade placed on the opposite side from that which is normal (the normal side being the side that is on the blade side away from the handle). A contrabevel chisel has its bevel placed on the side of the blade nearest the handle.

monangle chisel A chisel with one bend in its shank.

stright chisel A chisel with no bends in its shank.

triple-angle chisel A chisel with three bends in its shank.

Wedelstaedt chisel A chisel with a long curved blade continuous with its shank.

cingulum A lobe or eminence on the lingual surface of an anterior tooth.

clamp A device used to stabilize an apparatus or to apply compression to a part or parts, retainer.

cervical clamp A gingival clamp.

cotton roll rubber dam clamp A special type of rubber dam clamp with wide wings to hold cotton rolls.

Ferrier No. 212 clamp A gingival clamp.

gingival clamp A rubber dam clamp used to retract gingival tissue to provide access to the area of a tooth immediately occlusal or incisal to the gingival attachment.

Hatch gingival clamp An adjustable gingival clamp.

rubber dam clamp Any of a variety of devices made of spring steel for use in stabilization and management of a rubber dam.

cleoid A carving instrument, the blade of which is spade shaped and has a sharp tip.

compact *adj.* Densely and firmly united; pressed together; dense; solid; condensed.

v. To pack, make dense, unite closely, or condense.

composite resin See *resin—composite resin.*

compound An impression material also sometimes called modeling compound or impression compound. Composition is a matter of trade secrecy. Softens with heat and sets hard when cool. Used to stabilize separators, rubber dam clamps, and matrices.

condenser Any of a variety of instruments used to condense or compact a restorative material into a prepared cavity. The term *plugger* is obsolete.

amalgam condenser An instrument used to condense plastic (freshly mixed) amalgam into a prepared cavity.

automatic condenser See *condenser—mechanical condenser.*

back-action condenser A triple-angle instrument with three bends in its shank, allowing it to function with a pulling force.

bayonet condenser A binangle condensing instrument with its nib offset from the long axis of the handle.

condenser point The nib of a condensing instrument. Also, any of a variety of nibs that may be mounted on a cone socket handle or the handpiece of a condensing device.

electromallet condenser An electric-powered condenser designed by R. C. McShirley. Used with a variety of points and handpieces.

foil condenser A condenser used to insert and compact gold foil or other cohesive golds into prepared cavities.

hand condenser A condenser that depends on hand action to compact the restorative material in a prepared cavity. Condensing force may be augmented by hand malleting.

Hollenback condenser See *condenser—pneumatic condenser.*

mechanical condenser (automatic mallet) A mechanical device that is activated by hand pressure. As force is applied it becomes spring loaded, the condensing blow being released according to controlled adjustment. Supplied with a variety of points.

pneumatic condenser (Hollenback) A condenser, invented by Dr. George M. Hollenback, that delivers condensing blows pneumatically. Supplied with a variety of points.

contact A point or area where two teeth touch each other.

occlusal contact A point or area where the occlusal surfaces of two opposing teeth touch.

proximal contact The area where two adjacent teeth touch.

convenience form See *form—convenience form.*

convenience point See *point—convenience point.*

coping A thin form, usually a casting, that covers the prepared surface of a tooth. May serve as an understructure for another casting or for support as an integral part of a tooth-colored restoration.

core A cast gold foundation, usually having an extension (post) into an endodontically treated root canal. (May also designate a foundation of another material.)

coronal Pertaining to the crown of a tooth.

extracoronal Outside the crown.

intracoronal Within the crown.

corrosion The destruction or breaking down of a metal surface.

crown The part of a tooth covered by enamel.

clinical crown The part of a tooth extending occlusally or incisally from the depth of the gingival crevice.

cusp A rounded or conical eminence on or near the masticating surface of a tooth.

cuspid (canine) One of four pointed teeth, one located in each quadrant of the human dentition immediately distal to the lateral incisor. The term *canine* is being accepted and brought into wider use.

dam A moisture barrier.

rubber dam A sheet of thin rubber or latex used to isolate teeth in an operative area.

rubber dam clamp See *clamp—rubber dam clamp.*

rubber dam napkin See *napkin, rubber dam.*

decalcification The loss or removal of mineral salts from a calcified tissue.

decay Decomposed enamel and/or dentin. An objectionable term used as a synonym for *dental caries,* or *carious material.*

dental pulp See *pulp, dental.*

dentin (adj., **dentine**) The calcific tissue of a tooth formed by the odontoblasts. It forms the body of a tooth and is covered by cementum on its root and enamel on its crown. It surrounds the dental pulp.

dentin wall That portion of a prepared cavity wall located in dentin.

secondary dentin Dentin formed on the walls of the

pulp cavity after complete formation of the normal dentin.

dentinocemental junction See *junction—dentinocemental junction.*

dentinoenamel junction See *junction—dentinoenamel junction.*

diamond point See *point—diamond point.*

die Reproduction of a form. For operative dental purposes, designates reproduction of a tooth or cavity prepared to receive a restoration. Usually made of a metal or a hard stone that also may be metal-plated.

direct Used to identify a procedure executed directly in or on a tooth without the use of intervening steps performed on a die.

discoid A carving instrument, the blade of which is round or disk shaped.

disk A thin, circular object. Designates any of many materials used as rotary instruments in dentistry for cutting or polishing. The abrasive agent may be impregnated in its structure, luted on one or both sides as on diamond disks, or on one side only as on finishing disks.

distal Located away from the median line in a dental arch.

dovetail Designates a mortise form or enlarged portion of a cavity preparation placed primarily as a retentive factor to the restoration.

  lingual dovetail The dovetail form placed in the lingual surface of an anterior tooth.

  occlusal dovetail The dovetail form placed in the occlusal surface of a posterior tooth.

dowel See *endopost*

drill A cutting instrument used to create holes.

  bibevel drill A drill with two bevels on its cutting end.

  twist drill A drill with one or more spiral grooves extending form the cutting end to the smooth shaft.

drilling Establishment of a hole with a drill usually for placement of a pin. (Not acceptable as a term relating to use of other than a drill. Does not apply to use of other rotary instruments such as burs, stones, and so forth.)

Eames's technique See *technique—Eames's technique.*

embrasure The space between two teeth emanating from the proximal contact area. May be subdivided into *buccal, lingual, labial, occlusal,* or *incisal embrasure,* designating a portion of an embrasure.

enamel The hard, transluscent tissue that overlays the dentin of the anatomical crowns of teeth. It is formed by the ameloblasts and contains less organic matter than any other tissue in the body.

  enamel prism Enamel rod. The structural unit of tooth enamel, hexagonal in shape, extending from the dentin to the external surface of the tooth in an irregular or wavy direction.

  enamel rod See *enamel prism.*

  enamel, undermined Enamel that has lost its den-

tinal support either through advancement of dental caries or by instrumentation during cavity preparation.

endopost A metal rod cemented into a prepared hole (channel) that follows the pulp or root canal of the tooth. It is extended coronally to provide retention for restorative materials used to restore the crown.

engine, dental An apparatus consisting of an electric motor that, by means of a continuous belt carried by a series of pulleys and elbows, powers a dental handpiece used with rotary instruments.

epithelial attachment The attachment of the gingiva to the tooth.

erosion Noncarious loss of tooth structure, generally attributed in part to chemical and/or mechanical causes. Not all causative factors are known.

esthetics The aspect of the restorative art that is concerned with those factors pleasing in appearance or in harmony with existing tissues or structures.

eugenol Refined oil of cloves; colorless or pale yellow in color (darker if old), with a pungent, spicy odor and taste.

excavator Generally denotes a *spoon excavator,* a paired hand instrument with a slightly curved blade that is sharpened on all sides and that has a rounded end. Its primary purpose is the removal of carious material in treatment of carious lesions.

  discoid excavator An excavator that has a round, or disk-shaped, blade.

exposure, pulp An opening through dentin into the pulp chamber.

  carious pulp exposure The exposure of a dental pulp by means of dental caries.

  surgical pulp exposure also **mechanical pulp exposure** The exposure of dental pulp, intentionally or accidentally, by means of instrumentation.

extension An enlargement of; may pertain to inclusion of an additional area of a tooth in a restoration, such as a *groove extension,* but also used to designate increased depth or breadth—that is, *gingival extension.*

extension for prevention Placement or establishment of the outline form of a prepared cavity beyond the area of a defect or carious lesion for the purpose of inhibiting recurrence of the caries process.

extracoronal Outside of or surrounding the crown of a tooth or what remains of it.

fabricate To form, build, or make, as a restoration.

facepad See *napkin, rubber dam.*

facial Relating to, pertaining to, or toward the cheeks or lips.

field, operating or **operative** The general area or region in which a procedure is being performed.

file *n.* Any of various instruments that have on one side of the blade a series of cutting edges, or teeth. Used for finishing metallic restoration.

  v. To finish the surface of a restoration by means of a file.

filling An undesirable synonym for an intracoronal restoration.

finger One of the digits of the hand, usually not including the thumb.

    finger position Refers to the position or function of a finger or fingers during a particular operation.

    finger rest Use of one or more fingers to provide stability or a fulcrum during instrumentation.

finish *v.* To complete, as the final steps in placement of a restoration: correcting of occlusion, trimming of margins, and final polishing.

    n. The type or quality of surface established on a restoration.

    satin finish A finish free of scratches or pits but lacking high sheen or luster.

finishing strip See *strip—finishing strip.*

fissure A deep groove or cleft.

    developmental fissure A fault or incompletely closed developmental groove in the enamel of a tooth.

floor of cavity See *cavity—cavity floor.*

foil An extremely thin sheet of metal, such as gold, platinum, or tin. Generally, unless otherwise specified, refers to gold foil.

    cohesive foil Degassed (annealed) gold foil rendered capable of being welded cold.

    foil cylinder A cylinder of gold foil formed by folding part of a sheet of gold foil into a strip, which is then rolled into a cylindrical form.

    gold foil Pure gold that has been refined and ultimately beat into thin sheets. It is supplied in such forms as sheets, cylinders, and ropes.

    noncohesive foil Gold foil that has been rendered incapable of being welded cold owing to a layer of gas molecules (such as ammonia) or other impurities on its surface. If the foil has not been permanently contaminated, it may be rendered cohesive by degassing (annealing).

    platinum foil Pure platinum in very thin sheets.

    tinfoil Tin in very thin sheets.

force That which changes or tends to change the state of rest or motion in a body; the state of rest or motion of a body.

    condensing force That force used to condense or compact a restorative material.

    line of force The direction in which a force is applied.

form The physical shape or appearance of a thing.

    anatomical form The normal shape, form, or conformation of part of the anatomy.

    convenience form The shape of a prepared cavity in which those factors that are incorporated into prepared cavity design (1) enhance proper instrumentation and (2) facilitate easier starting or placement of the restorative material.

    outline form The boundary or periphery (cavosurface margin) of a prepared cavity.

    resistance form The internal shape established in a prepared cavity to enable the restoration to withstand the forces of masticatory stress.

retention form In a prepared cavity, the internal shape, which prevents the restoration from being dislodged by pulling, lateral, or tipping forces during function as well as masticatory stress.

foundation A term used to designate a pin-retained material formed to enhance succeeding restorative procedures—for example, pin-retained amalgam or composite formed to enhance preparation and retention of a cast restoration.

gingiva* The fibrous tissue covered by mucous membrane that immediately surrounds a tooth and is continuous with its pericemental ligament (periodontal membrane).

    attached gingiva That portion of the gingiva that extends from the depth of the gingival sulcus to the mucogingival junction.

    free gingiva That portion of the gingiva coronal (incisal or occlusal) to the epithelial attachment; the outer wall of the gingival sulcus.

    interdental gingiva The gingival tissue located between two contacting teeth.

    interproximal gingiva See *gingiva—interdental gingiva.*

    marginal gingiva That portion of the gingiva that is located on the buccal, labial, and lingual aspects of the teeth.

gingival Pertaining to or in relation to the gingiva.

    gingival attachment See *epithelial attachment.*

    gingival retraction Displacement of the free gingiva to facilitate restorative procedures.

    gingival sulcus or **crevice** See *sulcus—gingival sulcus.*

    gingival third The apical one third of the clinical crown of a tooth.

gold One of the noble or precious metals, yellow in color, malleable, ductile, and noncorrosive. Used in dentistry in pure form and in various types of alloys.

    gold file See *file.*

    gold foil See *foil—gold foil.*

    gold inlay An intracoronal restoration cast of gold alloy, cemented into a prepared cavity.

    gold knife See *knife, gold.*

    inlay gold An alloy, the principal metal of which is gold, used for cast restorations.

    mat foil A form of pure gold manufactured as a sandwich of mat gold between layers of gold foil.

    mat gold Pure gold manufactured as a powder by electrolytic precipitation, sintered, and then formed into strips.

grasp A term used to denote how an instrument is held, as in pen grasp, finger grasp, palm grasp, and so forth.

    palm and thumb grasp The holding of an instrument in the palm of the hand and grasped by the forefingers while the thumb is used for stability as a rest on another object.

---

*Boucher, C. O., editor: Current clinical dental terminology, ed. 2, St. louis, 1974, The C. V. Mosby Co.

pen grasp The holding of an instrument in the same manner as a properly held pen or pencil in writing. The upper part of the instrument handle rests against the base of the index finger while the ends of the thumb and index finger and the side of the end of the middle finger all support the lower part of the handle.

inverted pen grasp Similar to pen grasp, but the instrument is pointed toward the operator rather than away from him.

groove A sulcus or channel.

developmental groove Linear depressions in enamel that are formed by the joining of two lobes of the crown during its development.

supplemental grooves Smaller or secondary grooves in addition to developmental grooves found in enamel.

handpiece An instrument used to hold a working point, such as a rotary instrument or condensing point. In either case it is usually connected to a source of energy by which it may be activiated.

air-turbine handpiece A handpiece used for rotary instruments powered by compressed air.

contra-angle handpiece A binangled handpiece.

high-speed handpiece A general term used to designate a handpiece that is capable of operating at speeds in excess of 12,000 r.p.m.

ultrahigh-speed handpiece A handpiece that is capable of operating at speeds above 100,000 r.p.m.

miniature handpiece A small headed contra-angle (binangle) handpiece for use with short rotary instruments in confined areas.

right-angle handpiece A monangle handpiece.

straight handpiece A handpiece with no bends, its rotary instrument operated in line with its long axis.

hatchet A hand cutting instrument with a flat blade mounted so that its flat sides are in a plane common with the handle.

bibevel hatchet A hatchet, usually with a very small blade beveled on both sides of its end. May have a monangle or a trip-angle shank.

enamel hatchet A hatchet with a binangle shank. The blade end has a single bevel that may be right or left, and the blade is mounted in a flat plane with the handle.

Jeffery hatchets Hand cutting instruments that are not true hatchets because their blades are not in a flat plane with their handles. However, their blades are long and beveled on one side of the cutting ends and function similarly to normal hatchets.

off-angle hatchet Hand cutting instrument that is not a hatchet in the strictest sense but is like an enamel hatchet in that its blade is rotated on its long axis.

hoe A monangle instrument also called a monangle chisel; like a straight chisel but with a shorter blade and one bend in its shank.

horn, pulp See *pulp, dental—pulp horn*

hydrocolloid A colloid sol in water for use as an elastic impression material.

irreversible hydrocolloid (alginate) A hydrocolloid that, when mixed, sets by chemical action.

reversible hydrocolloid A hydrocolloid, the state of which may be controlled by temperature, liquefied by heat, and gelled by cooling.

hygroscopic Able to absorb water.

impression A negative or imprint of an object or part.

incipient In the first stage; beginning.

inlay An intracoronal restoration, usually cast gold or fired porcelain, cemented into a prepared cavity.

instrument A device or tool used especially for scientific or professional purposes.

cutting instrument An instrument used to cut, cleave, or plane enamel and dentin during treatment procedures.

diamond instrument Any of many shapes of rotary instruments made abrasive by diamond chips bonded into the cutting surface.

hand instrument An instrument held by hand, nonpowered, to perform a function during treatment of a tooth.

instrument formula Description of a hand instrument by means of formulas devised by G. V. Black.

instrument parts, hand Blade, handle, nib, or shank.

blade The working part of a hand instrument, beveled on its end to form a cutting edge.

handle (shaft) The part of the hand instrument by which it is held or grasped during its use.

nib The working point of a condensing instrument, the flat surface (end) of which is called its face.

shank The part of a hand instrument that connects the blade (or nib) with the handle.

instrument parts, rotary Head, neck, and shank.

head The part of a rotary instrument that does the cutting by means of a series of blades or an abrasive material. Abrasive rotary instruments are generally termed *points*.

neck The part of a rotary cutting instrument that tapers from the shank to the head.

shank The part of a rotary cutting instrument (bur) that is sealed in a handpiece.

plastic instrument A hand instrument for use in manipulation of a plastic restorative material.

rotary instrument Any of many types of instruments held by a handpiece driven by a source of power (air, electricity, or water); for example, bur, diamond point, Carborundum, stone, or disk.

instrumentation The use of instruments in treatment. The performance of a procedure or operation.

intracoronal Within or contained within the remaining normal substance of the crown of a tooth.

invest To surround, enclose, or embed in an investment material (gypsum).

junction A joining together or line of demarcation between two areas or parts.

   cementoenamel junction The line of junction of enamel and cementum; also called cervical line.

   dentinocemental junction The line or area of junction of dentin and cementum in the root of a tooth.

   dentinoenamel junction The line or area of junction of enamel and dentin in the crown of a tooth.

knife, gold An instrument used to remove excess material from a restoration.

labial Relating to, pertaining to, or toward a lip.

Lentulo spiral A wire spiral used in a handpiece to insert cement into a prepared pinhole.

lesion A pathologic change in structure, form, or function of a tissue or part. Hurt, loss, or injury.

   abrasion lesion An area of destruction in a tooth, caused by abrasion.

   carious lesion An area of destruction in a tooth, caused by dental caries.

   erosion lesion An area of destruction in a tooth, caused by erosion.

ligate To tie with a ligature.

ligature A strin, cord, or wire used to tie or stabilize something, as a rubber dam with dental floss.

line Boundary or demarcation.

   cement line Cement exposed between an inlay and tooth structure.

   cervical line See *junction—cementoenamel junction.*

   finish line The edge, margin, chamfer, or cavosurface angle of a preparation for a restoration.

   line of force See *force—line of force.*

linen strip See *strip—finishing strip.*

liner, cavity See *varnish, cavity.*

lingual Relating to, pertaining to, or toward the tongue.

loupe, binocular A device, consisting of two lenses and framework, worn for magnification of areas of operation.

mallet A hammerlike instrument.

   automatic mallet See *condenser—mechanical condenser.*

   electromallet An electronic device for condensing restorative materials.

   hand mallet a small hammer with a cushioned head to apply force in condensing cohesive gold or amalgam and for seating cast restorations.

mandrel A shaft, operated in a handpiece used to hold a rotary device such as a disk, stone, or rubber cup for finishing and polishing.

   Moore mandrel A mandrel with a split square head, the shape allowing finishing disks with metal centers to be quickly snapped on or off.

   sproule mandrel A mandrel that retains a disk by means of an indexed pin that slips into the neck (core) of the mandrel.

margin The junction of a restoration with the cavosurface angle of the prepared cavity.

mask, rubber dam See *napkin, rubber dam.*

mat gold See *gold—mat gold.*

matrix An artificial wall to form and retain restorative material as it is inserted and built up in a prepared cavity. A mold into which something is to be formed.

   amalgam matrix Usually a very thin metal strip that is adapted to a prepared cavity to contain and form the amalgam as it is packed into place.

   matrix retainer A device used to tighten and/or retain a matrix band to or around the crown of a tooth.

   plastic matrix Usually a very thin plastic strip used to retain materials as they are placed into prepared cavities.

   platinum matrix Platinum foil adapted closely to a die in the fabrication of a baked porcelain restoration.

mesial Pertaining to, or toward, the median line in the dental arch. Pertaining to, relative to, or toward the median line (midline).

microleakage The penetration and/or interchange of fluids and other matter between a restoration and the tooth.

mulling Final kneading or mixing of amalgam after it has been triturated and excess mercury expelled; usually performed manually.

napkin, rubber dam A piece of cloth or flannel cut to fit over a patient's face; interposed between the rubber and the face. A facepad.

Nealon's technique See *technique—Nealon's technique.*

nib The working tip or end of a condensing instrument corresponding with the blade of a hand cutting instrument.

noncohesive Incapable of coherence, or sticking together.

occlusal Pertaining to, relating to, or toward the chewing surfaces of posterior teeth.

odontalgia Toothache.

odontotomy, prophylactic also **odontomy** Restoration of developmental pits and grooves (fissures) to prevent dental caries.

onlay See also *overlay.* An occlusal rest that is extended to cover the entire occlusal surface of a tooth.*(Current dental literature seems to favor use of the term *onlay* as synomomous with *overlay.*)

operating field See *field, operating* or *operative.*

operative procedure See *procedure—operating procedure*

operation A procedure, act, or series of acts performed on a patient to effect relief or cure.

overhang Excess restorative material extended over and/or past a prepared cavosurface margin.

overlay See also *onlay.* A cast restoration that restores the occlusal surface of one or more cusps but not a cast or crown or three-quarter crown.

---

*Boucher, C. O., editor: Current clinical dental terminology, ed. 2, St. Louis, 1974, The C. V. Mosby Co.

pad, rubber dam See *napkin, rubber dam.*

pattern A form created to make a mold, as for a cast inlay or crown.

pickling Cleansing of a casting in acid.

pin A metal rod.

Markley pin See *cemented pin.*

pin casting A casting that includes one or more pin extensions to provide retention.

pinhole A hole drilled into dentin to receive a retention pin.

retention pin A metal rod extended into dentin to aid in stabilization and/or retention of a restoration.

cemented pin A retention pin cemented in a prepared hole.

friction-retained pin A retention pin placed in a prepared hole and retained by the elasticity of the dentin.

self-threading pin A retention pin placed in a prepared hole and retained by the interlocking of spiral threads on the pin and those created in dentin as the pin is screwed into place.

sprue pin A length of metal, wax, or plastic to which a wax pattern is attached to provide an opening to the void created in the investment mold after the pattern and sprue are eliminated (burned out).

pinledge also **pinlay** A cast restoration, usually on the lingual surface of an anterior tooth, that relies on retention pins to hold it in place. The pins are integral parts of the casting.

pit A small depression, usually connected to one or more developmental grooves, in enamel. Also, a void or defect in a restoration.

pit and fissure cavity See *cavity—pit and fissure cavity.*

plane A flat surface, real or imaginary, the position of which may be determined by three points with which it intersects.

axial plane An imaginary plane parallel with the long axis of an object. May designate a plane passing buccolingually (buccolingual axial plane) or mesiodistally (mesiodistal axial plane).

plastic A material capable of being molded to a desired form. Restorative materials, such as freshly triturated amalgam, are said to be plastic when they are soft prior to insertion and condensation into a prepared cavity. Also, the state of certain restorative materials when they are freshly mixed or prepared prior to their becoming hard, or set.

pliers Any of many pincer-type tools that function by means of gripping or squeezing an object.

contouring pliers An instrument used to place contour in metal matrix bands, metal shells, etc.

cotton pliers A tweezerlike instrument for use primarily to hold cotton pledgets or other small objects.

plug Archaic. To place a "filling" or restoration. To close a cavity.

plugger (archaic) See *condenser.*

point An intersection of two or more lines. In restorative dentistry, may be any of various small rotary instruments.

abrasive point A mounted stone or diamond abrasive instrument for use in a handpiece.

condenser point The nib of a condensing instrument. Also, any of various small condensing instruments for use in a mechanical condenser or in a cone socket handle.

contact point The area of contact of one tooth to another in the same arch.

convenience point A small point, pit, or hole to facilitate retention of the first increment of a restorative material placed in a prepared cavity.

diamond point An abrasive rotary instrument in any of many shapes, usually for use in preparation of a tooth for a restoration.

starting point See *convenience point.*

polishing The art of finishing the surface of a restoration to a high luster. To make smooth and glossy.

porcelain, baked A fused mixture of feldspar, silica, and other minor ingredients, resulting in a glasslike material, semitranslucent, that is used for various dental restorations

synthetic porcelain (misnomer) See *cement, silicate.*

porosity The presence of voids within a material.

post See *endopost.*

preparation The form established by instrumentation on or in a tooth designed to receive a restoration.

cavity preparation An intracoronal form established in a tooth by instrumentation to receive and retain a restoration. The cavity preparation is individualized according to the location, type, and extent of the lesion and the biomechanical factors necessary to restore and maintain proper health, form, and function.

prism, enamel See *enamel prism.*

procedure A series of steps designed to accomplish a specific objective.

order of procedure An organized system of steps followed to execute a particular technique to achieve an objective.

operating procedure The steps necessary to accomplish or complete a surgical objective or desired result.

restorative procedure The series of steps used to properly and efficiently restore the oral cavity to health, form, and function.

prophylactic odontotomy See *odontotomy, prophylactic.*

pulp, dental Connective tissue that fills the pulp cavity enclosed in dentin of a tooth. It is composed of a vascular network, nerves, the peripheral layer of odontoblasts with their protoplasmic processes extending into dentinal tubules, and other cellular and fibrous constituents.

pulp canal Root canal. That portion of the dental pulp that extends from the pulp chamber to the apex of the root.

pulp capping See *capping, pulp.*

pulp cavity The cavity within a tooth, enclosed by dentin containing the dental pulp.

pulp chamber The portion of the dental pulp contained within the crown of the tooth.

pulp horn The tip, small filament, or extension of the pulp into a lobe or part of the crown of a tooth.

pulp tester An instrument or device usually electrical, used to determine whether or not a dental pulp is vital, or to aid in evaluation of its normalcy.

pulp amputation See *pulpotomy.*

pulpal Pertaining to, relating to, or located toward the dental pulp.

pulpotomy A procedure for removal of the coronal portion of a vital dental pulp.

punch, rubber dam An instrument that provides a variety of sizes of holes and a punch for placing holes in rubber dam according to individual requirements of a particular case.

reduce To make smaller. Usually refers to removal of material from a specific area.

reduction An area from which material has been removed.

remineralization See *capping, pulp—indirect pulp capping.*

resin A general term denoting organic substances that occur naturally or are synthetic and that are usually translucent or transparent, and soluble in ether, chloroform, and so forth but not in water. The various types of resin are named according to their chemicophysical properties—for example, acrylic resin, autopolymer resin, synthetic resin, styrene resin, and vinyl resin.

acrylic resin In direct dental restorations, an autopolymerizing methyl methacrylate resin that sets at body temperature and is tinted to harmonize with tooth structure.

composite resin Any of several filled resin restorative materials generally formed of some type of epoxide molecule. The fillers may consist of glass, silica, or trisodium phosphate.

self-curing resin Any of several resins that set by means of autopolymerization.

restoration A general term used to identify any mechanically fabricated device, removable or fixed, to replace any missing or damaged portion of a tooth, an entire tooth, some teeth, all the teeth, and/or oral tissues; a repair, made on an oral tissue or parts, that replaces or reestablishes proper form, function, and health.

cusp restoration The inclusion of a cusp in the preparation for a restoration and in the final restoration. (Terms such as shoeing, capping, or tipping of cusps are not desirable.) The terms *onlay* and *overlay* are also used as synonyms.

inconspicuous Class 3 restoration A gold restoration in a proximal surface of an anterior tooth, for which the cavity is prepared and the restoration inserted from the lingual aspect. The labial extension of such as restoration is minimal to assure that there will be no display of metal to casual observation.

invisible restoration A misnomer for an inconspicuous Class 3 restoration.

temporary restoration A restoration intended to serve only a short period of time.

permanent restoration A restoration designed to serve for an extended period of time.

provisional restoration A restoration used for diagnostic purposes.

restorative Pertaining to efforts to replace form, function, and health in oral parts or tissues.

restorative preparation Preparation of a tooth to receive a restoration.

retention That aspect of preparation of a cavity that will maintain stability of the restoration against being tipped or unseated form the tooth. See *form—retention form.*

pin retention See *pin—retention pin.*

retraction The pulling or pushing away of tissues or parts to facilitate access and/or vision to a particular part or area.

gingival retraction Displacement of the free gingiva to expose the gingival margin of a restorative preparation. May be accomplished by means of clamps, surgically or chemically, or chemophysically (cotton and astringent).

rod A thin, straight, cylindrical object.

enamel rod or **enamel prism** The structural unit of tooth enamel, hexagonal in shape, 4 or 5 microns in diameter, extending from dentin to the external surface of the tooth in an irregular (wavy) direction.

rotary cutting instrument See *instrument—instrument parts, rotary.*

rubber dam See *dam—rubber dam.*

rubber dam clamp See *clamp—rubber dam clamp.*

rubber dam punch See *punch, rubber dam.*

satin finish See *finish—satin finish.*

saw An instrument with a serrated cutting edge.

gold saw A sawlike instrument used to reduce surplus gold from the contact area in the beginning stages of finishing a cohesive gold restoration.

self-curing resin See *resin, self-curing.*

separator An instrument used to move teeth apart or out of contact during the restoration of a contact area.

Ferrier separator One of a set of instruments designed by W. I. Ferrier for separation of teeth. It has double bows, which, when stabilized by compound, facilitate balanced function of the instrument.

True separator An instrument designed by Harry A. True for separation of teeth. It has a single bow to allow greater access to the area being restored.

shoulder The gingival wall of an extracoronal restorative preparation.

silicate cement See *cement—silicate cement.*

silver amalgam See *amalgam—silver amalgam.*

slice A flat plane produced in some techniques of cavity preparation. Removal of a convex area from the surface of a crown, usually the contact area.

spatula An instrument used to mix a material.

spatulate To mix or manipulate with a spatula the components or ingredients of a material into a homogeneous mass.

spatulation The process of using a spatula in mixing.

spatulator, mechanical A device that mixes materials by means other than a hand spatula.

speed Rate of motion.

    low speed A relative term to designate rotary motion of a handpiece of usually less than 12,000 r.p.m.

    high speed A relative term that generally designates rotary speeds slower than 100,000 r.p.m.

    ultrahigh speed A term used to designate speeds of 100,000 r.p.m. or more. (Falling into disuse, the term *high speed* generally implying ultrahigh speeds.)

spherical alloy A class of alloys used for amalgam. The particles are spherical in shape.

spoon See *excavator.*

sprue See *pin—sprue pin.*

starting point See *point—convenience point.*

stone An abrasive instrument, usually rotary.

    Arkansas stone A very fine-grain stone used to sharpen instruments. Some are in the form of rotary instruments.

    Carborundum stone A silicon carbide stone.

    dental stone A gypsum product used to make casts and dies.

    diamond stone See *point—diamond point.*

    sharpening stone A stone used to sharpen instruments.

stopping, temporary A gutta-percha compound used to temporarily seal prepared cavities.

strip *n,* A long, thin, narrow piece of a material.

    v. To remove material as with a finishing strip, or electrically to reduce the size of a metal casting.

    abrasive strip See *strip—finishing strip.*

    celluloid strip A thin, narrow piece of celluloid used to contour and retain quick-setting Class 3 restorative materials.

    finishing strip A long, narrow strip of linen or plastic, abrasive on one side, for finishing proximal areas of restorations.

    lightning strip A strip of steel, abrasive on one side, for contouring proximal areas in early stages of finishing a restoration.

    linen strip See *strip—finishing strip.*

subgingival Pertaining to a point or area located in the area between the crest of the free gingiva and the gingival attachment. Also, within the confines of the gingival sulcus.

sulcus A groove, furrow, or trench, as a groove on the surface of a tooth.

    gingival sulcus The groove or space formed by the free gingiva (gingival cuff) and the tooth occlusal or incisal to the gingival attachment. Sometimes known as gingival crevice.

surface The exterior of an object.

    occlusal surface The functional, or chewing, surface of a tooth.

    proximal surface A surface of a tooth that contacts of races another tooth in the same arch.

    smooth surface An area on a tooth that does not include developmental pits or grooves.

swage To shape or form material or metal onto a die by burnishing, hammering, or forcing with a counterdie, in order to adapt the material closely to the die surface.

tarnish Loss of luster of a metal surface; discoloration.

technique Degree of skill used in performance of a procedure. Also the skillful completion of a procedure. May also denote a particular procedure.

    Eames's technique A procedure, advocated by Dr. Wilbur Eames, utilizing the concept of placing amalgam with an alloy-mercury ratio of 1:1.

    Nealon's technique A method of building up an autopolymerizing resin in a prepared cavity, with a brush used to apply powder and liquid.

toilet of cavity The final cleansing of a cavity preparation prior to insertion of restorative materials.

trauma An injury, damage, hurt, or wound caused by external force.

trimmer, gingival margin A hand cutting instrument, binangled and double-paired, with left and right curved blades having cutting edges not perpendicular to the blade. The cutting edges are designed for one type to plane distal margins (the tip of the cutting edge away from the handle) and mesial margins (the cutting edge near the handle).

trituration The making of amalgam by mixing silver alloy with mercury.

    hand trituration The making of amalgam using a hand mortar and pestle.

    mechanical trituration The making of amalgam by means of a powered mechanical device.

undercut The portion of a prepared cavity that does not permit a material placed in the cavity to be removed without distortion.

undermined enamel See *enamel, undermined.*

varnish, cavity A clear solution of copal, resin, or rosin dissolved in acetone, ether, or chloroform used to coat the walls of prepared cavities to reduce microleakage and to seal dentinal tubules, thereby reducing pulp irritation and tooth discoloration.

vitalometer See *pulp, dental—pulp tester.*

wall The side of a cavity.

    cavity wall One of the enclosing sides or component walls of a prepared cavity.

Wedelstaedt chisel See *chisel—Wedelstaedt chisel.*

INDEX